CHILDREN ADAPT

A Theory of Sensorimotor-Sensory Development Second Edition

Elnora M. Gilfoyle
Dean, College of Applied Human Sciences
Colorado State University
Fort Collins, CO

Ann P. Grady
Director, AccessAbility Resource Center
The Children's Hospital
Denver, CO

Josephine C. Moore
Professor, Department of Anatomy
University of South Dakota Medical School
Vermillion, SD

SLACK International Book Distributors

In Canada:
McGraw-Hill Ryerson Limited
330 Progress Avenue
Scarborough, Ontario
M1P 2Z5

In Australia and New Zealand:
MacLennan & Petty Pty Limited
P.O. Box 425
Artarmon, N.S.W. 2064
Australia

In Japan:
Igaku-Shoin, Ltd.
Tokyo International P.O. Box 5063
1-28-36 Hongo, Bunkyo-Ku
Tokyo 113
Japan

In Asia and India:
PG Publishing Pte Limited.
36 West Coast Road, #02-02
Singapore 0512

Foreign Translation Agent

John Scott & Company
International Publishers' Agency
417-A Pickering Road
Phoenixville, PA 19460
Fax: 215-988-0185

Editor: Cheryl Willoughby
Production Manager: David Murphy
Publisher: Harry C. Benson

Photography: Ann P. Grady, MA, OTR, FAOTA, Tia Brayman, Steve Kast
Drawings: Margaret Johnson Bowles, MA, OTR
            Josephine C. Moore, PhD, OTR
Typing and Editing: Ruth McNeal

Printed in the United States of America

Library of Congress Catalog Card Number: 86-043125

ISBN 1-55642-187-7

Published by: SLACK Incorporated
               6900 Grove Road
               Thorofare, NJ 08086

Last digit is print number: 10   9   8   7   6   5   4   3   2   1

This book is dedicated to two special people, both our teachers—one as a friend and colleague and the other as a child from whom we learned.

Mary R. Fiorentino, OTR, FAOTA
1917-1986

"A teacher touches not only her students but her students' students, and soon a whole generation."
—Mary R. Fiorentino Commemorative
Symposium, 1987

Grant G. Sholar
1974-1984

"It is Life. That lasts forever and we are all a part of Life."
—Buscaglia, 1982

Contents

Preface

Preface to the Second Edition

During the past nine years since the publication of the first edition, *Children Adapt* has been useful to rehabilitation personnel and educators. Also, it has been used by students who are preparing for roles as therapists or teachers. The use, as both a reference and textbook, has led to additions in format as well as our undertaking improvements.

Changes in this edition are in five major areas. For use as a text, each chapter has stated learning objectives, self-study questions, and identification of key points. New material, gleaned from research and publications, has been inserted throughout the text. Notable changes are included in the chapter, "Highlights of Nervous System Development and Function," and in three chapters discussing the theory and its application to rehabilitation programs. Additions to the text comprise the third change. For example, a chapter is included to provide an overview of rudiments of theory building so that the reader has a reference point from which to analyze spatiotemporal adaptation as a grounded theory. A theoretical framework to relate theory to practice has been developed for this edition. An additional change is a reconsideration of some of the ideas that resulted in modification of terminology and organization of material. The final change was the omission of the chapter, "Development of the Personality." In general, the revisions in the second edition reflect development toward a more parsimonious expression of our theory.

The task of revision has been aided by reviewers who made suggestions for change, students in universities and post-graduate courses who continue to question and challenge, by clinicians who have applied theory to practice and have cogently provided feedback, and by researchers who have developed hypotheses to test the theory. Special recognition is given to our colleagues at The Children's Hospital in Denver, Colorado State University, as well as those from the American Occupational Therapy Association and the American Occupational Therapy Foundation with whom we have had many hours of dialogue. As before, our families have encouraged and supported us throughout this endeavor.

Preface to the First Edition

Children Adapt was conceived in 1973 at a developmental workshop sponsored by the Colorado Occupational Therapy Association. The faculty, Mary Fiorentino, Pat Komich, and the authors of this book shared ideas regarding a developmental approach to pediatric rehabilitation. Recognizing their common interest, plus the need to identify a framework for evaluation and treatment of children, the authors set out to write this text.

The content has undergone its own growth, development, and maturation over the past six years. Many "writings," hours of searching, and days of sharing have been integrated into the present manuscript. Children have been our prime teachers, for their actions provided the stimulus to seek answers, modify concepts, and adapt our beliefs.

Concepts presented in this book provide a perspective regarding the development of movement. We have attempted to answer the question of how children learn to function.

We present our theory of development, as well as present a philosophical base for pediatric occupational therapy and a model for designing individual therapeutic programs for children. The core of the concepts, theory, and philosophy is in the adaptation process.

This book, like all children, developed with a great deal of understanding and love. To those who provided the book with "parenting" we want to say a very special thank-you. *Children Adapt* would not have become a reality without the understanding, help, support, patience, encouragement, and sacrifices given to us from Lou Shannon, and Gene and Sean Gilfoyle.

Although we have taken the step to organize and write the materials, many persons have contributed to the evolution of the principles and concepts. We appreciate the therapists and staff with whom we have worked, especially the occupational and physical therapists at The Denver Children's Hospital. These friends and colleagues have been a major source for knowledge sharing and encouragement. The participants of our workshops and our occupational therapy students from Colorado State University have listened, questioned, and provided feedback that has contributed to our growth and adaptation of beliefs. To these friends and colleagues we are grateful. Special appreciation is given to Maggie Johnson for her creative art work, to Mary Fiorentino and Pat Komich for their stimulating idea exchange and assistance with the creation of concepts, and to Wilma West and Jean Ayres who have been prime contributors to the development of pediatric occupational therapy and provided us with stimulus and opportunities for integration of ideas.

But most of all, we want to thank the children—our teachers—particularly the children pictured in this book:

Aron	Kris
Brad	Kristen
Cindy	Kris and Grant
David	Laura
Emily	Meg
Eric	Michael
Grant	Mike and Tim
Heather	
Jeff	

and, of course, Sean

Foreword

Occupational adaptation is the functional adjustment of humans to environmental demands for productive performance. *Children Adapt* focuses specifically on the adaptation of children to environmental demands. Adaptation/adaptive performance is facilitated by the integrity of the central nervous system and the interaction of individuals with human and nonhuman objects in the environment elicited by need requirements and the attempt to fulfill them. Occupational performance components in sensory, motor, psychological, social and cognitive spheres of development support the achievement of competence in occupational performance in the areas of self-care, work, education, play and leisure. Occupational performance comprises the elements of role behavior required as a part of social culture.

Spatiotemporal adaptation theory refers to a set of interrelated concepts regarding the sensorimotor components of human functioning and conceptual categories that explain the adaptation process for the development of performance skills required for self-care, work/education, and play/leisure occupations. Occupations are conceived and described both as "means" for development when spatiotemporal distress provokes dysfunction and "ends" of the developmental process when the growth process proceeds without disruption.

The basic premises of spatiotemporal adaptation theory have been expanded in the second edition of *Children Adapt* to place the theory into the context of theory development in the field of occupational therapy. These premises include the following:

1. Development is a function of nervous system maturation;
2. Adaptation depends upon attentiveness and active participation with purposeful events in the environment;
3. Purposeful events (activities and behaviors) are perceived as providing the experiences to enhance maturation;
4. Higher level responses are believed to result from integration with lower level function with adaptation spiraling through primitive, transitional and mature phases of development;
5. Environmental experiences may present situations of spatiotemporal stress; and
6. Spatiotemporal distress may provoke dysfunction as the process of adaptation is disrupted (Gilfoyle, Grady, and Moore, 1981).

While more emphasis is placed on the development of the theory as dynamic and interactive, the practical aspects of its application in practice are described. In its discussion of assessment process, *Children Adapt* emphasizes the need to collect and review present and past information, interview and consult family members and others in addition to the child patient, and collect standardized and non-standardized evaluation procedures to create the data base for conducting treatment procedures to ameliorate dysfunctional performance and facilitate functional adaptation.

The treatment/rehabilitation process in the application of the theory is also dynamic and places the therapist, client, and family in partnership. The therapist may need to structure the environment and engage the motivation of the client, promote purposeful experience, and guide appropriate actions with the major goal of facilitating children's potential to achieve competence in their social roles in the environment.

Goals of prevention, performance modification, remediation, compensation, and maintenance can be achieved through application of the theory. Through early intervention, therapists can minimize or eliminate potential stress factors. Change can be facilitated in the self-system. Skill levels can be corrected or improved. Substitute actions can be taught and acquired appropriate functions can be practiced for retention.

This second edition of *Children Adapt* moves the development of the theory of spatiotemporal adaptation to a more complex level with clearer understanding of its relevance to human development, to the philosophical base of occupational therapy, and to its application in practice.

Lela A. Llorens, PhD, OTR, FAOTA
Professor, Chair, and Graduate Coordinator
Department of Occupational Therapy
San Jose State University
San Jose, CA

CHAPTER 1

Theory Construction

Objectives

The reader will be able to

1. define the terms **theory**, **model**, and **frame of reference**;
2. list elements and purposes of theory;
3. compose and contrast theory, model, and frame of reference;
4. delineate characteristics of a profession's model;
5. define **grounded theory** and list its elements;
6. identify interrelationships of a profession's model with theory and frame of reference; and
7. discuss major points gleaned from the literature that provide scientific evidence for spatiotemporal adaptation theory.

Introduction

Children Adapt presents a threefold approach to the theory-based practice of occupational therapy: (1) the process by which the theory evolved and basic elements of theory are included to expand knowledge of theory construction in a practice profession; (2) the theory itself is presented to elucidate the understanding of normal and abnormal sensorimotor development; and (3) the relationship between theory and practice.

The domain of the theory encompasses the sensorimotor basis for adaptation of developmental and purposeful actions in children through a transactional process of movement with environmental events. Developmental and purposeful nature of children's sensorimotor adaptations influences, and is influenced by, the psychosocial aspects of behavior. Reciprocal development of these interdependent aspects of behavior promotes integration and creation of a unique "self." Psychosocial aspects of development are integral to the adaptation process; however, the theory presented in this text focuses on the sensorimotor aspects of development.

The theory presented in this book explains how children adapt components of environmental events for development of performance skills. A clinician's understanding of the adaptation process provides the basis for therapeutic reasoning necessary for evaluation and program planning for children with special needs. An analysis of the theory unfolds in the succeeding chapters. For a complete understanding of the theory and its use in therapeutic practices, an overview of theory construction is presented in this chapter. As you proceed with the following chapters, you may find it helpful to return to this chapter to establish how parts of theory fit into the whole.

Robert Dubin[1] proposes that a theorist is one who observes a portion of the world and seeks to bring order to that experience. As Dubin explains, the idea of order is in the mind of the theorist; therefore, the locus of theory is the human mind. Our need to bring order and a sense of understanding to how children learn to perform skilled activities resulted in the construction of a theory as presented in this text.

Development of theory must be suited to its use, and the use for spatiotemporal adaptation theory is to provide a sense of understanding about developmental processes of acquiring movement skills. An understanding of developmental processes can assist with an explanation and prediction of the development of children with handicapping conditions. Understanding how children learn movement skills is the necessary basis for clinical reasoning to implement rehabilitation processes designed to bring about change in a child's sensorimotor behaviors. Therefore, a major use of theory is its relationship to practice. Another significant use of this and other theories is its role in the development and critique of research for creation and application of knowledge. Through research and theory analysis, unique features of rehabilitation disciplines and their applications may be identified and explained.

Theory Definition

Most authors and theorists agree that theory can be defined as an interrelated set of ideas or constructs. However, there are various definitions, purposes, and rudiments of theory. Also, there are different terms, such as **theoretical model, model of practice, conceptual model,** and **frame of reference,** used to describe ideas that form a basis for therapeutic practice. An orientation to terminology is presented, providing a comprehensive view of how the term **theory** is used in the presentation of spatiotemporal adaptation. Appendix 1-A summarizes four perspectives on theory building.

Reynolds [2] proposes that theory is developed to promote scientific knowledge. He believes scientific knowledge is a system for description and explanation and becomes a set of laws with well-supported empirical generalizations. As a vital component of scientific knowledge, theory is a set of definitions. Dance [3] states that theory is a set of constructs, while Glaser [4] proposes that theory is an interrelated set of ideas that explains or predicts something and, as such, becomes a strategy for handling data in research. Dubin[1] believes theory presents order to experience and is the major source for delineation of hypotheses for testing. Each author emphasizes the concept of theory as a set of interrelated ideas, assumptions, or constructs that presents a systematic view of phenomena to provide order for explanation. Theory is interrelated with research and provides a source for further research toward the development of scientific knowledge.

Spatiotemporal adaptation theory provides an interrelated set of constructs concerning sensorimotor components of human performance. Conceptual categories and properties of spatiotemporal adaptation explain a spiraling process of incorporating spatiotemporal environmental events for the development of performance skills.

Purpose of Theory

There is agreement in the literature about the purpose of theory. Reynolds, Dance, Dubin, and Glaser state that theory provides a sense of understanding to phenomenon, enables prediction, and explains behavior. Reynolds proposes that the purpose of theory is validity of an idea, while Glaser states that theory is developed to advance knowledge by guiding research and is useful for practical applications by providing a perspective about behavior.

Theory Components

According to Reynolds[2], rudiments of theory include the idea itself, taxonomy, defined concepts, empirical generalizations, and theoretical statements. Dubin[1] delineates the components of theory as its "things" or "variables" which he terms "units," with the interactions of units being the subject matter for attention. Theory also has stated boundaries that define its geography, limits, propositions, empirical indicators, and hypotheses. Dance[3] presents the idea that attributes of theory include its range and occurrence of phenomena described, parsimony (referring to economy of concepts), assumptions and relationships characterizing the theory, and elegance (referring to succinctness of expression). In contrast to theory that evolves from deductive reasoning, Glaser[4] presents a discussion on theory building that he terms "grounded theory." He proposes that theory is best generated from data obtained through the general method of comparative analysis. Therefore grounded theory is developed through inductive reasoning. According to Glaser, elements of theory are (1) conceptual categories and their conceptual properties, and (2) hypothesis or generalized relations among categories and properties. A category stands independently as a major concept or construct of the theory. A property serves as an aspect of the category. Both category and property are concepts indicated by data.

Through comparative analysis, differences and similarities among groups generate categories and relationships among categories. Glaser explains that hypotheses, as rudiments of theory construction, have at first "the status of suggested, not tested, relations among categories and their properties."[4p39]Hypothesis is a belief used as the basis for action, and through research action, hypotheses are verified.

Spatiotemporal adaptation has been developed through the methodology of comparative analysis. Clinical observations and audiovisual recordings of children functioning within the environment were analyzed to identify similarities and differences throughout early developmental years (birth through age six). Data from these studies, as well as data from literature, served as the basis for delineating categories and their properties. Also, an analysis of functioning behaviors of children with handicapping conditions was compared with the analysis of children with no known pathology. Spatiotemporal adaptation is presented as a grounded theory, with the succeeding chapters presenting an explanation, introducing the conceptual categories and properties, and relating theory to practice.

Theory—Frame of Reference—Model

Because this book centers around theory and its relationship to practice, it is helpful in understanding the concept of theory to compare it to the concepts of model and frame of reference. An explanation of the relationships of these concepts assists a reader in practical application of theory to practice.

Some authors use the term **model** or **theoretical model** interchangeably with the term **theory**. Model refers to the philosophical belief system, content, and internal structure of a profession. According to Mosey,[5] a profession's model is the typical way in which a discipline perceives itself, its relationships to others, and its association with society. Mosey emphasizes that a profession's model includes a description of its philosophical assumptions, ethical code, theoretical foundation, domain of concern, tools of profession, and nature and principles of practice. A model of a profession, such as the medical model, educational model, or occupational therapy model, defines and delineates broad concepts and boundaries of a profession as understood by the particular profession and society.[5] A profession's model can also be identified as its paradigm. Theories are developed to explain, to provide order to specific aspects of the profession's model, and to guide the development of the profession's academic discipline. For example, the occupational therapy model has its foundation in the occupational nature of human beings, in the use of occupations as therapeutic media, and in the development of occupational behavior.[6] In relationship to model, the theory of spatiotemporal adaptation is specific to one aspect within the occupational therapy model. Spatiotemporal adaptation theory explains development of sensorimotor skills in children and discusses adaptation of movement for developmental and purposeful actions.

Just as theory has a direct relationship to model, frame of reference is another concept pertinent to practice. Mosey[5] presents an excellent description of the concept of frame of reference. She describes a frame as a set of interrelated definitions that provides a description of a particular aspect of a profession that links the model with practice. For example, the occupational therapy model is concerned with the development of human occupational behavior; therefore, a developmental frame of reference is pertinent to that domain of concern related to the developmental behavior of human beings. To that end, spatiotemporal adaptation theory provides one developmental frame of reference which serves to link theory to practice in occupational therapy, but it can also be applied to practice in other health and education disciplines.

A profession's model or paradigm provides unity for general directions and boundaries of a profession as a discipline; frames of reference present guidelines for specific aspects of practice, and theories describe interrelated constructs that explain and predict behaviors, as well as provide strategies for research. A model of occupational therapy organized around philosophical assumptions of the occupational nature of human beings is the unifying force for the profession. A system of theories and frames of reference are necessary to substantiate the various aspects of the profession. Spatiotemporal adaptation is presented as one theory pertinent to occupational therapy. We view our theory as a theory of process and a theory **in** process, as it is an ever-developing entity, not a finished product.

Related Research

A brief review of information gleaned from literature is summarized to orient the reader to the basis of the theory presented in **Children Adapt**. Scientific evidence gleaned from literature that had most influence upon theory development is summarized here according to intrauterine, maturational, and environmental factors.

Intrauterine Developmental Factors

1. Movement begins during early fetal development with the reflex activity of the fetus being the foundation for sensorimotor behaviors.[7-9]
2. Sensorimotor behaviors develop as an expanding total pattern, generalized to localized, cephalocaudal, and proximal to distal.[7,9-11]
3. Generalized reactions involving the head and trunk develop prior to the localized reactions of the body.[11-13]
4. Generalized withdrawal reactions develop and remain prepotent over pursuit reactions.[14,15]
5. In the newborn, exteroceptive and proprioceptive reflexes and withdrawal reactions dominate, with the exception of pursuit reactions of the mouth.[14,15]
6. Specific localized reactions are components of earlier, more primitive total response patterns.[7,10,11]
7. A newborn has a crude form of visual perception indicated by preference to patterns.[17]

Maturational Factors

1. The central nervous system has a hierarchal, functional organization, which is responsible for voluntary sensorimotor activity.[8,12]
2. Different levels of the central nervous system do not function in isolation, as all parts of the nervous system are influenced by and influence activities of other parts.[18,19]
3. Maturation proceeds in a cephalocaudal, generalized to localized, and proximal to distal direction.[7,19]
4. Most of the cortex is not functioning as a control for behavior at birth.[19]
5. Behavior patterns of early infancy are believed to be primarily under subcortical control.[19-21]
6. Maturation of the nervous system is not uniform; therefore, several maturational levels occur simultaneously in relation to different body segments until the whole is established.[19]
7. Higher cortical development of skill continues to be centered in the superior spinal segments throughout the maturational process.[19]
8. Coordinated movements are a result of various feedback mechanisms of the nervous system.[7,18,22-26]
9. Nervous system activity is adaptive and does not seem to depend on any specific group of circuits; therefore, specific patterns of neuronal activity may not be attributed to particular functions of the nervous system.[13]
10. The brain becomes aware of movements through sensorimotor links, builds up patterns of movements, and is able to anticipate the purpose for which a movement will be used.[7,8,14]

Environmental Factors

1. Development is dependent upon organized integration, environmental experiences, and adaptation.[7,16,27,28]
2. Knowledge and action can be viewed as both the product and/or process of individual environmental transactions.[27-29]

3. Life begins with certain neurological and anatomical structures; however, these structures do not account for functioning itself.[30]
4. Higher functioning results from adaptation to the postnatal environment, and feedback from new experiences is associated with already acquired prenatal and postnatal adaptations.[29,30]
5. Infants are part of an environment that demands little from them; however, as infants mature, they place increasing demands on the environment and the environment on them.[31]
6. There is an evolving interplay of self and environment as individuals both create and are created by their environments.[31,32]
7. When movement remains smooth, a person can encounter discontinuity of the environment that is neither "too harsh nor too perfect, but good enough."[13 p192]
8. A "good enough" environment meets, challenges, and contradicts an individual's needs for development; therefore, an organism calls forth a developmental dialogue or internal conversation to cope with conflicting and changing messages from the environment.[31,33]
9. Reflexes/reactions of an infant undergo modifications as a result of environmental contact and are integrated into acquired behaviors. Higher level behaviors are modifications of older, more primitive patterns.[7,9,29,30]
10. Behavior that an infant possesses is the beginning of the adaptation process, which continues to occur throughout life.[28,30]
11. Movement provides a means by which a child can interact with the environment.[8]
12. During environmental interactions, purposeful movements are made by a child to increase his awareness of space, to manipulate the environment, and to communicate with persons and objects within the environment.[8]
13. Sensorimotor activity is important as an integrating mechanism for linking together the developmental progress of physical, intellectual, emotional, and social components.[8, 30]
14. Through existence of a sensory feedback mechanism, movement of a child influences his ongoing development, for the level of developmental maturity reached by a child allows progressively more complex sensorimotor behaviors to be exhibited.[8,27]
15. Temporal (timing) components of the environment are concomitant features of the dynamics of sensorimotor actions and, in production and control of movement, timing is crucial for skilled performance.[34]
16. Early movement control involves a spatial reaction to gravitational forces. Once postural reactions are present, sensorimotor control requires graded spatial responses in a structured environmental time frame.[35]
17. Individuals have a spatial frame of reference that is culturally constituted and accumulated through experiences.[36]

Key Points

1. Theory is an interrelated set of concepts that explains, predicts, and provides a sense of understanding to phenomena.
2. Theory is a source for research and expansion of scientific knowledge.
3. Theory must be suited to its use for explaining, predicting, and presenting strategies for research.

4. Theory is useful for practical applications, as it provides a perspective about behavior and a framework for rehabilitation practices.

5. Spatiotemporal adaptation theory provides an interrelated set of constructs that concerns sensorimotor components of human functioning and conceptual categories that explain the adaptation process of the development of performance skills. The theory provides a source for further research related to the nature and use of occupations as therapeutic media.

6. Spatiotemporal adaptation theory was developed from comparative analysis of data of both children with handicaps and children with no known pathology. Spatiotemporal adaptation is presented as a grounded theory.

7. Grounded theory presents conceptual categories and their properties and presents hypotheses for testing.

8. A model describes the philosophical assumptions of a profession and includes the ethical code, domain of concern, tools of practice, and nature and principles of the profession's practice.

9. Frame of reference delineates a particular aspect of a profession and links a profession's model with practice.

10. The occupational therapy model has its foundation in the occupational nature of human beings, in the use of occupations as therapeutic media, and in the development of occupational behavior.

11. Literature has provided scientific information that served as a basis for development of the spatiotemporal adaptation theory. Information from the literature was organized into intrauterine, maturational, and environmental factors that support the interplay of self and environment, the sequential nature of development, and the hierarchical, functional organization of the central nervous system.

Self-study Guidelines

1. Define theory, discuss the purposes of theory, and delineate its elements.
2. What is the relationship of theory to practice?
3. List characteristics of a profession's model.
4. What is the relationship of theory to model?
5. What is the relationship of frame of reference to model?
6. Why is the development of grounded theory considered an inductive reasoning process?
7. What is the relationship of theory to research?
8. Summarize intrauterine, maturational, and environmental factors that provide background for the development of the theory of spatiotemporal adaptation.

References

1. Dubin R: Theory Building. (Rev Ed) New York, The Free Press, A Division of MacMillan Publishing Co., 1978.
2. Reynolds PD: A Primer in Theory Construction. Indianapolis, Bobbs-Merril Educational Publishing, Inc., 1982.
3. Dance FEX: Human Communication Theory. New York, Harper & Row Publishers Inc., 1982.

4. Glaser BG, Strauss AL: The Discovery of Grounded Theory. New York, Aldine Publishing Co., 1967.

5. Mosey AC: Occupational Therapy, Configuration of a Profession. New York, Raven Press, 1981.

6. Kielhofner G (Ed): A Model of Human Occupation: Theory and Application. Baltimore, Williams & Wilkins, 1985.

7. Smoll F: Developmental kinesiology: Toward a subdiscipline focusing on motor development. In Kelso J, Clark J (Eds): Development of Movement Control and Co-ordination. New York, John Wiley & Sons, 1982.

8. Holt K: Movement and child development. In Clinics in Developmental Medicine, No. 55. Philadelphia, J.B. Lippincott Co., 1975.

9. Ian E, Fisher D: Newborn stepping: An explanation for a "disappearing" reflex. Dev Psych 18(5):760-775, 1982.

10. Jacobs MJ: Development of normal motor behavior. Am J Phys Med 46:41-50, 1967.

11. Twitchell TE: Normal motor development. In The Child with Central Nervous System Deficit. Children's Bureau Publication, No. 432. U.S. Dept. of Health, Education and Welfare, Washington, D.C., U.S. Government Printing Office, 1965, pp 85-89.

12. Twitchell TE: Attitudinal reflexes. In The Child with Central Nervous System Deficit. Children's Bureau Publication, No. 432. U.S. Dept. of Health, Education and Welfare, Washington, D.C., U.S. Government Printing Office, 1965, pp 77-84.

13. Szumski AJ: Mechanisms underlying normal motor behavior. Am J Phys Med 46:52-86, 1967.

14. Jones B: The importance of memory traces of motor efferent discharges for learning skilled movements. Dev Med Child Neurol 16:620, 1974.

15. Munn WE: The Evolution and Growth of Human Behavior. Ed 2. Boston, Houghton Mifflin Co., 1965.

16. Bruner JS: Course of cognitive growth. Am Psychol 19:1-15, 1964.

17. Fantz, RL: Visual perception from birth as shown by pattern selectivity. In Whipple HE (Ed): New Issues in Infant Development. Ann NY Acad Sci 118:793-814, 1965.

18. Taylor E (Ed): Selected Writings of John Hughlings Jackson. London, Hodder and Stoughton, 1932, p 64.

19. McGraw MB: The Neuromuscular Maturation of the Human Infant. New York, Hafner, 1966.

20. Andre-Thomas: The neurological examination of the infant. Clinics in Developmental Medicine, No. 1. Philadelphia, J.B. Lippincott Co., 1964.

21. Bjeintema JD: A neurological study of newborn infants. Clinics in Developmental Medicine, No. 28. Philadelphia, J.B. Lippincott Co., 1968.

22. Buchwald JS: Exteroceptive reflexes and movement. Am J Phys Med 46:121-128, 1967.

23. Buchwald JS: General features of nervous system organization. Am J Phys Med 46:88-113, 1967.

24. Buchwald JS: Proprioceptive reflexes and posture. Am J Phys Med 46:104-113, 1967.

25. Eldred E: Peripheral receptors: Their excitation and relation to reflex patterns. Am J Phys Med 46:69-87, 1967.

26. Fisher E: Factors affecting motor learning. Am J Phys Med 46:511-516, 1967.

27. Newall K, Barclay C: Developing knowledge about action. In Kelso J, Clark J(Eds):

The Development of Movement Control and Co-ordination. New York, John Wiley & Sons, 1982, pp 175-179.

28. Piaget J: The Grasp of Consciousness: Action and Concept in the Young Child. Cambridge, Massachusetts, Harvard University Press, 1976.

29. Piaget J: Success and Understanding. Cambridge, Massachusetts, Harvard University Press, 1978.

30. Flavel J: The Developmental Psychology of Jean Piaget. Princeton, Van Nostrand, 1963.

31. Daloz L: Effective Teaching and Monitoring. San Francisco, Jossup-Bass, 1986, p 1347.

32. Kegan R: The Evolving Self: Problem and Process in Human Development. Cambridge, Massachusetts, Harvard University Press, 1982.

33. Winnicott D: The Maturational Process and the Facilitating Environment. New York, International Universities Press, 1965.

34. Wade M: Timing behavior in children. In Kelso J, Clark J (Eds): The Development of Movement Control and Co-ordination. New York, John Wiley & Sons, 1982, pp 239-249.

35. Jones B: The development of intermodal co-ordination and motor control. In Kelso J, Clark J (Eds): The Development of Movement Control and Co-ordination. New York, John Wiley & Sons, 1982, pp 105-106.

36. Reed K: Models of Practice in Occupational Therapy. Baltimore, Williams & Wilkins, 1985, pp 175-177.

Appendix 1-A
Perspectives on Theory Building

Theory Construction (Reynolds)

The Idea	Concepts	Definition	Quantification	Statements
1. Paradigms 2. Paradigm variations 3. Kuhn paradigm	1. Defined by primitive or derived terms 2. Concrete = specific to time or place Abstract = independent of time or space	Operational—determines existence of concept in concrete setting	1. Refer to object 2. Refer to characteristics, situations/state —nominal —ordinal —interval —ratio	1. Relationship between two or more concepts —existence —relational —associational —causal 2. Forms —laws "truth" —axioms independent origin of all other statements —propositions idea —hypotheses compare against data collected —empirical generalizations pattern based on data

Grounded Theory (Glaser and Strauss)

Insight	Conceptual Categories	Conceptual Properties	Hypotheses	Integration	Comparative Analysis
1. Experience 2. Others' experiences 3. Other theories	Stands by itself as a conceptual element of the theory	Aspect or element of the category	Generalized relations among categories and properties	Generalizing concepts to situations-patterns	1. Substantive-empirical area of inquiry 2. Formal-conceptual area of inquiry

Perspectives on Theory Building *Appendix 1-A cont.*

	Order	Concepts	Laws of Interaction	Boundaries	System State	Propositions	Empirical Indicators	Hypotheses
Covering Law Theory (Dubin)	Need to find order—exists in the mind	1. Units—things or variables which interact —enumerative —associative —relational —statistical —summative	Linkages among units —categoric —sequential —determinant —negative-null hypothesis	Limits theory holds	Conditions under which units interact differently	1. Predictions re: values of units 2. Truth statement about a fully specified model	An operation used to measure values on a unit	Predictions about values on a unit in which empirical indicators are used for each unit in the proposition

	Concepts	Definitions	Postulates
Theory (Mosey)	Words or phrases—label similarity between seemingly varied phenomena —simple—observable —construct—abstract —variable—measurable	1. Abstract—without reference to specific 2. Functional—action, purpose 3. Operational—relative to measurement	Relationship between two or more concepts —hierarchical —temporal —spatial —quantitative —correlative

References

Dubin, R. *Theory building* (1978). New York: The Free Press.
Glaser, B., Strauss, A. (1967). *The discovery of grounded theory.* New York: Aldine Publishing Co.
Mosey, A. *Occupational therapy: Configuration of a profession* (1981). New York: Raven Press.
Reynolds, P. *A primer in theory construction* (1971). Indianapolis: The Bobbs-Merrill Co., Inc.

CHAPTER 2

Theory of Spatiotemporal Adaptation

Objectives

The reader will be able to

1. define and explain spatiotemporal adaptation as a grounded theory;
2. define terminology specific to the theory;
3. explain the four conceptual categories of the theory as well as properties of each category;
4. identify and discuss principles of spiraling continuum as used with spatiotemporal adaptation theory;
5. discuss movement and environment as a system of relationships culminating in acquisition of performance skills;
6. describe "stress" as a positive factor of adaptation as well as an important developmental phenomenon; and
7. describe "distress" as a negative factor for development and relate the impact of distress upon dysfunction.

Introduction

Theories frequently develop from clinical practice in an attempt to organize information and explain phenomena. Spatiotemporal adaptation theory, which explains the sensorimotor basis for emergence of developmental and purposeful actions in children through an adaptation process, grew out of observations and comparative analyses of children functioning normally and those attempting to function with a disability. We noticed that a child with a disability, or developmental delay, used movement patterns that resembled performance patterns of much younger children who were considered to be functioning normally. Not only were abnormal postures and movements controlled by primitive reflex patterns and primitive movement sequences, but the ways in which children attempted to move from one position to another and the approach they chose to adapt movement to handling objects reflected adaptive patterns we had seen at chronologically and maturationally lower levels of development. We began observing normal children more closely, using photographic and video media to gather data for more detailed analysis. We were interested in observing the children's process to determine how they progressed from one level of competence to another, so we could discover the antecedents to change. We expected to uncover ideas for evaluation and treatment of children with dysfunction—and we did.

In general, normally functioning children revealed the extent to which normal performance varies, depending upon the adaptive competence of a child and demands of the environment. Almost invariably, a child who was just beginning to accomplish a developmental milestone or task would lose the ability whenever the activity required increased precision, change in speed, or challenge to gravity; was accompanied by talking, thinking, or doing something else simultaneously; or was influenced by fatigue. Instead of using their most mature levels of performance to adapt to space and objects, children in transition tended to call forth previously acquired patterns to adapt. These older patterns were more stable and less dexterous, but children could adapt these to accomplish their goals successfully, at least from their perspective. As we observed each child's performance, we noted that it "lacked quality" because the seemingly more mature, most efficient patterns of movement were not being used. The child appeared to add an extra step to the process by seeking stability through weight shifts or change in holding patterns before actually engaging in activity. Efficiency that comes from smoothly coordinating both initiation and control of movement simultaneously was not possible for these children during transitional phases of development. Even when the end result of task accomplishment was the same, the mode of accomplishment was immature.

We were also impressed with the intimate relationship between the state of a child's central nervous system development and the importance of environmental challenges to the system. Transitional situations appeared stressful for children because they had to work so much harder to accomplish tasks. Movements appeared uncoordinated, and failure often preceded success. But in fact, the children responded positively to challenge, seemed to enjoy engaging in the process—however difficult—and used the situation as part of the maturational process. By attempting activities that appeared to be beyond their adaptive competence, children seemingly related components from previous behaviors to requirements of a new challenge, differentiated those components needed for the new activity, and adapted them to develop a more mature approach. Through this adaptation process, children used the challenging situations and adapted by "calling forth" their already developed capabilities to gain competence in movement patterns required for more difficult tasks. The interaction was a transactional process between children and their environment. We visualized this adaptation process, of moving between more primitive and more mature functioning, as a spiraling continuum with a child functioning between using old patterns to gain new patterns and new patterns to change old patterns of behavior.

However, normal challenging or stressful situations presented a different set of problems for children who had disability. Most notably, these children were not able to make use of normally stressful situations to enhance their development. With central nervous system dysfunction impeding their development, children could not make use of challenges from the environment to create new patterns of movement, but instead continued to use primitive patterns even in new situations. For some children, these abnormal patterns of movement ultimately became a way of adapting to the world.

From these observations, we saw possibilities for evaluation and treatment of children with dysfunction. Although there were treatment approaches available that controlled sensory information and/or motor performance of children, we determined that by incorporating concepts from spiraling adaptation, a clinician could expand, explain, and enhance available treatment approaches. Application of such adaptation concepts as changing postural or spatial demands of a situation, or changing movement or temporal considerations of an activity, or both, meant that we could link together the facilitation emanating from therapeutically controlled sensory and motor intervention with situations requiring higher level adaptation performance. A result of controlling the spatiotemporal demands by linking sensorimotor intervention methods with selected situations increases both the quality and maturational level of a child's functioning within the limits of the original problem.

Explanation of Theory

Spatiotemporal adaptation theory proposes that children acquire sensorimotor skills through a transactional process as they develop movement patterns to adapt to their environments of space and time. Adaptation occurs through developmental and purposeful sequences of activity with developmental sequences emanating essentially from innate, genetically determined behavior, and purposeful sequences evolving from a child's intention to accomplish a goal. Both developmental and purposeful sequences make use of neuromuscular functions to produce movement. Developmental sequences direct maturation of automatic responses, which culminate in patterns of controlled movement, used primarily for moving about in space and for developing reaching and grasping. Purposeful sequences make use of developmental patterns of movement by adapting them to new experiences motivated by intention. As basic functions are adapted to increasingly complex developmental or purposeful activities, higher level functions emerge.

Integration of previously acquired movements with requirements of new environmental challenge is an ongoing spiraling process. Spiraling adaptation emphasizes association/differentiation of previously acquired (old) patterns with new experiences and newly acquired (new) patterns with previous experience, as a transactional process between functions of movement inherent in the person and purposes for movement that lie within the person and environment. Function-to-purpose and purpose-to-function continuum (Figure 2-1) forms the basis for the spiraling process of adaptation with more complex movement sequences emerging from the more primitive acquired actions as a result of environmental interactions.

Environment provides a source of stimulation for functional change in bodily structures as children adapt to the demands of their surroundings. Environmental challenges present spatiotemporal stress situations, which are temporary states characterized by an inability for children to adapt their highest levels of movements to new or more complex events. With stress situations, lower level functions are called forth to adapt; thus, children resolve these stressful situations by linking lower level functions to purposes of new experiences in order to successfully meet that particular environmental challenge. However, a child's response to spatiotemporal stress is not only relevant to

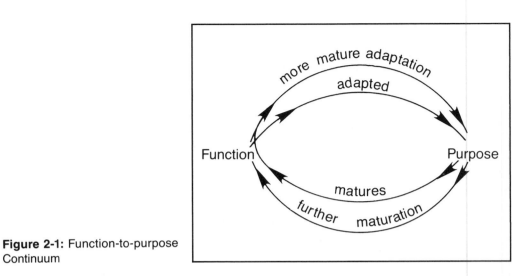

Figure 2-1: Function-to-purpose Continuum

resolving the immediate situation, but sets the stage for higher level functional abilities to develop. As the central nervous system matures, along with challenges from the environment, higher level functions mature and are adapted to new experiences through the association-differentiation process.

The natural phenomenon for children to "call up" previously acquired patterns to adapt under stress is evident with children who have disabilities or dysfunctional movement patterns. Spatiotemporal adaptation theory proposes that children with dysfunction are unable to make use of stress to move to higher levels of development, probably because of problems associated with delayed or lack of central nervous system maturation. The process is one of maladaptation characterized by the continued use of lower level functions and an inability to associate-differentiate old with new and new with old.

Spatiotemporal adaptation has previously been described as being most closely related to grounded theory. Using the grounded theory framework, conceptual categories and properties will be presented and explained. Four categories have been identified: (1) Movement, (2) Environment, (3) Adaptation, and (4) Spiraling Continuum. Although each category stands alone, dynamics of the theory come from interaction among the categories.

Movement

Movement in infancy creates one of the first possibilities for a child to adapt to an ever-changing environment and, through adaptation, to change primitive movements to more effective, efficient, mature action patterns. In early postnatal life, movement is initiated from within all levels of the central nervous system by genetically programmed behavioral patterns or drives. These genetic drives enable the child to obtain meaningful goals without using conscious effort—i.e., without having to think through the actual movement patterns involved or using cortical energy to remember these patterns. A child's pursuit of the upright posture and locomotion is central to the concept of a genetically programmed development sequence. With goal-oriented drives, a child can interact with the environment in a meaningful way, and through interaction, express and gradually adapt genetic potential through experiential learning. Normal movement is considered a goal-oriented activity consisting of a repetitive, yet constantly changing, adaptive process.

Movements are adapted to a specific purpose almost as soon as they are initiated. Through the adaptation process, repertoires of movement strategies are established so that the purpose of movement begins to direct the initiation of movement in terms of spatial and temporal orientation.[1] A child's development of smooth, coordinated reach, combined with a neat pinch grasp for obtaining small objects, is an example of the emergence of purposeful sequences. Moore[2] discussed the nervous system's genetic and purposeful potential, and these concepts will be further elaborated in subsequent chapters.

Movement puts a child into changing relationships with the environment and provides varied experiences for interaction and perception of immediate surroundings, including self in space, persons in space, objects and object relationships, movement of objects in space, and effect of self-movement on object movement. As a child gains competence in movement, purposeful movement supports cognitive and social development. Movement links sensorimotor adaptation with psychosocial development by ways in which movement is used for play and its contributions to learning; or for communication and its relationship to verbalizing or writing thoughts; or for emotional response, such as nonverbal or verbal expression of feelings; or for social interaction, particularly seeking or separating from others. Adaptation of movement to goals of cognitive and social development serves to promote integration of the sensorimotor adaptive processes into the system as a whole. Movement initially provides power for a child to experience cognitive and social situations. Eventually, environmental situations provide the challenge for more discrete and automatic movement to support more complex thinking and acting.

Properties of Movement in this theory are **structure, function,** and **purpose.** Structures and functions are bodily processes used to adapt to the environment. Purpose provides the motivation for initiating and adapting movement. Structures include bones, joints, muscles, and neural mechanism. Structures are essentially present at birth, although they change to some extent as the system matures and functional capacities inherent to the structures develop. Functions are inherent to structure in the sense that the structure determines what functions, or in this theory what movements, are possible. For example, bone and joint structures allow movement only in certain directions and through certain ranges. Muscles as structures move body segments within bone/joint limitations. However, differences in the ways in which movements are used depend upon functions that exist within muscle structures. For example, some muscles develop more as a stabilizing force in postural control because they are shorter and located proximally with broad attachments; other muscle structures develop mobilizing functions for volitional movement because they are longer, thinner, and designed for faster reciprocal actions. Nerves, or neural mechanisms, are structured to transmit information and develop networks that link neuromuscular functions within the system and with the environment. Location, size, and myelination of nerves determine conduction velocity of the pathway and, therefore, the way in which it transmits information and type of information transmitted. Although neuromusculo-skeletal functions are determined by possibilities that exist within the structure, they are facilitated by both genetic potential and stimulation from the environment. Development of functions promotes changes in the structures themselves; for example, growth of bony structures, muscle fibers, myelination. Functions are initially developed as they are being initiated and are adapted to genetically programmed developmental sequences.

Purpose provides direction for movement and, as a goal of movement, is key to the manner in which functions are programmed to achieve certain purposes. A purpose is that which can be done with something and identifies a specific outcome that is intended to result. Whereas function describes an inherent relationship with structure, without implying conscious intent on the part of a developing child, purpose can be described as an uncompelling, but intentional, action on the part of a child. Intentionality makes action meaningful to a child and brings about change in structures and functions.

Purposes are endless in nature and number. Each purpose requires a certain variation in basic movement pattern available to serve that particular purpose; i.e., picking up a bead, peg, or pencil requires a similar, but slightly different, variation of the basic prehension pattern. During development, functions are combined to form new and usually more complex movement patterns in order to meet challenges for a purposeful response to the environment. As functions are adapted to purposes, the functions and their structures mature. More mature adaptations in the form of discrete, efficient, coordinated movements emerge and, as a result, more challenging intentions can be pursued. Functions are programmed in such a way that automatic patterns of complex movement develop and become available whenever the purpose for that particular movement presents itself. Function-to-purpose continuum is a transactional process between the functions of movement inherent within a child and the purposes of movement that lie within a child and the environment.

Relationships between functions of movement and purposes of movement are influenced by a child's motivation to move and adapt movement. Intrinsic motivation particularly influences the development of movement through emergence of genetically programmed developmental sequences. Both intrinsic and extrinsic motivation influence the environmentally programmed purposeful sequences of movement. According to White[3] people have an inherent urge to explore and master the environment, which he termed **effectance motivation.** Effectance motivation can be likened to intrinsic motivation, both terms emphasizing that people perform for the value of action. Intrinsic motivation enhances an exploratory and experimental attitude that leads to a competent interaction with the environment.[4] Deci and Porac[5] noted that intrinsic motivation is goal-directed toward the behavioral completion itself, whereas extrinsic motivation is directed toward an external reward for completion of behaviors. The theory in this text proposes that participation with purposeful sequences is both intrinsically and extrinsically motivated. Intention and intrinsic motivation to explore and master the world are primary elements of purposefulness of movement and common characteristics of purposeful sequences that are developmental in nature. Developmental and purposeful nature of movement serve to motivate the self-system for modification or change.

Environment

Movement is not a self-contained process that takes place independently. Development of movement, and in fact how we move, has a great deal to do with the nature of environment and our transactions with it. Movement and environment can be likened to a system of relationships. When a person's movement remains smooth, he or she encounters the environment as neither "too harsh nor too perfect, but just good enough."[6] p192 According to Winnicott[7] a "good enough" environment meets and challenges a person's need to grow and develop, and there is a developmental dialogue or internal conversation to meet and adapt to stimulation from the changing environment. A person's movement is both a product and process of the self-environment interplay as individuals both create and are created by the environment. Winnicott speaks to a human's surroundings as a facilitating environment that "makes possible the steady progress of the maturational processes . . . but the environment does not make the child. At best, it enables the child to realize potential."[7 p85]Movement and environment are viewed in terms of a single whole that is set to work as a system of relationships that promote adaptation and integration. Within the system, movement provides the power for the child to experience, the environment provides the motivation to experience, and adaptation provides the process.

The category **Environment**, as used in reference to spatiotemporal adaptation theory, is all-inclusive. Environment is the complete setting or surrounding—that is, the milieu—including self, other persons, objects, the earth, space, and relationships within space. Environment is everything with which an individual interacts.

Transactions with the environment take place within dimensions of space and time. As used in the theory of spatiotemporal adaptation, **space** and **time** are properties of the category **Environment**. Space, or spatial, refers to the area surrounding an individual, including the supporting surface for the body, gravitational and three-dimensional space surrounding the body, and space occupied by the body or by other persons or objects within the area. Spatial dimensions encompass the environment in which a person exists and functions. Time, or temporal aspects of adaptation, is defined as duration, regulation, memory, and sequence of a person's actions, body movements, or movements to other persons or objects within the area. Temporal dimensions encompass planning and professing of actions in relation to stationary or moving objects.

Within the context of the spatiotemporal milieu, environment has four major functions: the **holding function**, which serves to embed the infant and support the body; the **facilitating function**, which provides the source of stimulation, arousal, intent, and motivation to move; the **challenge function,** which helps a child reach higher levels of the self's potential; and the **interactive function**, which promotes an interplay between self and environment. The value of one's environment is in the dynamic integration and balance of these four functions. Through environmental functions, individuals acquire a spatiotemporal awareness and an ability to be aware of and oriented to spatiotemporal components of the environment, learn rules of social interactions, and develop behavioral flexibility or adaptability to successfully interact with one's environment. Transactions with the environment culminate in one's spatiotemporal orientation.

Humans are unique in their abilities to possess spatiotemporal orientation to life's experiences. Spatiotemporal orientation is the way in which a person perceives and interprets his own situation within space and, at a specific time, adapts to and with that situation.[8] Spatiotemporal orientation concerns itself with past, present, and future, and requires that each individual have a kinesthetic awareness, or clear picture, of his own body and its place in space, at rest, or in motion.[9] Spatiotemporal orientation also requires that an individual can assess the spatial positioning of objects in the environment and relate his own spatial position to them.[10]

Literature indicates several studies on spatial and temporal adaptations.[8-11] Application of findings and theories related to space and time has led to the belief that spatial and temporal elements of the environment cannot be separated in the developmental process of acquiring skills. Therefore, the following assumptions about space and time can be integrated into a single construct termed **spatiotemporal environmental assumptions**.

1. Each person has a unique spatiotemporal orientation to environmental experiences.
2. Spatiotemporal orientation to one's milieu begins in infancy and develops through transactions between movement and environment.
3. Orientation and organization of space and time are influenced by an individual's psychosocial and sensorimotor components, including a person's cultural and social roles.
4. A person's use of space and time is a product of balancing holding, facilitating, challenging, and interacting functions of the environment.
5. Spatiotemporal characteristics of environmental events are critical factors for adaptation, resulting in purposeful actions and goal-directed events.

Through the movement-environment system of relationships, the uniqueness of self is continually evolving from specific transactions between child and environment; however, there are certain commonalities in the transactional process that characterize human development, including adaptation.

Adaptation

Adaptation is a dynamic process of expanding a child's repertoire of movements and activities. Through adaptation, more complex movements evolve, which provide a child with increased abilities to expand environmental interactions. Increased movement provides a child with a sense of competence to move about within the environment and engage in goal-directed, purposeful experiences. Adaptation is defined as the continuous, ongoing state or act of adjusting those bodily processes required to function within a given space and time. As stressed by Kegan[10], adaptation is not a coping process or a process of adjusting the body to events as they are. Instead, adaptation is an active process of organizing and relating self with environment. Kegan[10] also believes that the relationship of self and environment gets more organized through the ongoing active adaptation processes, which accounts for increasing differentiation of self from environment and increasing integrations of environmental experiences.

As a category, **Adaptation** has three properties: **sensorimotor-sensory process**, **developmental nature**, and **purposeful nature**. Each of the properties is introduced in this section with additional discussions in succeeding chapters.

Sensorimotor-sensory process includes assimilation, accommodation, association, and differentiation. **Assimilation** is the sensory process of receiving information external to, and within, the system. To illustrate, a ball is seen as coming toward one's self and the hands are felt as being inside one's pockets. Sensory information is "taken in" or assimilated into the system. As information is received by the self-system, an individual will modify his posture and adjust the position of the hands in preparation for catching the ball. One's response or motor process of adjusting the body to react to incoming stimuli is termed **accommodation**. The third component, **association**, is an organized process of relating sensory information with the motor act being experienced, as well as calling up previously acquired behaviors for relating present and past experiences with each other. For example, the visual stimulation of the moving ball is related with the accommodation of the body, and the present act of catching the ball is related with past experiences of ball catching. **Differentiation** is the process of discriminating those essential elements of a specific behavior that are pertinent to a given situation, distinguishing those that are not, and thereby modifying or altering the behavior in some manner, e.g., discriminating the forearm pattern necessary to catch the ball by distinguishing the amount of elbow flexion and supination necessary, and thus modifying the forearm position for more efficient ball catching.

Association and differentiation of adapting to different situations become integrated into the self-system, providing a repertoire of actions that can be used by an individual for a variety of environmental transactions. Integration of the situation or experiences provides a child with abilities to exercise choice and make decisions based on the most efficient and effective way to respond. Outcomes from the adaptation process include developmental and purposeful sequences of behavior.

Assimilation, accommodation, association, and differentiation processes of the sensorimotor-sensory property is a variation of the adaptation paradigm introduced by Piaget[12] and of Moore's[2] concepts of sensorimotor-sensory association.

The term **sensorimotor-sensory** emphasizes the relationship of sensory input, motor output, and the importance of feedback for association and differentiation. Thus movement, environment, and adaptation must be judged from this view, as the three categories are viewed as a dynamic whole that becomes perfected when set to work as a sensorimotor-sensory unit. Sensorimotor-sensory shall be referred to in this text as SMS. A discussion of the SMS property, as related to spiraling, appears later in this chapter.

Sequential maturation of the central nervous system is inherent in the developmental nature of adaptation, which is characterized by predictable changes proceeding in a cephalocaudal, generalized to localized, and proximal to distal direction. The developmental nature of adaptation enhances growth, maturation, and development of the structures and functions required for pursuit of upright and upper extremity abilities.

Development's sequential nature, a quality of the adaptation process, describes the innate drive to proceed along a predictable sequence for acquisition of higher level sensorimotor skills. During development, children seem to utilize certain innate functions that encourage them to seek out those events or activities most related to the specific developmental phase needing reinforcement or development. Thus, the objective of an event provides the stimulus to reinforce needed functions for higher level performance.

Seeking and interacting with environmental events is the purposeful nature of adaptation. As movement patterns are adapted to environmental events, there is an arousal of a child's intention. Intention is the initial reaction to stimulus and promotes the purposefulness of adaptation. Adaptation becomes purposeful when the nature of, and participation with, the activity/event facilitates meaningful responses for one's nervous system. Responses become meaningful when sensory feedback associated with actions provides directions and efforts that are more mature or at a higher level than those previously experienced. Thus the purposefulness of adaptation processes augments sensorimotor-sensory integration and results in the emergence of purposeful sequences of movement required for skilled performance.

Spiraling Continuum

Adapting lower level primitive patterns of posture and movement to higher level complex skills is the spiraling continuum process of spatiotemporal adaptation theory.

The process is illustrated by the ever-widening and upward continuum of a spiral (Figure 2-2). The continuum illustrates the ongoing process of development, while the spiral effect emphasizes integration of old with new. The spiraling process of spatiotemporal adaptation has both developmental and purposeful sequences and matures as a result of environmental experiences and modification of self's maturing nervous system to eventually encompass the highest levels of complex performance skills. Spiraling includes integration of sensory input, motor output, and sensory feedback. Assimilation is likened to sensory input, accommodation viewed as motor output, and association differentiation components are the vital aspect of sensory feedback that occurs as a person functions within the environment.

When the environment provides a new experience, a child adapts to that experience with an acquired behavior and integrates sensory feedback from the new experience with actions of a previously acquired behavior. Through integration, one's self-system organizes information from the experience. Integration of new with old is dependent upon and results in modification of the nervous system. Association and differentiation of information further facilitates higher level performance. Therefore, maturation results from the spiraling process of sensorimotor-sensory adaptation and integration of environmental experiences.

Inherent within the spiraling process of adaptation is the development of perception.

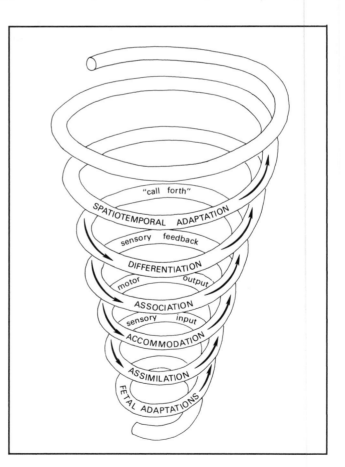

Figure 2-2: Spiraling Continuum of Spatiotemporal Adaptation

Perception is an individual's sensory judgment or feeling about information received by the system and the system's accommodation to it. The perceptual process functions to automatically direct the selection of movement patterns for specific activities and plays a major role in programming developmental patterns for specific skilled purposes. As an infant, sensory stimuli are received by the system; as stimuli are integrated with experiences, the system becomes aware or acquires a sensory awareness. Awareness of sensation associated with environmental experiences ultimately leads to sensory perception as a result of highly complex SMS integration and by means of the spiraling process. Adaptation and integration, combined with the use of perception, forms one aspect of cognition.

The spiraling continuum of spatiotemporal adaptation emphasizes four important principles:

1. **A child's adaptation process with new experiences is dependent upon past acquired behaviors**. To illustrate, a child begins to walk using a reciprocal pattern that is dependent upon the reciprocal patterns that developed with crawling and creeping.

2. **With integration of past experiences with new experiences, the past behaviors are modified in some manner and result in a higher level behavior**. For example, once reciprocation is integrated with standing, a child acquires an ability to walk, and locomotion is by walking rather than by the lower level creeping behavior.

3. **Integration of higher level behaviors influences and increases the maturity of lower level behaviors**. To illustrate, as walking is practiced and reciprocation repeated, a child's creeping pattern matures further because, by walking, the child develops more extension with rotation, allowing simultaneous weight shift and forward movement, thereby smoothing out reciprocal patterns.

4. **Lower level functions or performance patterns may emerge during adaptation whenever the environmental demands exceed the functional capabilities of the child, resulting in a spatiotemporal stress reaction**. To illustrate this principle, consider a child who has recently acquired an ability to walk. A child meets a step or an incline that demands higher level balance reactions; thus, environmental demands exceed the child's functional capacities. To adapt to these demands, a child calls up lower level skills, such as creeping, to negotiate the obstacle or incline. Therefore, in the spiraling continuum of spatiotemporal adaptation, a child does not acquire totally new behaviors; rather, new behaviors are higher level modifications of the old level reactions.

There are two properties of the **Spiraling Continuum** category—stress and distress. Stress is presented in detail in this chapter, with the property, distress, being introduced here. Chapter 8, which discusses dysfunction and relates the theory to abnormal development, provides additional discussion regarding distress.

Stress. In the process of adapting, a child encounters a variety of experiences that represent stress. The way a child meets and handles these stress experiences has a direct impact upon results of adaptation. Therefore, stress may be considered a positive or a negative factor of development. As a positive factor, stress produces a temporary state that results in higher level functions and maturation; as a negative factor, stress is a persistent state that results in maladaptation and interferes with maturation.

Hans Selye[13] describes stress as a relationship between an organism's biological system and changes through which one goes in adjusting to demands of the environment. Selye defines stress as a phenomenon characterized by an alteration of the system's equilibrium. The result of stress is an adjustment made to the environment, with a return to normal functioning or equilibrium, following a stress impact. A child will experience stress impact when acquired or learned ways of coping with situations no longer suffice. In the spiraling process of adapting, a child alters learned performances in some manner to resolve the "stress" situation. Alteration of performance results in resolution of the stress situation, modification of learned patterns, and higher level functioning—a positive outcome.

For example, as a child is adapting functions to purposes, the challenge of the process and demands of the environment may exceed his or her functional capacities; the child may experience spatiotemporal stress. In a stress situation, aspects of lower level posture and movement strategies may influence the adaptation process. The use of lower level strategies is often apparent during the course of normal development when a child meets a new experience. In Figures 2-3, 2-4, and 2-5, influences of the lower level prone extension posture (pivot prone) can be observed in early sitting and walking postures. Scapular adduction, shoulder retraction, and elbow flexion pattern of the lower level prone extension posture facilitates the necessary trunk extension for early sitting and standing. When a child first assumes sitting and standing, she will utilize a pattern similar to a prone extension posture to facilitate trunk extension necessary to maintain vertical postures of sitting and standing. As vertical postures are repeated, lower level reactions are differentiated so that essential elements are integrated to form higher level adaptations. With the above example, the essential elements of postural extensor tone are differentiated from the prone extension pattern and integrated into the higher level adaptation of trunk stability in vertical postures (Figure 2-6).

Effects of stress upon a child's spatiotemporal adaptation is further illustrated in Figures 2-7 and 2-8. Figure 2-7 illustrates a baby adapting with a beginning form of the Landau reaction (note the extension patterns of the body). In Figure 2-8 he is blindfolded, which temporarily changes one parameter of his sensory integration patterns, and temporary alteration of sensory integration interrupts the midline stability of the Landau reaction. The baby adapts to his stress situation with a lower level pattern of asymmetrical stability.

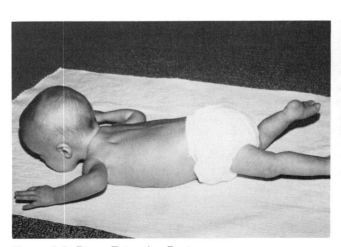

Figure 2-3: Prone Extension Posture

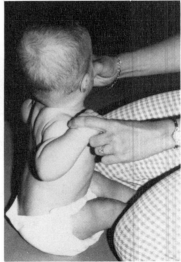

Figure 2-4: Early Sitting

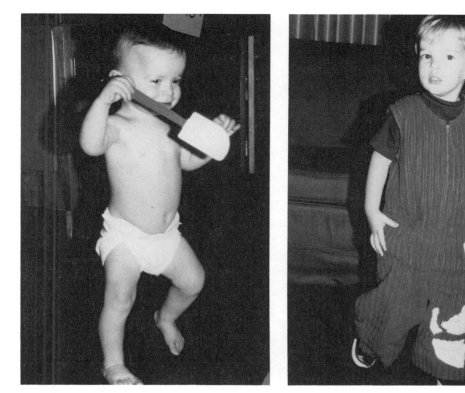

Figure 2-5: Primitive Walking   **Figure 2-6:** Standing/Walking

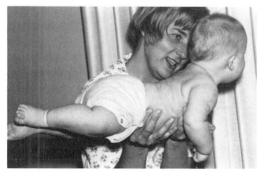   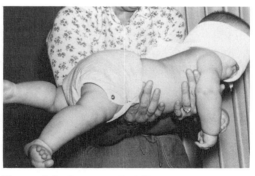

Figure 2-7: Vertical Righting   **Figure 2-8:** Asymmetrical Posture

The boy in Figures 2-9 and 2-10 demonstrates the stress phenomenon while performing higher level actions. While walking on a balance beam with his eyes open, the boy is able to adapt with a mature equilibrium reaction (Figure 2-9). In Figure 2-10, he is walking the balance beam with his eyes closed, which alters his sensory integration, and he adapts with a lower level immature equilibrium reaction (note the asymmetrical upper extremity pattern). In both sets of figures the changing integration that occurs with vision occluded results in spatiotemporal stress, and the boy adapts with a more primitive pattern of posture and movement.

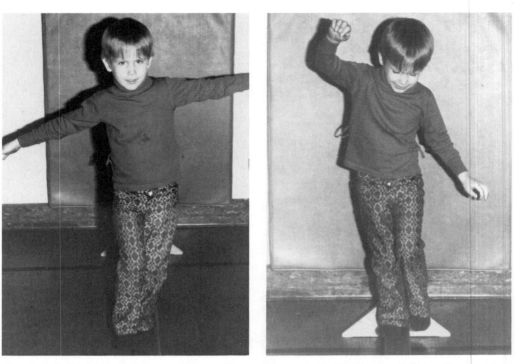

Figure 2-9: Walking on Balance Beam - Eyes Open

Figure 2-10: Walking on Balance Beam - Eyes Closed

"Stress—the internal drummer, so to speak—truly lies within us, and so also does the solution of the human predicament. The answer is already there; we just need to learn how to call it forth."[14pp14-15] Calling forth previously acquired behaviors in order to adapt to stress experiences is inherent within the spiraling continuum of spatiotemporal adaptation.

Spatiotemporal stress is the "internal drummer" phenomenon of the normal developmental process. When the phenomenon occurs, the system "calls forth" previously acquired older patterns to adapt to demands of the situation. Calling forth acquired patterns to adapt expends only the needed energy to maintain the system's hemostasis. Although the system is confronted with change, the amount and degree of change is not past the point for "homeostatic energy expenditure."[15] Therefore spatiotemporal stress, as a normal developmental phenomenon, is not anxiety provoking to the self-system. Rather, spatiotemporal stress is a motivating force that stimulates us to adapt to the constant changes of our existence.

Environmental factors that create spatiotemporal stress are gravity, complexity of movement, and requirements of the action. Gravity is a significant force to move against for purposes of developing strategies that support function. In addition to facilitating and strengthening posture and movement strategies, gravity demands that organized strategies be continually available for adaptation to developmental sequences and purposeful sequences. Gravity becomes a significant factor in eliciting selected strategies for adapting to the demands of the environment. The system monitors changes in body position in relation to gravitational input, and postural adjustments are automatically made. A child is free to attend to activities without expending cortical energy on balance or posture. However, during periods of development and adaptation of strategies, gravity may produce stress rather than promote balance. A child will either seek a more secure posture to perform desired activity, or pause to practice balance at a higher level of postural control before attempting activities at that level. In either case, **gravitational stress** is a factor for change in both higher and lower level performance.

A related factor known to produce stress is the **complexity of movement** required to complete an action. A movement strategy adapted to any situation demands smooth blending of stability and mobility functions to produce coordinated flow. A movement strategy adapted to a complex situation requires even more careful monitoring of movement combinations in order to produce the most efficient and accurate strategy. As long as movement flow and countermovement control are automatically monitored and blended, a child employs his or her acquired highest levels of posture and movement for desired actions. However any situation that interrupts monitoring and blending of muscle functions, such as changes in feedback or demands for more intricate movement, may produce spatiotemporal stress. A child will either call forth a more secure posture to support more intricate movement or will choose a less complex movement strategy to complete the desired action.

A third related factor of spatiotemporal stress is found in the **requirements of the action or skill** itself. If complexity of an action or skill increases in terms of spatial, temporal, cognitive, or emotional demands, stress may interrupt automatic use of more recently established sequences or performance skills. A child may call forth a previously acquired behavior to adapt to increased demands from the environment.

Factors contributing to spatiotemporal stress are interrelated, and several factors are often responsible for change. Gravity usually plays a major role in stress during adaptation of developmental sequence skills when mastery of spatial demands predominates. The gravity factor continues to re-emerge, along with the complex movement factor, when movement is being matched to temporal demands of purposeful sequential skills. Complexity of movement is particularly stressful during the time when performance skills are developing. Requirements of the action and event become the intervening variable when performance behaviors are expanding and being adapted to skills.

The following example citing modification of on-hands behavior is presented to illustrate the role of spatiotemporal stress in facilitating normal development:

1. In prone, a child can assume and maintain the on-hands position; however, she lacks the ability to shift weight onto one upper extremity in order to reach out and grasp a toy (Figure 2-11).
2. To reach out for a toy, a child calls forth previously acquired on-elbows position and gains the stability required to shift weight to one upper extremity and to reach out successively (Figure 2-12).
3. A child repeats the sequence frequently, moving to an on-hands position to practice a new behavior and back to on-elbows to play. By repeatedly assuming the new on-hands posture, and perhaps occasionally going to hands and knees, a child develops functions necessary to stabilize and move in the on-hands position (Figure 2-13).
4. With more control in the on-hands position, a child responds differently to a stimulus to reach for a toy. Rather than resume on-elbows posture to reach, a child differentiates the concept of shifting weight and reaching, and adapts it to the on-hands position. Newly developed stability in on-hands position supports the

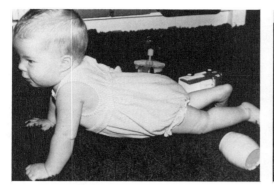

Figure 2-11: On Hands

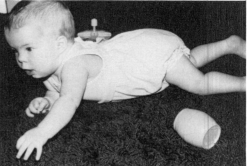

Figure 2-12: On Elbows Reaching

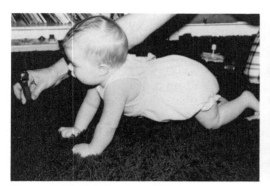

Figure 2-13: On Hands and Knees

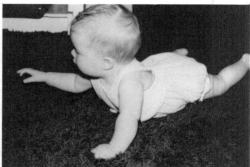

Figure 2-14: On Hands Reaching

weight shift, and a new reaching behavior emerges at a higher level of development (Figure 2-14).

From this illustration, the role of stress as a developmental motivator is apparent. Stress factors that caused the child to alter posture in order to function also provided the purpose for function to be associated with new experiences, differentiated and adapted so that higher level behaviors change and development proceeds.

During the normal developmental process, spatiotemporal stress primarily occurs in three situations: (1) when adapting to new experiences, (2) when the sensorimotor-sensory integrative process is temporarily altered in some manner, and (3) during transition of one behavior to another. In these three situations, a child may attempt to adapt with his or her highest level of learned performance. When the method of coping does not suffice, the system will subsequently "call forth" older patterns to resolve the situation and enhance maturation.

Throughout development, the self-system learns to manage stress experiences of the environment and ultimately develops methods of coping. Thus, adaptation of developmental and purposeful sequence skills is dependent upon spatiotemporal stress. As a result, the system matures. Adapting children thrive on spatiotemporal stress experiences that can be managed and controlled by the self-system.

Distress. Stress that is out of control and cannot be managed is termed **distress**. Distress as a property is defined as a negative factor for development, characterized by an alteration of the system's equilibrium, and resulting in purposeless performance and maladaptation. With distress there is a lack of return to the system's normal functioning level or equilibrium. When the environment provokes distress, homeostasis is affected, purposeless (meaningless) behaviors prevail, and maladaptation occurs.

During the spiraling process of adapting spatiotemporal components of environmental experiences, distress may occur. When the system experiences spatiotemporal distress, lower level behaviors cannot be adapted to new experiences and higher level behaviors do not emerge. Integration of lower and higher level behaviors and/or activities does not occur. Therefore, functions are not adjusted to, or with, purposes, and movement patterns are not linked with environmental events or adaptation to higher level skills.

Spatiotemporal distress may result from (1) abnormal assimilations, e.g., abnormal sensory reception, sensory deprivation, or sensory overload (jamming); (2) abnormal accommodations, e.g., purposeless sensorimotor patterns, abnormal neuromuscular characteristics (tone, range, control, speed, etc.); and (3) abnormal association/differentiation, e.g., faulty sensorimotor-sensory integration.

Origins of spatiotemporal distress are numerous. There are hereditary factors; chromosomal abnormalities; unexplained birth defects; fetal distress or lack of expected development in utero; prematurity or dysmaturity; difficulties before, during, or after birth with residual brain lesions; retardation; acquired problems from trauma or disease affecting the central nervous system or peripheral systems; and abuse, neglect, or environmental deprivation. There is also a large idiopathic category of developmental disabilities for which diagnosis is not available to explain the origin of the problem, but the problem of spatiotemporal distress still exists for the child, family, educator, and health-care professional. Although information about origins of a child's distress/dysfunction is valuable for purposes of evaluation, planning, monitoring, and predicting progress and prognosis, the most valuable source of information available for analysis of spatiotemporal distress is the child herself.

Spatiotemporal distress affects every aspect of a child's progress toward maturity. Relationships within the family and world outside, feelings of competence and autonomy, and others' responses are built upon performance expectations held by the child, and by others.

Since so much of measurable performance is built upon spatiotemporal adaptation, especially for a young child, interruptions in the process or failure to develop according to expectations has a reverberating effect upon the SMS process, neurophysiologically and emotionally.

Summary

The theory of spatiotemporal adaptation has been constructed through comparative analysis of differing groups of children performing within the environment. Factors from the literature were synthesized and integrated with clinical data to provide the basis for identification of conceptual categories and their properties. Four categories—movement, environment, adaptation, and spiraling continuum—have been discussed as major constructs inherent in the theory. Appendix 2-A presents the categories and their properties.

The theory was developed to explain how children learn sensorimotor skills and to provide guidelines for evaluation, planning, and implementation of services for children with special needs. Another major purpose for the theory is a source for research.

Spatiotemporal adaptation theory proposes that children learn and develop movement patterns through the spiraling continuum of spatiotemporal adaptation. Adaptation occurs through primitive, transitional, and mature phases of development, with each phase having distinct purposes for evolution of skilled movements. Skilled movements are acquired through developmental and purposeful sequences emanating from innate, genetically determined functions and a child's innate desire to accomplish a goal. The spiraling nature of adaptation emphasizes the association/differentiation of previously acquired patterns with new experiences and newly acquired experiences as an ever-widening, ongoing, transactional process of self and environment. The theory proposes that children with dysfunction or disability cannot make use of the spiraling process, thus maladaptation occurs.

Succeeding chapters provide detailed explanations about the conceptual categories and their properties. The following chapter presents the neuroscience base to substantiate the spiraling adaptation process and theory categories. Chapters 4, 5, 6, and 7 discuss and illustrate the conceptual categories and properties of posture and movement strategies, and adaptation of movement to developmental sequences and purposeful sequences. Elaboration of the effects of distress and dysfunction in children and application of theory to practice are presented in Chapters 8, 9 and 10.

Key Points

1. Adaptation is a sensorimotor-sensory process, dependent upon the interaction between movement and environment, as well as the interrelationship of movement, perception, and cognition. Adaptation results from the transactions with environmental space and time (spatiotemporal).
2. Spatiotemporal adaptation can be described as a "grounded theory" that has four categories: movement, environment, adaptation, and spiraling continuum. Each category has properties that further illustrate the uniqueness of the theory.
3. Spatiotemporal adaptation is an ongoing process of adjusting the bodily processes to, and with, the events of the environment.
4. Spatiotemporal adaptation is a variation of the adaptation paradigm introduced by Piaget, with assimilation, accommodation, association, and differentiation as components of the process of adaptation. These components are reflected in the sensorimotor-sensory process (SMS) of environmental transactions.
5. Spatiotemporal adaptation is a spiraling process of adapting posture and movement strategies to developmental sequences and to purposeful sequences. Patterns gained through the spiraling process are differentiated and adapted to goal-directed events within the environment, culminating in performance skills. The system of relationships of movement-environment is the essential ingredient in the purposeful process of developing performance skills.
7. Intrinsic motivation is a biologically inherent urge to explore and master the environment and, as such, is the common characteristic of the nature of purpose.
8. The uniqueness of a person is intrinsic to both process and product of spatiotemporal adaptation.
9. Spiraling Continuum is a conceptual category illustrating the ongoing process of development and integration of past and present events. Therefore, children do not acquire totally new behaviors; rather, new behaviors are higher level modifications of older, lower level behaviors.

10. Lower level functions may emerge during adaptation, when the environmental demands exceed the functional capacities of a child, resulting in spatiotemporal stress.
11. Spatiotemporal stress is a natural phenomenon and a vital stimulus for development, as integrating lower level functions with new experiences results in higher level adaptation.
12. In stress situations children may "call up" lower level posture and movement strategies to adapt to the demands of the environment.
13. Gravity and complexity of activity are major stress factors.
14. In distress situations maladaptation occurs.

Self-study Guidelines

1. Define the components of a spatiotemporal adaptation process and give examples of each component.
2. Relate sensorimotor-sensory (SMS) process to the components of adaptation.
3. Compare and contrast spatiotemporal stress and distress.
4. Describe spiraling continuum as a category of the theory and identify four principles.
5. Explain spatiotemporal adaptation as a grounded theory and describe each conceptual category and its properties.

References
1. Goodgold-Edwards S: Motor learning as it relates to the development of skilled motor behavior: A review of the literature. Phys Occup Ther in Peds 4:5-16, 1985.
2. Moore JC: Proceedings 1987 Sensorimotor Symposium: Movement and Learning. San Diego, California, San Diego State University.
3. White R: The urge toward competence. Am J Occup Ther 25:271-274, 1971.
4. Florey LL: Intrinsic motivation: The dynamics of occupational therapy theory. Am J Occup Ther 23:319-322, 1969.
5. Deci EL, Porac J: Cognitive evaluation theory and the study of human motivation. In Leyser MR, Greene D (Eds): The Hidden Costs of Reward. Hillsdale, New Jersey, Erlbaum, 1978.
6. Daloz L: Effective Teaching and Mentoring. San Francisco, Jossey-Boss, 1986.
7. Winnicott D: The Maturational Process and the Facilitating Environment. New York, International Universities Press, 1965.
8. Kielhofner G: A Model of Human Occupation. Baltimore, Maryland, Williams & Wilkins, 1985, p 18.
9. Newall K, Barclay C: Developing Knowledge about Action. In Kelso J, Clark J (Eds). The Development of Movement Control and Co-ordination. New York, John Wiley & Sons, 1982, pp 175-179.
10. Kegan R: The Evolving Self: Problem and Process in Human Development. Cambridge, Massachusetts, Harvard University Press, 1982.
11. Reed K: Models and Practice in Occupational Therapy. Baltimore, Maryland, Williams & Wilkins, 1985, pp 155-179.

12. Flavell J: The Development Psychology of Jean Piaget. Princeton, New Jersey, Van Nostrand Co., 1963.
13. Selye H: The Stress of Life. New York, McGraw-Hill Book Co., 1956.
14. Fitzgerald S: Stress: The internal drummer. The Denver Post, March 11, 1979, pp 14-15.
15. Moore JC: Concepts from the Neurobehavioral Sciences. Dubuque, Kendall Hunt Publishing Co., 1973, p 38.

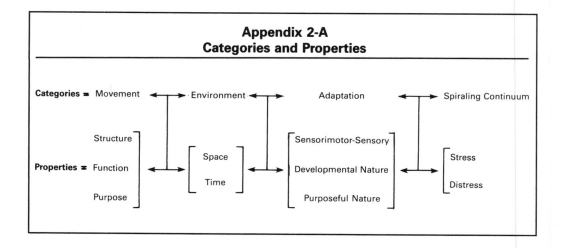

**Appendix 2-A
Categories and Properties**

CHAPTER 3

Highlights of Nervous System Development and Function

Objectives

The reader will be able to

1. become familiar with anatomical structures and functional components of the central nervous system;
2. acquire an understanding of the hierarchy of developmental sequences of the nervous system;
3. be able to define pertinent terminology and explain functional relationships of the integrated nervous system;
4. gain an overview of the concept "neuroplasticity" and its importance for rehabilitation; and
5. gain an understanding of the concept of "individual differences" and its relationship to rehabilitation.

Introduction

Structural Subdivisions of the Central Nervous System

Prior to a discussion of the developmental aspects of the human organism, an introduction to the nervous system is presented to familiarize the reader with the seven basic levels, the hierarchy of developmental sequences, pertinent terminology, and important functional relationships of the integrated nervous system (Table 3-1 and Figure 3-1). Level one represents the spinal cord and the 31 pairs of spinal nerves. This is the least complex level of the central nervous system (CNS). Level seven, the telencephalon [tel = distant + encephalon = brain] or the cerebral hemisphere, is the most highly developed, the most complex, and the last area of the CNS to reach full functional maturity. The numbering system from one through seven roughly parallels ontogenetic

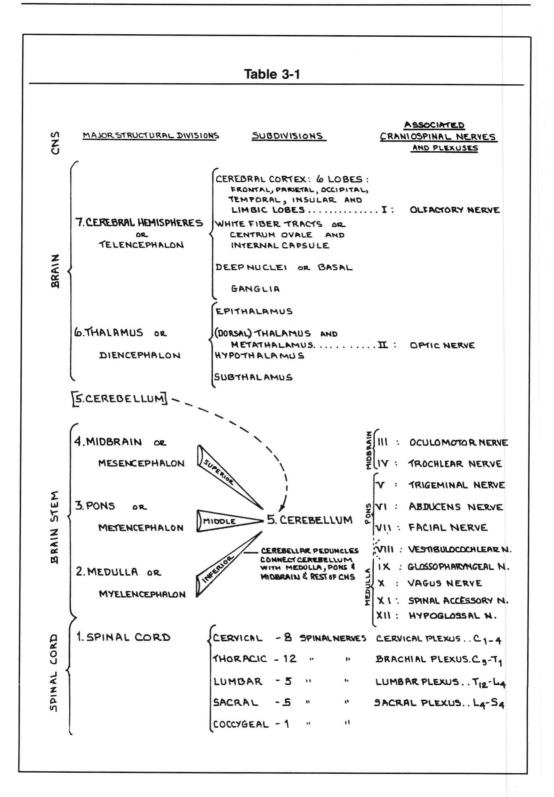

Table 3-1

CNS	MAJOR STRUCTURAL DIVISIONS	SUBDIVISIONS	ASSOCIATED CRANIOSPINAL NERVES AND PLEXUSES
BRAIN	7. CEREBRAL HEMISPHERES OR TELENCEPHALON	CEREBRAL CORTEX: 6 LOBES: FRONTAL, PARIETAL, OCCIPITAL, TEMPORAL, INSULAR AND LIMBIC LOBES .... I : OLFACTORY NERVE	
		WHITE FIBER TRACTS OR CENTRUM OVALE AND INTERNAL CAPSULE	
		DEEP NUCLEI OR BASAL GANGLIA	
	6. THALAMUS OR DIENCEPHALON	EPITHALAMUS	
		(DORSAL) THALAMUS AND METATHALAMUS .... II : OPTIC NERVE	
		HYPOTHALAMUS	
		SUBTHALAMUS	
	[5. CEREBELLUM]		
BRAIN STEM	4. MIDBRAIN OR MESENCEPHALON	SUPERIOR	MIDBRAIN: III : OCULOMOTOR NERVE / IV : TROCHLEAR NERVE
	3. PONS OR METENCEPHALON	MIDDLE → 5. CEREBELLUM	PONS: V : TRIGEMINAL NERVE / VI : ABDUCENS NERVE / VII : FACIAL NERVE / VIII : VESTIBULOCOCHLEAR N.
	2. MEDULLA OR MYELENCEPHALON	INFERIOR — CEREBELLAR PEDUNCLES CONNECT CEREBELLUM WITH MEDULLA, PONS & MIDBRAIN & REST OF CNS	MEDULLA: IX : GLOSSOPHARYNGEAL N. / X : VAGUS NERVE / XI : SPINAL ACCESSORY N. / XII : HYPOGLOSSAL N.
SPINAL CORD	1. SPINAL CORD	CERVICAL - 8 SPINAL NERVES	CERVICAL PLEXUS .. C_{1-4}
		THORACIC - 12 " "	BRACHIAL PLEXUS . C_5-T_1
		LUMBAR - 5 " "	LUMBAR PLEXUS .. T_{12}-L_4
		SACRAL - 5 " "	SACRAL PLEXUS .. L_4-S_4
		COCCYGEAL - 1 " "	

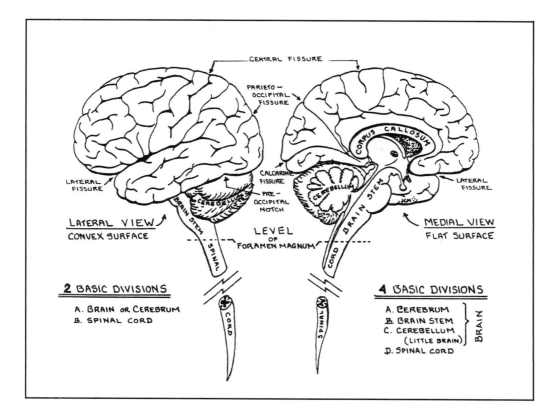

Figure 3-1: Lateral and medial views of the Central Nervous System illustrating the structural relationships of the brain, brain stem, cerebellum and the spinal cord.

development as well as the phylogenetic appearance of these structures in evolution. Also, postnatal growth and development parallels this sequence, in that the lower levels mature and function much earlier than higher levels. For example, the spinal cord pathways are fully myelinated, thus they become functionally mature by 1½ to 3½ years of age, depending upon the sex of the child; it should be noted that the CNS pathways of females tend to myelinate and function somewhat earlier than males.[1,2] Maturation continues for many years, with certain parts of the neocortex not completely myelinated until sometime in the fourth decade of life, or even later (Figure 3-2).[1-4] It is important to keep in mind that any insult to the developing organism can delay myelination, and hence maturation, of the CNS.[1,2,5,6,7,8,9]

Peripheral Nervous System

Figures 3-3 and 3-4 illustrate the peripheral nerves which are associated with the seven major levels of the CNS. These nerves enable the CNS to communicate with the organism's external environment (somatosensory and motoneurons or nerves) and its internal environment (viscerosensory and visceromotor neurons of the autonomic nervous system [ANS]). Even though all of the somatic nerves are sensorimotor in composition, different terms are used to express their origins. Nerves associated with the

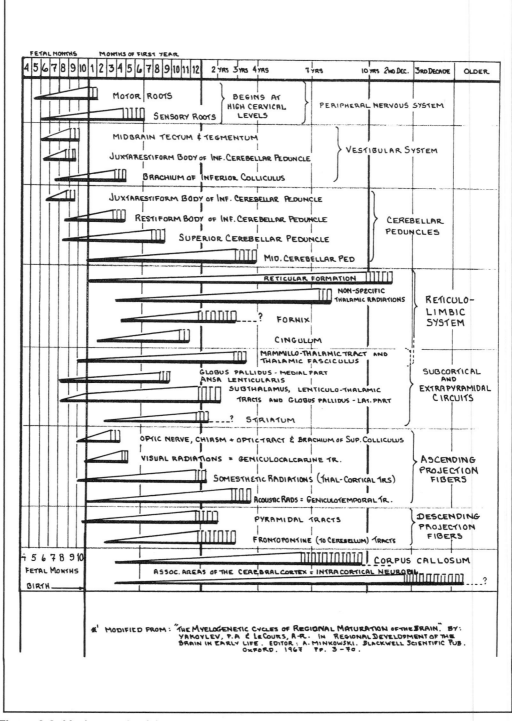

Figure 3-2: Myelogenesis of the nervous system

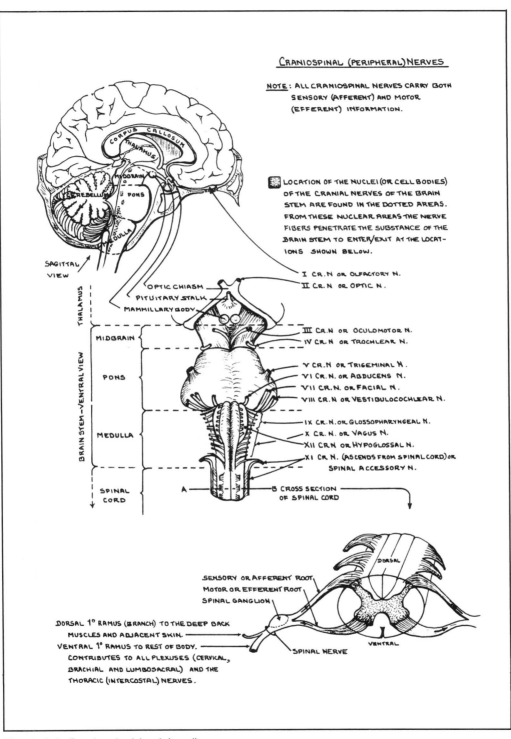

CRANIOSPINAL (PERIPHERAL) NERVES

NOTE: ALL CRANIOSPINAL NERVES CARRY BOTH SENSORY (AFFERENT) AND MOTOR (EFFERENT) INFORMATION.

LOCATION OF THE NUCLEI (OR CELL BODIES) OF THE CRANIAL NERVES OF THE BRAIN STEM ARE FOUND IN THE DOTTED AREAS. FROM THESE NUCLEAR AREAS THE NERVE FIBERS PENETRATE THE SUBSTANCE OF THE BRAIN STEM TO ENTER/EXIT AT THE LOCATIONS SHOWN BELOW.

I CR.N OR OLFACTORY N.
II CR.N OR OPTIC N.
III CR.N OR OCULOMOTOR N.
IV CR.N OR TROCHLEAR N.
V CR.N OR TRIGEMINAL N.
VI CR.N. OR ABDUCENS N.
VII CR.N. OR FACIAL N.
VIII CR.N OR VESTIBULOCOCHLEAR N.
IX CR.N. OR GLOSSOPHARYNGEAL N.
X CR.N. OR VAGUS N.
XII CR.N OR HYPOGLOSSAL N.
XI CR.N. (ASCENDS FROM SPINAL CORD) OR SPINAL ACCESSORY N.

CORPUS CALLOSUM
THALAMUS
MIDBRAIN
CEREBELLUM
PONS
MEDULLA
SAGITTAL VIEW

THALAMUS
BRAIN STEM – VENTRAL VIEW
OPTIC CHIASM
PITUITARY STALK
MAMMILLARY BODY
MIDBRAIN
PONS
MEDULLA
SPINAL CORD

A
B CROSS SECTION OF SPINAL CORD

DORSAL
SENSORY OR AFFERENT ROOT
MOTOR OR EFFERENT ROOT
SPINAL GANGLION
VENTRAL
SPINAL NERVE

DORSAL 1° RAMUS (BRANCH) TO THE DEEP BACK MUSCLES AND ADJACENT SKIN.
VENTRAL 1° RAMUS TO REST OF BODY. CONTRIBUTES TO ALL PLEXUSES (CERVICAL, BRACHIAL AND LUMBOSACRAL) AND THE THORACIC (INTERCOSTAL) NERVES.

Figure 3-3: Craniospinal (peripheral) nerves

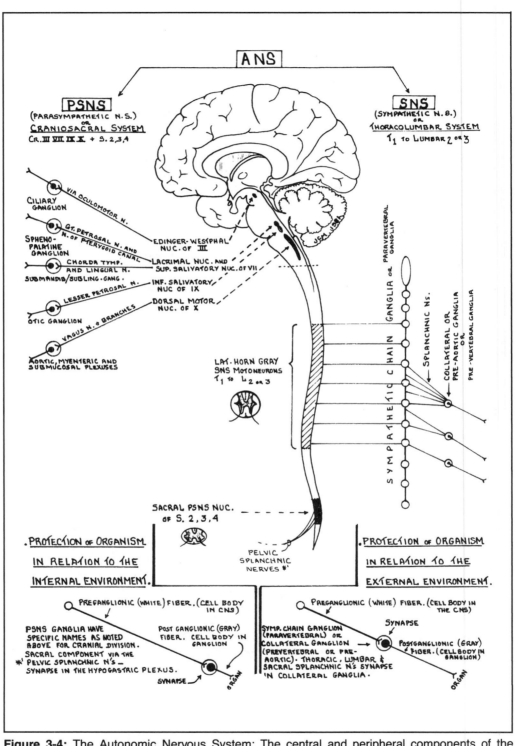

Figure 3-4: The Autonomic Nervous System: The central and peripheral components of the parasympathetic and sympathetic divisions and the major functions of each system.

spinal cord are called spinal nerves. There are 31 pairs of spinal nerves, reflecting the 31 functional embryonic segments of the spinal cord and the associated somites of the body wall structures. Of the 31 pairs, 8 are cervical, 12 thoracic, 5 lumbar, 5 sacral, and 1 coccygeal. From these various levels, the spinal nerves form into four functional plexuses; i.e., C 1-4 is the cervical plexus; C 5-T 1, the brachial plexus; T 12-L 4, the lumbar plexus; and L 4 to S 4, the sacral plexus (Figure 3-3, Table 3-1).

Peripheral nerves which are associated with cranial vault structures (brain stem and brain) are called cranial nerves. There are 12 pairs of cranial nerves (Cr.N.), numbered in sequence from "fore to aft" or as they appear on the base of the brain beginning anteriorly and counting posteriorly-inferiorly to the lowest level of the brain stem. The Ist Cranial Nerve (Cr.N. I) is the olfactory nerve. It is associated with the limbic lobe of Level 7. The IInd, Cr.N.II, or Optic nerve, is associated with the diencephalon or thalamus (level 6). The IIIrd (Oculomotor n.) and the IVth (Trochlear n.) are associated with the midbrain (level 4). The Vth (Trigeminal n.), VIth (Abducens n.), VIIth (Facial n.), and part of the VIIIth (Vestibulocochlear n.) are associated with the pons (level 3). The rest of the VIIIth, the IXth (Glossopharyngeal n.), the Xth (Vagus n.), the XIth (Spinal Accessory n.), and the XIIth (Hypoglossal n.) are all associated with the medulla (level 2) which is the lowest level of the brain stem (Table 3-1).

Central Nervous System -The Triune Brain

Previously the CNS was presented as seven hierarchal levels, recognizing its **structural** levels. Because this structural approach is based upon standardized terminology, it enables everyone to have a basic shorthand for expressing the exact location of a given structure, or the site of a lesion, within a designated level or area of the CNS. However, there is another method for understanding the CNS, based upon its phylogenetic subdivisions, which is useful as the approach parallels nervous system development and maturation. This concept is based upon Paul D. MacLean's triune brain, which divides the CNS into three major areas, or the archi-(oldest), paleo-(intermediate), and neo-(newest) components of the nervous system (Figures 3-5, 3-6).[10,11] Also, the major structural units of the CNS can be further subdivided into their respective archi-, paleo-, and neo-components (Table 3-2). The system is useful for understanding how the entire nervous system develops both phylogenetically and ontogenetically, as well as how different areas function in relation to the others. Likewise, it helps in understanding why some areas, i.e., the newer ones, are more vulnerable to insult than the older areas.

Archi-areas or systems are phylogenetically old. In ontogeny they are the first to develop and function. Many of the archi-areas are primarily concerned with visceral and endocrine functions, maintenance of homeostasis, as well as enabling the organism to be awake, alert, and attending or asleep. Also, these areas have a great deal to do with basic reflexes, such as postural adaptations and/or balance and spatiotemporal orientation.

Paleo-areas are intermediate in age. These structures develop and function next. They are primarily concerned with protective responses in relation to the general and special sense, patterns of locomotion, and survival mechanisms. The paleo-areas function with, and are integrated into, the older archi-systems and later the neo-systems; i.e., in the mature nervous system all three systems function in concert or as an integrated whole. Even though a great deal of "overlap" exists in all areas among these three functional subdivisions, the neo-areas primarily inhibit or dominate the older paleo- and archi-systems.[12-14]

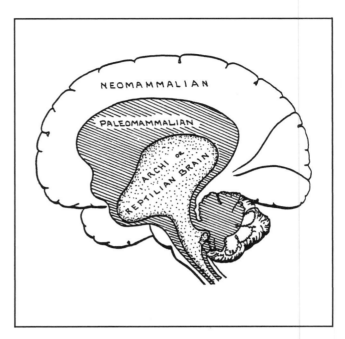

Figure 3-5: The triune brain, conceptualized by Paul D. MacLean, illustrating the archi-reptilian brain, the paleomammalian and the neomammalian brain.

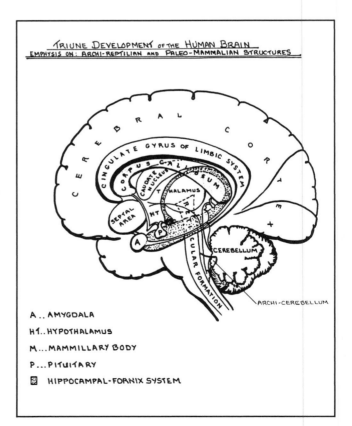

Figure 3-6: Relationships of the archi-reptilian and paleo-mammalian structures of Paul D. MacLean's triune brain.

Table 3-2

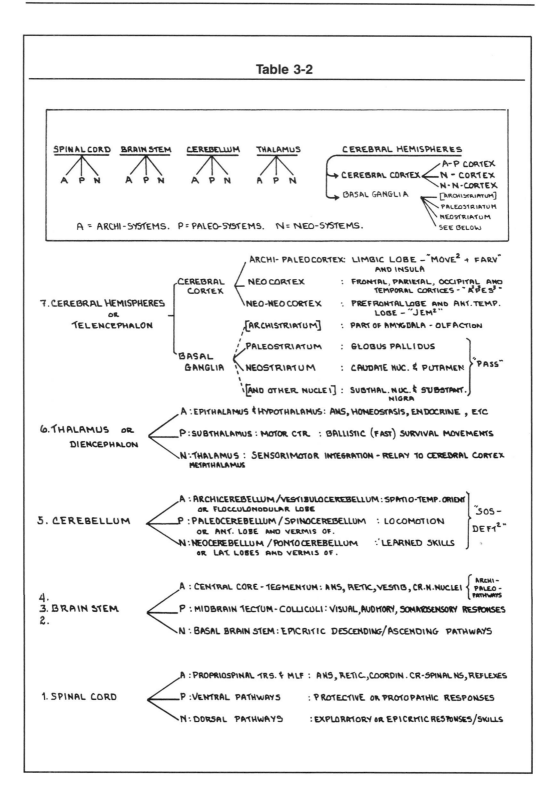

SPINAL CORD   BRAIN STEM   CEREBELLUM   THALAMUS   CEREBRAL HEMISPHERES

A P N   A P N   A P N   A P N

CEREBRAL CORTEX — A-P CORTEX / N - CORTEX / N - N - CORTEX

BASAL GANGLIA — [ARCHISTRIATUM] / PALEOSTRIATUM / NEOSTRIATUM / SEE BELOW

A = ARCHI-SYSTEMS.   P = PALEO-SYSTEMS.   N = NEO-SYSTEMS.

7. CEREBRAL HEMISPHERES or TELENCEPHALON

CEREBRAL CORTEX
- ARCHI-PALEOCORTEX: LIMBIC LOBE – "MOVE^2 + FARV" AND INSULA
- NEOCORTEX : FRONTAL, PARIETAL, OCCIPITAL AND TEMPORAL CORTICES – "A^{3}PES^3"
- NEO-NEOCORTEX : PREFRONTAL LOBE AND ANT. TEMP. LOBE – "JEM^2"

BASAL GANGLIA
- [ARCHISTRIATUM] : PART OF AMYGDALA - OLFACTION
- PALEOSTRIATUM : GLOBUS PALLIDUS
- NEOSTRIATUM : CAUDATE NUC. & PUTAMEN } "PASS"
- [AND OTHER NUCLEI] : SUBTHAL. NUC. & SUBSTANT. NIGRA

6. THALAMUS or DIENCEPHALON
- A : EPITHALAMUS & HYPOTHALAMUS: ANS, HOMEOSTASIS, ENDOCRINE, ETC
- P : SUBTHALAMUS : MOTOR CTR : BALLISTIC (FAST) SURVIVAL MOVEMENTS
- N : THALAMUS : SENSORIMOTOR INTEGRATION - RELAY TO CEREBRAL CORTEX   METATHALAMUS

5. CEREBELLUM
- A : ARCHICEREBELLUM / VESTIBULOCEREBELLUM : SPATIO-TEMP. ORIENT. OR FLOCCULONODULAR LOBE
- P : PALEOCEREBELLUM / SPINOCEREBELLUM : LOCOMOTION OR ANT. LOBE AND VERMIS OF.
- N : NEOCEREBELLUM / PONTOCEREBELLUM : LEARNED SKILLS OR LAT. LOBES AND VERMIS OF.

} "SOS-DEFT^2"

4.
3. BRAIN STEM
2.
- A : CENTRAL CORE - TEGMENTUM: ANS, RETIC, VESTIB, CR.N.NUCLEI { ARCHI-PALEO-PATHWAYS
- P : MIDBRAIN TECTUM - COLLICULI: VISUAL, AUDITORY, SOMATOSENSORY RESPONSES
- N : BASAL BRAIN STEM : EPICRITIC DESCENDING/ASCENDING PATHWAYS

1. SPINAL CORD
- A : PROPRIOSPINAL TRS. & MLF : ANS, RETIC, COORDIN. CR-SPINAL NS, REFLEXES
- P : VENTRAL PATHWAYS : PROTECTIVE OR PROTOPATHIC RESPONSES
- N : DORSAL PATHWAYS : EXPLORATORY OR EPICRITIC RESPONSES/SKILLS

Neo-areas are phylogenetically recent. They are the last areas of the CNS to develop and function. These systems enable us to anticipate events, explore and appreciate the environment, and learn from experiences. Thus the neo-areas are concerned with skills, associated memories, judgment (foresight and hindsight), and emotional tone, as well as behaviors that enable one to function in a gregarious society.

Vulnerability of CNS Areas

As a general rule, neo-systems are more vulnerable to insult (both prenatally and postnatally) than are the paleo-systems, and the paleo-systems are more vulnerable than the archi-systems. However there are several major exceptions to this general rule: (1) any center (no matter whether it is archi-, paleo-, or neo-) that has a high metabolic demand is extremely vulnerable to hypoxic-ischemic episode; e.g., the inferior colliculi of the midbrain, the vestibular nuclei of the lower pons and medulla, and the hippocampal gyri of the limbic cortex; (2) any center or area that harbors the largest cells of the CNS (these cells also have a high metabolic demand) are vulnerable to hypoxic-ischemic episodes; e.g., the betz cells of the cerebral cortex, the pyramidal cells of the hippocampus of the limbic lobe, and the Purkinje cells of the cerebellum; (3) cells of the gray matter of the cerebral cortex, and small penetrating branches of the cerebral arteries are vulnerable to trauma and edema; e.g., the cortices of the cerebral hemispheres and the cerebellum; (4) cell bodies and axons (pathways), which are located in the border zones or watershed territories of the CNS. These are areas where the fine terminal branches of two or three arteries come together but do not anastomose or overlap sufficiently to supply these border zones during or following a hypotensive or hypovolemic episode (Figures 3-7 and 3-8).[5,8,9]

A lesion in one or more areas of the neo-systems can result in a loss of inhibitory control over the lower paleo-systems and archi-systems; the loss may result in a "release phenomenon." In other words, the lower or older functional systems are released from "higher" inhibitory control, and this release is usually expressed by abnormal movement patterns and/or a loss of various potential skills, loss of anticipatory and exploratory capabilities, various degrees of mental retardation, and/or diminished capacities concerned with sensations, judgment, emotional tone, and learning potentials.

Introduction to the Archi-, Paleo-, and Neo-Subdivisions of the Triune Brain

Figures 3-9 through 3-13 illustrate several major areas of the CNS, including the archi-, paleo-, and neo-subdivisions and the general functions associated with each area. Remember that a great deal of functional overlap exists between various archi-, paleo-, and neo-structures, especially as one ascends the CNS to higher levels, with levels six and seven (diencephalon or thalamus and telencephalon or cerebral hemispheres) having the greatest amount of structural and functional overlap. However, in order to understand the basic concepts concerning different areas, overlap has been kept to a minimum, and the illustrations have been simplified to show only the major archi-, paleo-, and neo-areas and their major functions.

Before discussing the functional subdivisions, one should note that even though each major area can be subdivided into archi-, paleo-, and neo-components, not all archi-

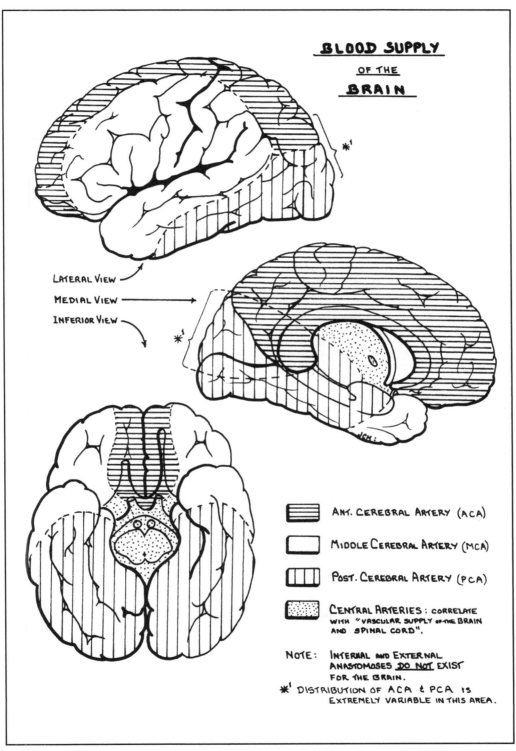

Figure 3-7: The vascular supply of the brain

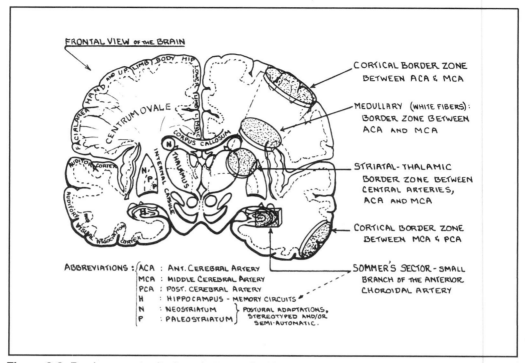

Figure 3-8: Border zone territories where terminal branches of two or three arteries approach one another but do not overlap. Hypoxic-ischemic episodes may result in neuronal cell death in one or more of these vulnerable areas. Amount of insult is extremely variable.

systems at all levels are functionally equivalent. For example, archi-systems of the spinal cord may be quite different functionally than archi-systems of the cerebral hemispheres. To explain, the cerebral hemispheres are phylogenetically new (neo) in contrast to the much older spinal cord, yet each structure has within it archi-, paleo-, and neo-subdivisions. In other words each major area, no matter how old or how recent, has within it functional archi-, paleo-, and neo-components. These major areas and their respective subdivisions are noted in Table 3-2.

Spinal Cord: Archi-, Paleo-, and Neo-Subdivisions

In Figure 3-9 the major pathways (white matter) of the spinal cord are subdivided into three functional areas. Note that the oldest or archi-pathways surround the centrally located cell bodies or the gray matter of the spinal cord. These archi-pathways, which are both ascending and descending, are the first to develop, myelinate, and function, beginning at high cervical levels. These pathways are concerned with autonomic or visceral functions such as bowel and bladder control, digestion, heart, respiration, and regulation of perspiration and vomiting. These pathways are also involved in intrasegmental and intersegmental reflex functions and the integration of these functions with various levels of the spinal cord and brain stem. One archi-pathway of major importance is the medial longitudinal fasciculus or MLF, which is one of the very first pathways to develop, myelinate, and function. This pathway's major function is to coordinate the cranial nerves of the brain stem with the spinal cord and spinal nerves, so that all of the

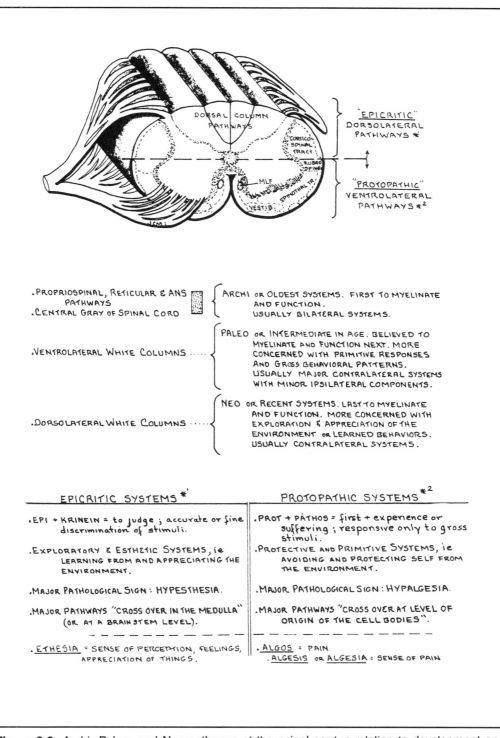

Figure 3-9: Archi- Paleo- and Neo-pathways of the spinal cord in relation to development and function.

peripheral nerves (cranial and spinal) function together in such activities as rooting, sucking, swallowing, visual searching, fixation and tracking, and communication. Many of these archi-systems are associated with the reticular formation of the brain stem, an area of the central core of the CNS that helps regulate autonomic functions, as well as the thresholds of motorneurons, interneurons, and sensory neurons.

The paleo-pathways are located in the ventral half of the spinal cord (Figure 3-9). For the most part these function as protective or protopathic systems, in that they relay information concerning pain, temperature, touch and pressure, and other senses, which enables the developing organism to learn about the environment by experiencing sensations that could be harmful to the system if not heeded. Other paleo-pathways in the ventral half of the spinal cord are concerned with spatiotemporal orientation. These pathways function with the older reticulospinal and vestibulospinal tracts and help regulate the thresholds of motorneurons so that the developing and mature nervous system can achieve and maintain antigravity postures. Another important paleo-pathway is the rubrospinal tract. This one develops and functions slightly later than the others noted. This tract enables the organism to assume progravity postures, especially in relation to grasping objects and bringing them towards the midline or the oral cavity.

The dorsal half of the spinal cord comprises both ascending and descending neo-pathways. These tracts develop last and take several years of postnatal growth before they reach full maturity. The ascending dorsal column-medial lemniscus (Figure 3-9) relays epicritic or kinesthetic types of sensory information; i.e., these pathways enable an organism to anticipate, appreciate, explore (or have conscious awareness of) the environment, and also learn from experiences in order to manipulate the world around them. Manipulation and other skilled movements are carried out by pyramidal or corticospinal tracts, which originate in the neocortex. These pathways, acting in concert with archi- and paleo-systems, endow an organism with a multitude of progravity skills, such as eating, writing, playing with and constructing things. All ascending and descending pathways of the archi-, paleo-, and neo-systems of the CNS have direct or indirect connections with the cerebellum; without cerebellar influence upon these pathways, a nervous system cannot develop and function normally.

Brain Stem

Levels two, three, and four comprise the brain stem (Figure 3-10). These major structural areas (medulla, pons, and midbrain) can be redivided longitudinally into the functional or archi-, paleo-, and neo-subdivisions. Each functional area is roughly equivalent to the way in which this part of the CNS develops and matures.

The archi-part of the brain stem is the central core (or tegmentum), located ventral (anterior) to the ventricular system of the brain stem. This oldest or primitive part consists of the brain stem reticular formation nuclei of the IIIrd through XIIth cranial nerves, the ascending and descending archi- and paleo-pathways of the CNS, and the oldest parts of the ANS concerned with reflex centers regulating eye movements, sleep-wake cycles, heart rate, respiration, perspiration, salivation, and vomiting.

Dorsal (posterior) to the brain stem ventricular system in the midbrain are the roof structures (stectum) or the superior and inferior colliculi. These are intermediate in age (paleo) and are important centers concerned with integration of visual, auditory, vestibular, and somatosensory stimuli, and responding to stimuli primarily at protopathic or protective levels of behavior. These tectal centers also play an important role in

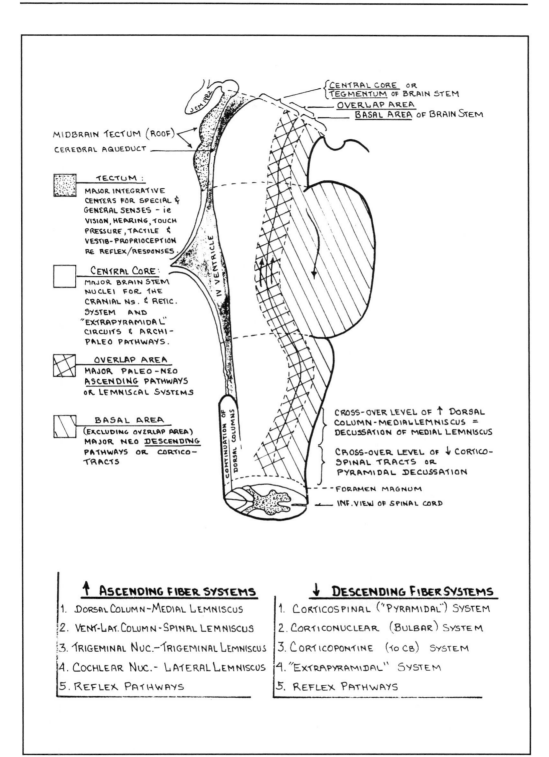

MIDBRAIN TECTUM (ROOF)
CEREBRAL AQUEDUCT

CENTRAL CORE OR
TEGMENTUM OF BRAIN STEM
OVERLAP AREA
BASAL AREA OF BRAIN STEM

TECTUM :
MAJOR INTEGRATIVE
CENTERS FOR SPECIAL &
GENERAL SENSES - ie
VISION, HEARING, TOUCH
PRESSURE, TACTILE &
VESTIB-PROPRIOCEPTION
RE REFLEX/RESPONSES.

CENTRAL CORE :
MAJOR BRAIN STEM
NUCLEI FOR THE
CRANIAL Ns. & RETIC.
SYSTEM AND
"EXTRAPYRAMIDAL"
CIRCUITS & ARCHI-
PALEO PATHWAYS.

OVERLAP AREA
MAJOR PALEO-NEO
ASCENDING PATHWAYS
OR LEMNISCAL SYSTEMS

BASAL AREA
(EXCLUDING OVERLAP AREA)
MAJOR NEO DESCENDING
PATHWAYS OR CORTICO-
TRACTS

IV VENTRICLE
CONTINUATION OF DORSAL COLUMNS

CROSS-OVER LEVEL OF ↑ DORSAL
COLUMN-MEDIAL LEMNISCUS =
DECUSSATION OF MEDIAL LEMNISCUS

CROSS-OVER LEVEL OF ↓ CORTICO-
SPINAL TRACTS OR
PYRAMIDAL DECUSSATION

FORAMEN MAGNUM
INF. VIEW OF SPINAL CORD

↑ ASCENDING FIBER SYSTEMS	↓ DESCENDING FIBER SYSTEMS
1. DORSAL COLUMN-MEDIAL LEMNISCUS	1. CORTICOSPINAL ("PYRAMIDAL") SYSTEM
2. VENT-LAT. COLUMN-SPINAL LEMNISCUS	2. CORTICONUCLEAR (BULBAR) SYSTEM
3. TRIGEMINAL NUC.-TRIGEMINAL LEMNISCUS	3. CORTICOPONTINE (to CB) SYSTEM
4. COCHLEAR NUC.- LATERAL LEMNISCUS	4. "EXTRAPYRAMIDAL" SYSTEM
5. REFLEX PATHWAYS	5. REFLEX PATHWAYS

Figure 3-10: Concepts for understanding the Longitudinal Organization of the Brain Stem in relation to Archi-Paleo-Neo pathways and nuclear areas.

spatiotemporal orientation, i.e., in maintaining the body in appropriate posture in time and space, in relation to the demands of the environment.

The roof of the pons, or the medullary velum of the IVth ventricle, is a very thin layer of tissue and of little functional importance. The cerebellum, which develops from the rhombic lip of the pons, will be discussed later. The "roof" or dorsal part of the medulla is actually an extension of the dorsal column or neo-pathways of the spinal cord. These neo-pathways, after synapsing (in nucleus gracilis and cuneatus) will become the medial lemnisci and will change their position to a more ventral location in the brain stem, lying immediately adjacent to the basal area or the newest (neo) part of the brain stem (Figure 3-10). [Note: In the spinal cord the archi-pathways are located centrally, adjacent to the gray matter, and this relationship is retained throughout the central core of the brain stem. The paleo-pathways, located in the central half of the spinal cord, shift their positions to become incorporated into the central core. The neo-pathways, found in a dorsal position in the spinal cord, become ventrally located in the brain stem.] The basal or ventral areas of the brain stem consist of phylogenetically recent descending pathways of the CNS, i.e., (a) the corticobulbar (or corticonuclear) tracts to cranial nerve nuclei, (b) corticopontine tracts to the cerebellum, and (c) the corticospinal tracts (and the ascending medial lemnisci which are located immediately dorsal to these pathways). These descending pathways are primarily responsible for voluntary control and coordination of skilled functions as well as relaying signals concerned with cortical functions to subcortical centers, such as the basal ganglia, thalamic, cerebellum, and other nuclear areas. Also, these pathways are important modifiers of incoming sensory stimuli; i.e., they can dampen or enhance the various sensory modalities which are being received and/or relayed by the sensory systems of the CNS.

Cerebellum

There are many ways to subdivide the cerebellum, both structurally and functionally. Perhaps the best way to understand this complex organ is to study it phylogenetically, as this method parallels its primary developmental sequence and functional subdivisions (Figure 3-11). The archicerebellum (also known as the vestibulocerebellum or flocculonodular lobe) develops first and is primarily concerned with spatiotemporal orientation (balance or equilibrium), especially in relation to antigravity postures and movements and vestibulo-ocular reflexes, which enables the eyes to "stay on target" while the head is moving. The paleocerebellum (also known as the spinocerebellum or the anterior lobe and adjacent vermis) is principally concerned with locomotion. The neocerebellum (pontocerebellum) consists of the rest of the cerebellum, i.e., the lateral lobes and the adjacent vermal or midline structures (Figure 3-11). The neo-areas function in concert with the neocortex of the cerebral hemispheres and other systems noted and are concerned with circuitry that is involved in learned (or skilled) functions as well as anticipatory and exploratory behaviors and one's ability to appreciate the environment.

Whether one discusses the cerebellum in terms of its developmental or archi-, paleo-, and neo-subdivisions, or as a total functioning organ, the parts, as well as the whole, endow the nervous system (NS) with **synergy**; i.e., smooth, orderly sequencing of direction, extent, force, timing, and tone that is involved in all patterns of movement. In order to carry out these functions, the cerebellum must be informed, moment by moment, of everything (whether it is sensory, motor, or integrative signals from other

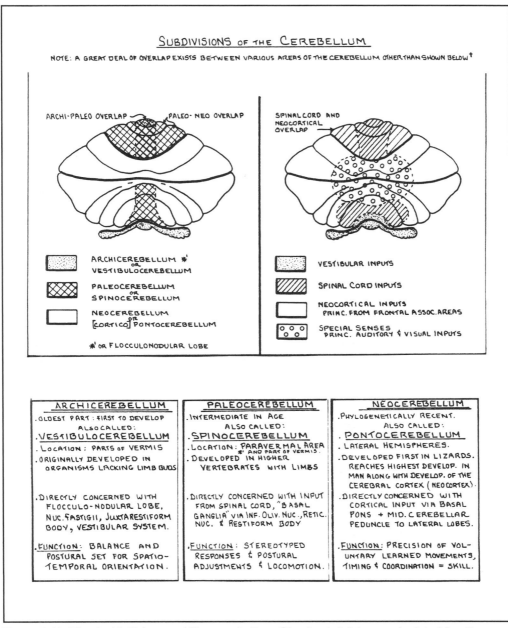

Figure 3-11: The Archi- Paleo- and Neo-cerebellum: Structural divisions and related functions.

centers) that is occurring both within and outside of the NS. Signals from the rest of the NS are constantly being relayed into the various parts of the cerebellum, via the three paired cerebellar peduncles associated with the medulla, pons, and midbrain, to be integrated with all other signals. Next, newly integrated signals are relayed out of the cerebellum, not only to new nuclear centers, but in many cases directly or indirectly to centers from which the original signals were generated. In this way the cerebellum continuously monitors everything, and in turn is able to coordinate all actions that have occurred, are occurring, or will occur in the next millisecond.

Diencephalon or Thalamus

The diencephalon [dia = through + encephalon = brain] or thalamus [a room, especially a bridal chamber] is located in the central depths of the brain (Figure 3-12). [Our forefathers who named this area apparently recognized the significance of this structure and thus named it the "thalamus"; i.e., a secluded room, deep within the brain, where millions of synapses occur.] Four main subdivisions are recognized: epithalamus, hypothalamus, subthalamus, and dorsal thalamus. The epithalamus [epi = above + thalamus] (pineal gland and associated afferent and efferent pathways) is primarily concerned with visceral or autonomic and hypothalamic regulation, growth hormone responses, and diurnal rhythms. The hypothalamus [hypo = under or below + thalamus] and associated afferent and efferent pathways is the master control center of the autonomic nervous system (ANS) and endocrine system. The hypothalamus, limbic, and reticular systems have numerous overlapping structures and functions, in that signals generated in one system always have direct effects upon the others. The subthalamus [sub = beneath + thalamus] is located at a junctional position between the midbrain inferiorly and the hypothalamic nuclei more anteriorly (Figure 3-12). This synaptic area has long been considered as a subcortical integrative center of the basal ganglia. It is believed to be involved in regulating ballistic movements (i.e., short, fast bursts of speed). The dorsal thalamus, commonly referred to as the "thalamus," comprises the largest group of nuclei of the diencephalon, including the metathalami [meta = beyond + thalamus] or the lateral and medial geniculate nuclei. The thalamus is the largest synaptic and integrative diencephalic nucleus located between the telencephalon and all of the lower centers of the CNS.

To subdivide the diencephalic nuclei into archi-, paleo-, and neo-components is difficult and misleading, except in a very general way. The epithalamus, hypothalamus, and subthalamus are phylogenetically older structures (archi-paleo), while the (dorsal) thalamus could be considered a neo-structure. However, the (dorsal) thalamus, of and by itself, can be further divided into archi-, paleo-, and neo-components. It is easier to think of the various nuclei of the (dorsal) thalamus as playing a major role in integrating and relaying (or feeding-forward) all kinds of archi-, paleo-, and neo-sensory and motor impulses from lower centers to various higher centers of the cerebral cortex. Likewise, thalamic nuclei act as a receptive center for feedback collaterals of descending fibers carrying impulses from the cerebral cortex, which are going to lower centers of the CNS (such as the basal ganglia, inferior olivary nuclear complex, cerebellum, reticular formation, as well as lower motorneurons, interneurons, and sensory tract cells). For example, visual afferent fibers from the eyes synapse in the lateral geniculate nuclei of the thalamus, before being relayed via the geniculocalcarine tracts (optic or visual radiations) to the visual cortices. Likewise, medial geniculate nuclei of the thalamus are synaptic centers for auditory impulses going to the auditory cortices via geniculotemporal tracts (auditory radiations). With few exceptions all ascending fibers and collaterals of descending fibers of the CNS, which are associated with cortical functions, must synapse in thalamic nuclei where they are integrated, before new impulses are relayed to their final synaptic destinations. Thus, the diencephalon participates in the functional integrity of numerous nuclear centers of the entire CNS, especially those concerned with cortical functions.

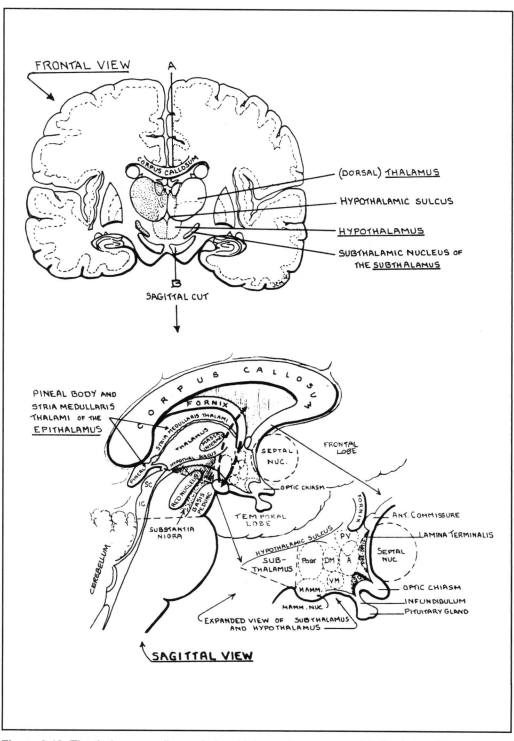

Figure 3-12: The thalamus or diencephalon: Major nuclear areas and their relationships within the brain. The metathalami (lateral and medial geniculate nuclei) are not illustrated. They are located laterally or deep to the pineal body.

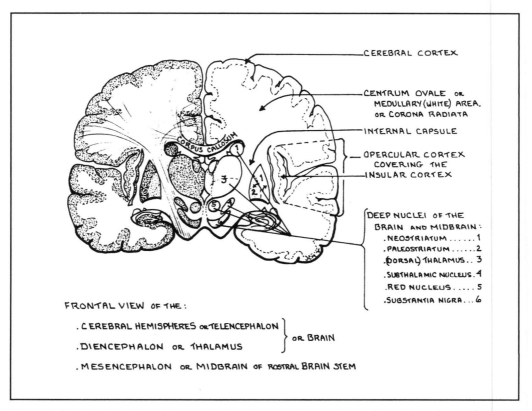

Figure 3-13: Relationships of the cerebral cortex, centrum ovale, and the internal capsule to the deep nuclei of the brain and rostral brain stem.

Telencephalon or Cerebral Hemispheres

The cerebral hemispheres or the telencephalon [tel = distant + encephalon = brain] consists of the cerebral cortices, subcortical white fiber traces (also known as medullated areas or central oval), plus the fibers of the internal capsule, and deep gray nuclei commonly referred to as the caudate nucleus, putamen, and globus pallidus (or corpus striatum), or by their newer terms, the neostriatum (caudate nucleus + putamen) and the paleostriatum (globus pallidus) (Figure 3-13). The neo- and paleo-striatum comprise the largest nuclear areas of the basal ganglia (Figure 3-14). (The basal ganglia, long considered a subcortical motor or kinetic center, will be discussed under "Functional Systems.")

The cerebral cortex can be subdivided phylogenetically into the archi-, paleo- and neo-components which roughly parallels the growth and development of the cortex in utero and postnatally. The insula and limbic cortices are older and comprise the archi-paleo-cortices, while the remaining areas are the neo-cortices, i.e., frontal, parietal, occipital, and temporal cortices (Figure 3-14). However, two areas of the neo-cortices—the prefrontal lobes and the anterior temporal lobes—are phylogenetically recent, thus the reason for referring to them as the "neo-neo" cortices (Figure 3-14). These areas have functional overlap with the rest of the neo-cortices, the limbic cortex, hypothalamus, and the reticular formation. The "neo-neo"cortices are the last areas of the CNS to myelinate and reach functional maturity.

In summary, the seven structural levels of the CNS and their related craniospinal nerves have been presented, followed by a discussion concerning the archi-, paleo-, and neo-subdivisions of these structural levels. One might think of the seven structural components as the horizontal or "man-made" divisions of the CNS, which are used to define specifically named areas. In contrast, the triune brain, along with the archi-, paleo-, and neo-subdivisions, represents a vertical or phylogenetic concept which is more closely related to ontogenetic development and function.

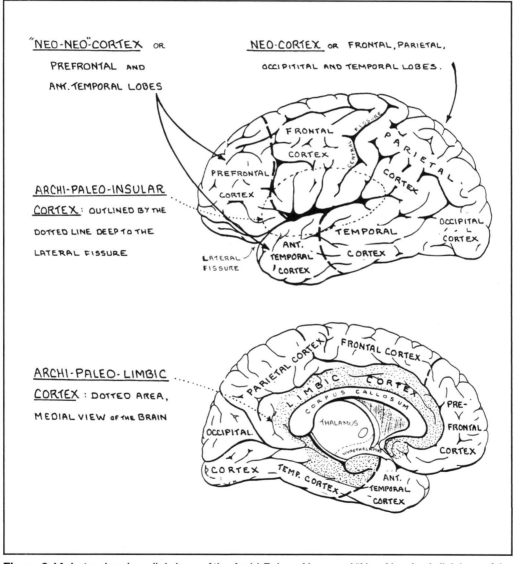

Figure 3-14: Lateral and medial views of the Archi-Paleo-, Neo-, and "Neo-Neo-I subdivisions of the cerebral cortex.

Prenatal and Postnatal Growth and Development

During prenatal and postnatal development, the archi-systems of the spinal cord, brain stem, and associated craniospinal nerves, and the archi-cerebellum, develop sufficiently to endow the newborn with basic survival reflexes, such as spatiotemporal orientation in relation to rooting, sucking, swallowing, and digestive processes; auditory processing of sounds; and the visual ability to fixate upon and track moving objects, especially those related to facial movements of parent or caretakers. Similarly, these archi-systems of the brain stem, spinal cord, and cerebellum endow the infant with a predominence of "extensor" or antigravity tone, over progravity or "flexor" tone, especially during the first few months of life. Figure 3-15 is a brief summary of the prenatal development of muscle tone and cutaneous sensibility. Note that three kinds of muscle tone are recognized in fetal development: (a) passive; (b) active, but not gravity dependent; and (c) active, gravity dependent. Generally speaking, development of muscle tone (passive and active) develops in a caudocephalic and distal to proximal sequence, a different developmental pattern in comparison to those systems illustrated in Figure 3-16. Figure 3-16 also gives a brief summary of the major developmental sequences relating to embryonic development, protective reflexes, and myelination sequences. Note that development of the CNS begins in the high cervical levels of the spinal cord and the lower brain stem, while the protective or primary reflexes of the body develop first in the oral-facial and cervical regions. Later development spreads both cephally **and** caudally and, at the same time, in a distal to proximal sequence. Why would different structural and functional systems develop and begin maturing in divergent locations instead of in one, as was once believed, i.e., the "cephalocaudal law" of development? For one, the cephalocaudal law of development was a very generalized and highly oversimplified concept. For another, these different developmental sequences are genetically endowed patterns of growth which have evolved to assure that the organism will have optimal survival advantages at birth, in spite of being very immature and helpless. For example, the oral-facial region and the hands will be the most sensitive to stimuli concerned with nursing, as well as nonverbal facial expressions for interacting with the mother. Muscle tone development (both passive and active) prepares a newborn for basic survival responses, such as head-raising and turning, should breathing be obstructed; sufficient tone to snuggle into a crib corner for support and comfort; or to interact with rhythmical movements to the cadence of the mother's voice or mimicry of her facial expressions. [1,2,15-19] One might think of these developmental systems as somewhat separate components initially; i.e., one group being cutaneous and protective and developing in one area, while muscle tone is developing in another area and CNS is developing in yet another area. As these various systems mature and spread out from their centers, they not only approach one another but eventually completely overlap. Thus, movement patterns generated from within the CNS or in response to external stimuli gradually become integrated into a smoothly coordinated system capable of interacting purposely with the environment, instead of reflexively.

During growth and development, note that older systems are not only modified by newer systems, but many of the newer systems are incorporated into and function with the older systems. Likewise, as the newest or neo-systems develop, these modify (primarily by inhibition) the older systems. In so doing, all systems eventually overlap and function together as an integrated whole. The unity of functional systems interacting

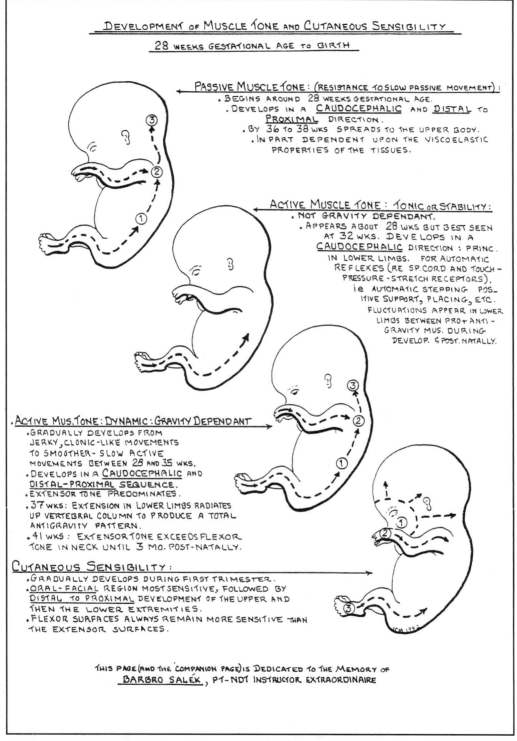

Figure 3-15: Development of muscle tone and cutaneous sensibility.

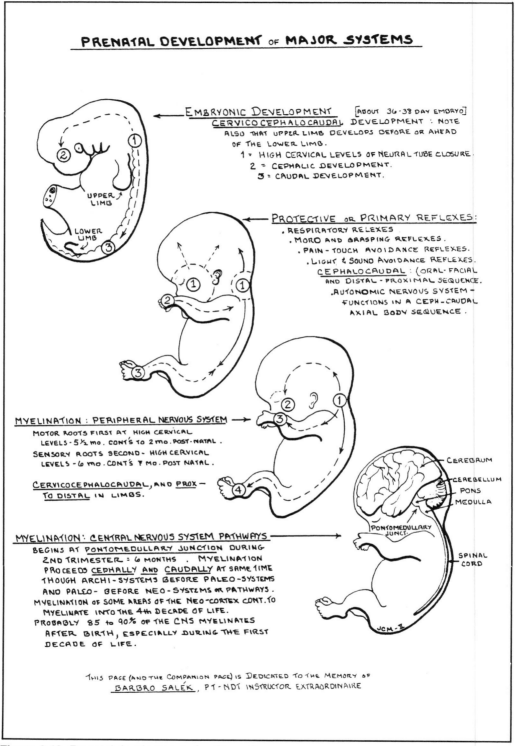

PRENATAL DEVELOPMENT OF MAJOR SYSTEMS

EMBRYONIC DEVELOPMENT [ABOUT 36-38 DAY EMBRYO]
CERVICOCEPHALOCAUDAL DEVELOPMENT : NOTE
ALSO THAT UPPER LIMB DEVELOPS BEFORE OR AHEAD
OF THE LOWER LIMB.
  1 = HIGH CERVICAL LEVELS OF NEURAL TUBE CLOSURE.
  2 = CEPHALIC DEVELOPMENT.
  3 = CAUDAL DEVELOPMENT.

UPPER LIMB
LOWER LIMB

PROTECTIVE OR PRIMARY REFLEXES:
 • RESPIRATORY REFLEXES
 • MORO AND GRASPING REFLEXES.
 • PAIN - TOUCH AVOIDANCE REFLEXES.
 • LIGHT & SOUND AVOIDANCE REFLEXES.
 CEPHALOCAUDAL : (ORAL-FACIAL
    AND DISTAL - PROXIMAL SEQUENCE.
 • AUTONOMIC NERVOUS SYSTEM -
    FUNCTIONS IN A CEPH-CAUDAL
    AXIAL BODY SEQUENCE.

MYELINATION : PERIPHERAL NERVOUS SYSTEM →
  MOTOR ROOTS FIRST AT HIGH CERVICAL
  LEVELS - 5½ MO. CONT'S TO 2 MO. POST-NATAL.
  SENSORY ROOTS SECOND - HIGH CERVICAL
  LEVELS - 6 MO. CONT'S 7 MO. POST NATAL.

  CERVICOCEPHALOCAUDAL, AND PROX -
  TO DISTAL IN LIMBS.

MYELINATION: CENTRAL NERVOUS SYSTEM PATHWAYS →
  BEGINS AT PONTOMEDULLARY JUNCTION DURING
  2ND TRIMESTER = 6 MONTHS . MYELINATION
  PROCEEDS CEPHALLY AND CAUDALLY AT SAME TIME
  THOUGH ARCHI-SYSTEMS BEFORE PALEO-SYSTEMS
  AND PALEO- BEFORE NEO-SYSTEMS OR PATHWAYS.
  MYELINATION OF SOME AREAS OF THE NEO-CORTEX CONT. TO
  MYELINATE INTO THE 4th DECADE OF LIFE.
  PROBABLY 85 to 90% OF THE CNS MYELINATES
  AFTER BIRTH, ESPECIALLY DURING THE FIRST
  DECADE OF LIFE.

CEREBRUM
CEREBELLUM
PONS
MEDULLA
PONTOMEDULLARY JUNCT.
SPINAL CORD
JCM-II

THIS PAGE (AND THE COMPANION PAGE) IS DEDICATED TO THE MEMORY OF
BARBRO SALÉK, PT-NDT INSTRUCTOR EXTRAORDINAIRE

Figure 3-16: Prenatal development of major systems.

with one another enables an organism to develop, mature, learn from, and adapt to, the ever-changing environment. Any insult to these systems, and especially the more vulnerable neo-systems, disrupts this unity and causes various kinds and degrees of dysfunction.

Figure 3-17 shows growth and development of the brain in utero; note that the brain quadruples in size during the second trimester and triples again during the last trimester. Also note that the older insular cortex (shaded in Figure 3-17) is gradually overgrown by the frontal, parietal, and temporal opercula [operculum = a small cover]. These fast-growing opercular areas are destined to become the major communication centers of the hemispheres. In postnatal development the insula lies deep to the opercula and only the lateral fissure remains (Figure 3-18). During the first year of life, the brain doubles in size; over the next 30 or more years, the brain gradually completes its full development. During the first year of life, the CNS is the most plastic or malleable. The neuroplasticity of the CNS remains pliable for life, even though it is recognized that it is the most plastic during infancy, early childhood, and pre-adolescence.

Ten major structural and functional changes occur during normal development of the NS.[2,5,6,7,14,20-24] These changes, listed below, take place in the CNS and account for the tremendous prenatal and postnatal growth of the brain.

1. During embryonic and early fetal development, an excess of neurons are produced at all levels of the CNS. As the fetus and neonate mature, many of these neurons are "pruned away" or die. The billions that remain are "tuned up" as part of the intricate circuitry and synaptic centers which will become the functional neurons of the NS.

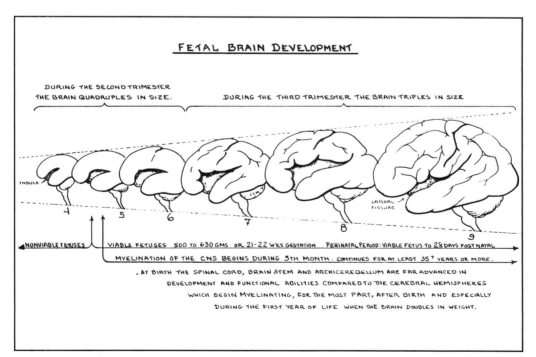

Figure 3-17: Fetal brain development.

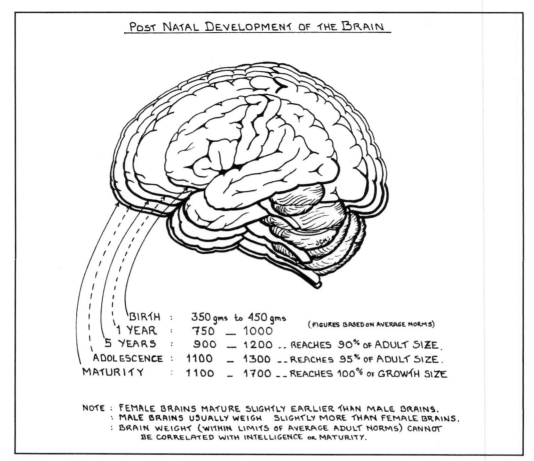

POST NATAL DEVELOPMENT OF THE BRAIN

BIRTH : 350 gms to 450 gms (FIGURES BASED ON AVERAGE NORMS)
1 YEAR : 750 — 1000
5 YEARS : 900 — 1200 .. REACHES 90% OF ADULT SIZE.
ADOLESCENCE : 1100 — 1300 .. REACHES 95% OF ADULT SIZE.
MATURITY : 1100 — 1700 .. REACHES 100% OF GROWTH SIZE

NOTE : FEMALE BRAINS MATURE SLIGHTLY EARLIER THAN MALE BRAINS.
: MALE BRAINS USUALLY WEIGH SLIGHTLY MORE THAN FEMALE BRAINS.
: BRAIN WEIGHT (WITHIN LIMITS OF AVERAGE ADULT NORMS) CANNOT
BE CORRELATED WITH INTELLIGENCE OR MATURITY.

Figure 3-18: Postnatal development.

2. There is an increase in both size and shape of the neuronal cell bodies.
3. There is a tremendous increase in both size and length of axonal processes.
4. Collateralization of axons occurs.
5. There is a tremendous increase in size, shape, and branchings of the dendritic tree.
6. There is a tremendous increase in the number of synapses as well as their locations.
7. There is a gradual increase in the amount of the different kinds of neurotransmitters.
8. Neuroglial cell proliferation takes place for up to 5 years postnatally.
9. There is a tremendous increase in myelination of axons and their collaterals.
10. There is increased vascularization in order to meet the structural, functional, and metabolic demands of the developing NS.

Growth and development of the embryo and fetus are governed by genetics and the internal environment in which the organism lives. As maturation progresses, a fetus begins to perceive more and more external environmental stimuli, such as voices or sound waves, perception of movement by the mother, the mother's heartbeat, and the gurgling of the intestinal contents. Also, around 5 to 6 months in utero, a fetus is capable of self-stimulation, i.e., rooting and sucking the fingers, kicking and turning, and later hiccuping. Both the genetic regulation of growth and development and the internal and external stimulation perceived by a fetus are necessary for normal maturation of one's NS.

A defect in the genetic code, or a decrease in or lack of normal amounts of stimuli (including oxygen and nutrients), may result in a nonviable fetus or an abnormal infant.[5,14,23,25,26] Normal postnatal growth and development, though still regulated in ways by genetics, becomes more dependent upon stimuli from the external environment. Without a certain amount of meaningful stimuli or interaction with one's environment, the CNS does not develop normally or reach its optimal potential. With a viable but abnormal CNS, purposeful stimulation and meaningful interactions with the environment become critical. Without therapeutic intervention, sensory deprivation is experienced, accompanied by a decrease in neuroplasticity. All of the ten major structural and functional changes (previously listed concerning normal growth and development) decrease instead of increase. Therapeutic intervention makes an impact as it prevents sensory deprivation, enables the system to remain plastic, experiences normal stimuli and movement patterns, and increases functional potentials of the baby. The nervous system can mature and eventually learn to survive and adapt in a more appropriate way to the environment through meaningful multisensory stimulation and the sequential reactions to all kinds of experiences.[2,5-7,19,21,23,24,27-32]

Seven Major Functional Systems of the CNS

Just as there are seven major structural divisions of the NS, the functional systems can be conceptualized by dividing them into seven components. Figure 3-19 is a schematic illustration of these seven functional systems. The companion page, Table 3-3, presents a brief summary of the anatomical areas associated with major functions of each system and mnemonics used to assist the reader in remembering the functions. Figure 3-19 presents the hierarchal organization of the functional systems with the older or more reflexive functions of the **S**ensory-**M**otor-**S**ensory (SMS) system illustrated at the bottom and the highest cortical functions shown at the top. Similarly, the archi-, paleo-, and neo-terminology is used to emphasize the way in which these systems develop and later function together as an integrated system. Centrally located in Figure 3-19 is the central core or archi-structures, hypothalamus, and reticular system. The synergic system, or cerebellum, is situated posteriorly to the central core of the brain stem, while the kinetic system, or basal gangli, lie slightly superior and anterior to the central core.

The cerebral hemisphere has been divided into three functional subsystems: (1) archi-paleo-limbic system; (2) neo-cortical system, the more posterior part of the frontal lobe, parietal and occipital lobes, and posterior half of the temporal lobe; and (3) "neo-neo"cortical system or the prefrontal and anterior temporal lobes. The concept of functional systems presents a very simplified view of the nervous system, one that is easy to understand, and at the same time based upon fundamental principals of nervous system functioning and dysfunction. Most of the mnemonics which are used for remembering these major structures and their functions are meaningful and are directly related to how various subsystems interrelate with one another for an integrated nervous system. For example, the mnemonic for the kinetic system (basal ganglia) is "PASS," which means **P**ostural **A**daptations which are either **S**tereotyped (genetically endowed)

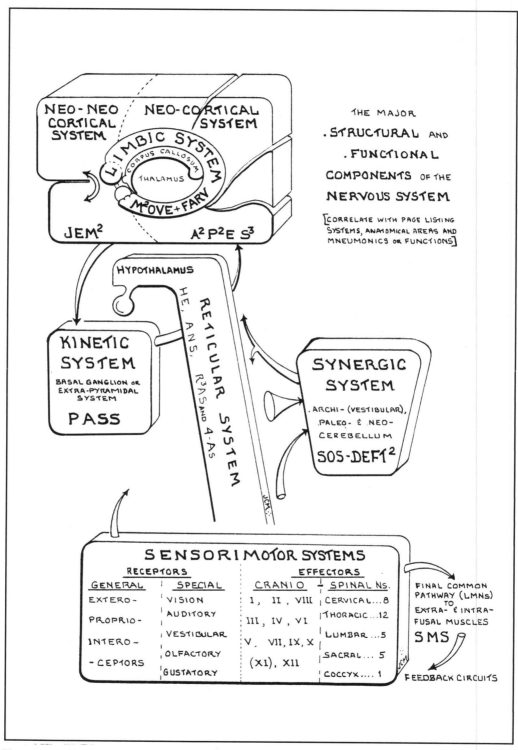

Figure 3-19: Schematic illustration of the seven functional systems of the CNS.

Table 3-3
The Major Structural & Functional Systems

	Systems	Anatomical Areas	Mneumonics or Functions
Skills & Aesthetic System / Perception and appreciation, / Intellect & higher cortical (3 Rs)	NEO-NEO-CORTICAL SYSTEM	Pre-frontal lobes and anterior temporal lobes	**JEM² CORTEX** / Judgment / Emotional tone / Motivation / Memory (circuits)
	NEOCORTICAL SYSTEM	Rest of Frontal lobes and Temporal lobes and Parietal and Occipital lobes	**A²P²ES³** / Appreciates and anticipates / Plans and programs and / Executes / Skills and / Survival Strategems
Affective System	**LIMBIC SYSTEM**	Cingulate Gyrus, Parahippocampal Gyrus and Hippocampus, Amygdala, Septal area: (Functions with JEM² cortex, A²P²ES³ cortex, Hypothalamus and Reticular system and Kinetic system).	**M²OVE and FARV** / Motivation and Memory (circuits) / Olfaction / Visceral / Emotional tone or 3-F's / [Feeding, Fighting & Reproduction] / Fear / Anger / Rage / Violence (continuum)
"Autonomic" Systems	**HYPOTHALAMIC and RETICULAR SYSTEM**	Hypothalamus and Pituitary gland Reticular formation of brain stem and adjacent areas of CNS	**HE:** Homeostasis and Endocrine system / **ANS:** Automatic Nervous System or Sympathetic & Parasympathetic Nervous System / **R³AS and 4 A's** / • Reticular Activating System / • Rhythm generator / • Regulates cell thresholds of sensorimotor neurons and ANS neurons / • Asleep or Awake / • Alert and Attending
"Background" Movement Patterns	**KINETIC SYSTEM**	Basal Ganglion or Extra-Pyramidal system: / Neostriatum / Paleostriatum / Subthalamic nucleus / Substantia nigra	**PASS** / • Postural (and/or Movement) / • Adaptations, which are / • Stereotyped or / • Semi-automatic learned responses
Coordination System	**SYNERGIC SYSTEM**	Cerebellum / Archi or vesibulocerebellum (Balance + Spat-tem Orient) / Paleo or Spinocerebellum (Locomotion) / Neo or Cortocoponto-cerebellum (learned skills)	**SOS-DEFT²** / Smooth orderly sequencing of: / Direction / Extent / Force / Timing and Tone / (in relation to equilibrium and movement)
"Tonic" System	**SENSORIMOTOR SYSTEM**	All craniospinal sensory receptors (general & special) and effectors (or LMNs) to muscles and glands	**SMS** / Sensory (receptors) / Motor (effectors) / Sensory (re-afferents or circuits) feedback

or **S**emiautomatic (learned). PASS is also related to the fact that movement patterns generated by the cerebral cortex must first PASS through the various circuits of the basal ganglia, where they are integrated with impulses from other centers, then are relayed via thalamic nuclei back to the motor centers of the cerebral cortex. Integrity of this feed forward-feed back loop of the "PASSage" of cortical impulses via the nuclei of the basal ganglia is critical for normal function, as well as being part of an anticipatory and preparatory system which enables humans to interact purposely with the environment. Another value for using mnemonics and subdividing the CNS into seven major functional systems relates to functional disabilities associated with each system, as a lesion of one (or more) of these seven systems results in a dysfunction of what the mnemonic means. For example, a lesion of the kinetic system (basal ganglia) disrupts **P**ostural **A**daptations which are **S**tereotyped and **S**emiautomatic and results in a dyskinesia [dys = difficult + kinetic = movement]. Thus the mnemonic is useful for knowing the major functions of a system as well as understanding the major functional disabilities associated with each system.

The seven functional components will be discussed beginning with the older or more reflexive systems and ending with the highest cortical functions.

I. Sensory-Motor-Sensory System

The CNS must be able to receive all kinds of stimuli, integrate these signals, and respond to them in a meaningful way. Also, feedback or re-afferent (sensory) signals are necessary for informing the CNS that the response is correct or needs to be modified. This fundamental system has been known as the S-M-S or the sensory-motor-sensory system (SMS—sensorimotor-sensory). The general sensory receptors (exteroceptors, proprioceptors, and interoceptors) and the five special senses (vision, vestibular, auditory, taste, and olfaction) are continually receiving a multitude of stimuli from the environment. These impulses are carried into the CNS over thousands of afferent nerves, where one of several things can occur: (1) if they are subliminal signals and/or not important for survival, they may be dampened or inhibited at the first or second synapse; (2) they may synapse onto tract cells and ascend or descend to other levels of the CNS; or (3) they may synapse on interneurons and lower motoneurons (LMN's) and cause a response. For every response, a multitude of re-afferent (sensory) signals inform the CNS that action is taking place, the quality of the action in relation to the goal, and the degree to which it is being accomplished. In the immature nervous system a great deal of SMS activity takes place in the older archi- and paleo-systems of the spinal cord, brain stem, and cerebellum. Repeated interactions with one's environment over time provides the system with experiences to "build up" gradually a memory storage of meaningful versus unimportant stimuli. As these older centers "build-up" memory storage, behavioral patterns become less excitatory or reactive to all kinds of stimuli. Also, responses which once were fractionated and gross become more coordinated and purposeful, and feedback from responses becomes smoother and more integrated. Eventually, every movement becomes purposeful in relation to environmental stimuli as higher centers develop and control these lower reflexive circuits.

II. Reticular System and the Hypothalamus

As the reticular formation of the brain stem and the hypothalamic nuclei gradually mature, they integrate their major functions with SMS systems. The hypothalamus is the master controller of **H**omeostasis, the **E**ndocrine system, and the **A**utonomic **N**ervous

System. The mnemonic "HE" and "ANS" can be remembered by the words "HE ANSwered"; i.e., the hypothalamus is forever answering to the constantly changing demands of the internal and external environment in order to maintain **H**omeostasis and regulate the **E**ndocrine system, as well as the **A**utonomic **N**ervous **S**ystem.

The reticular formation of the brain stem, located in the central core or tegmentum, consists of numerous recognized nerve cell groups, many of which extend throughout the entire length of the brain stem tegmentum. Axons of these cell clusters have rich arborizations, not only throughout the brain stem, but many axonal processes extend into the spinal cord, cerebellum, thalamus, and cerebral hemispheres. Hence the more inclusive term "reticular system" can be used to express the fact that the brain stem reticular formation influences and is influenced by all other areas of the CNS. Though the reticular formation is usually thought of as an archi-system, in reality it consists of archi-, paleo-, and neo-components. During the phylogenetic and ontogenetic development, paleo-components were "added" to and incorporated with the archi-systems. As neo-systems developed, these were incorporated into the older archi- and paleo-parts. Thus the reticular system, through its extensive interconnections with all other parts of the CNS, is able to play a key role in REGULATING a great number of functions which are critical for survival, learning, and memory. Likewise, the reticular system is similar to a huge spy network in that it is constantly being informed of all incoming stimuli as well as everything that has just occurred, is taking place, or will take place in the next several milliseconds. Thus the reticular system is in a perfect, centrally located position to be a regulator of many of the vital and very basic functions of our nervous system.

The mnemonic for the major functions of the reticular system is $R^3AS + 4$ A's. The three R's emphasize that this anatomical area is the **R**eticular (reticular = a diffuse network) system, it is a major **R**egulator of many vital CNS functions, and it is a **R**hythm generator. Functions are accomplished by the RAS, or the **R**eticular **A**ctivating **S**ystem. The four A's pertain to the sleep-wake cycles or the "**A**sleep, **A**wake, **A**lert, and **A**ttending continuum.

The sleep-wake cycles and the alert-attending responses are not only regulated by the reticular activating system (via its vast connections with the other areas of the CNS), but are intrinsically regulated by pontine and midbrain feed forward-feed back centers within the brain stem reticular formation. Also, the reticular activating system (RAS) can activate rather specific nuclear areas of the CNS, which in turn enables these centers to respond with greater sensitivity (or awareness) to environmental stimuli, especially if these stimuli are novel or threatening. This results in an alerting response and causes the individual to attend to the important stimuli and to dampen out other signals. With unimportant or repetitive stimuli the RAS dampens or inhibits incoming signals, either to the extent that sleep results or merely an awake state that is neither alert nor attending. Eventually the vast majority of stimuli received by the organism over time results in no overt reactions, because the CNS habituates to those environmental stimuli which are no longer novel. However, a normal developing and awake NS never appears to habituate to stimuli which are critical for survival.

The reticular formation appears to be the master controller of many of the basic rhythms of the CNS, such as alpha, beta, delta, and theta brain-wave rhythms, circadian sleep-wake cycles, and especially the 4 stages of sleep (REM and NREM) and the EEG rhythms associated with these stages.[20] Last but not least, the RAS plays a vital role in filtering out or inhibiting incoming sensory signals that are not important to the individual's function at any given moment in time. This is accomplished by regulating cell thresholds (either decreasing thresholds + excitation or increasing thresholds inhibition) of not only sensory neurons and tract cells, but also interneurons and ANS neurons. Also, the reticular system plays a vital role in regulating the thresholds of cranial and spinal lower motorneurons, especially in relation to antigravity postural adjustments and maintaining correct spatiotemporal orientation during activities in which the individual is engaged. Later in development as the progravity systems mature, the reticular system will have a background role in regulating both progravity and antigravity systems so that the individual can adapt both posture and movement patterns to any situation encountered.

III. Synergic System

The cerebellum develops in an archi-paleo-neo sequence. The oldest part or archi-cerebellum (also known as the vestibulocerebullum) functions with the vestibular system, develops first, and endows the infant with spatiotemporal orientation in relation to gravity, antigravity muscle tone, and auditory-visual orientation to sounds and visual stimuli. The paleocerebellum develops along with the brain stem and spinal cord and is principally concerned with all kinds of locomotion patterns. The neocerebellum is the last to develop, along with the cerebral hemispheres, and is principally concerned with learning skills. As each system develops and matures, the oldest, intermediate, and newest areas function together as an integrated whole. Like the reticular formation of the brain stem, the cerebellum also must be informed, at all times, of everything that is taking place both within the CNS and externally in relation to the multitude of stimuli (afferent and re-afferent) constantly being received by the individual. Thousands of impulses are continually being relayed into the various cortical areas of the cerebellum via the cerebellar peduncles. These signals are integrated and, for the most part, are inhibited prior to being relayed to the deep cerebellar nuclei, where they are re-integrated. Next, the final signals are sent via the superior cerebellar peduncle to various nuclear centers of the CNS. The cerebellum is very skilled (deft) at **S**ending **O**ut **S**ignals, hence the mnemonic SOS-DEFT. SOS-DEFT expresses the principal function of synergy that the cerebellum gives to the rest of the CNS. Synergy is the **S**mooth **O**rderly **S**equencing of the the **D**irection, **E**xtent, **F**orce, **T**iming, and **T**one of all the activities in which the individual is engaged. Interruption of the input/output circuitry of the cerebellum, or a cerebellar lesion per se, results in a "dys-surgery" or deficit in smooth, orderly, sequential movements in relation to the direction, extent of the movement, amount of force necessary, and timing and tone of that movement pattern. Archi-cerebellar lesions primarily affect the SOS-DEFT of trunk musculature in relation to midline postural adaptations. Paleocerebellar lesions principally affect SOS-DEFT of locomotion patterns, while neocerebellar lesions affect the SOS-DEFT of skilled movements, particularly in relation to the distal parts of the body; i.e., oral-facial and language functions and manipulative activities of the hands and feet.

IV. Kinetic System

The kinetic system (or the basal ganglia) consists of a group of subcortical nuclear centers known as the neostriatum (caudate nucleus and putamen), paleostriatum (globus pallidus) of the cerebral hemisphere, the subthalamic nuclei of the thalamus, and the substantial nigra of the midbrain (Figure 3-20). Just as the cerebellum endows the CNS with synergy (SOS-DEFT) in relation to motor behaviors, the kinetic system contributes the background movement patterns that are necessary for postural adapta-

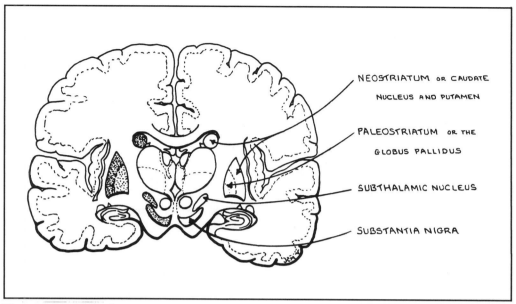

Figure 3-20: Midbrain.

tions and, later in development, the foundations upon which learned skills will be superimposed. As mentioned previously, the mnemonic for the kinetic system is PASS (**P**ostural **A**daptations which are either **S**tereotyped or **S**emiautomatic). The mnemonic also stands for the fact that impulses from higher cortical levels must first "PASS" through the various nuclei of the basal ganglia, where they are integrated, relayed to thalamic nuclei, and re-integrated with synergic impulses and other ascending sensory signals, before being relayed back to various cortical centers of the cerebral hemispheres. Thus, the cerebral cortex receives kinetic, synergic, sensory, and reticular input **prior** to sending impulses to the craniospinal LMN's, which finally results in an appropriate response. This cortical→kinetic→thalamic→cortical circuit is also part of an anticipatory and preparatory system which enables animals and humans to survive and interact purposely with the environment. Various lesions of the kinetic system and/or the circuitry involved result in dyskinetic syndromes; i.e., difficulties in **P**ostural **A**daptations which are both **S**tereotyped and **S**emiautomatic. Included in this dyskinetic syndrome may be an inability on the part of the CNS to anticipate and plan for the moment-to-moment movement sequences in advance of the actual movement taking place. Thus movement becomes spastic, choreoathetodic, rigid, or dysonic (depending upon the site of the lesion), and the individual is unable to perform normal movement patterns.

V. Limbic System of the Cerebral Hemispheres

Three functional subdivisions of the cerebral cortex were noted—i.e., the older limbic system (limbic cortex and associated nuclear areas), the neocortex, and the "neo-neo" cortex. The mnemonics for the limbic system are M²OVE + FARV. M²OVE is used to express the fact that the limbic system is believed to be the major area of the CNS that is responsible for moving us or providing the motivating force behind basic behaviors and personality traits. Thus, the word M²OVE is the key word not only for remembering the primary function of this system, but also the other functions. The **M** stands for **M**otivation or basic drives and also for **M**emory functions. This does not imply that memories are stored in the limbic system. [It is known that different kinds of memory are stored all over the CNS.] However various nuclear areas and circuits of the limbic system are critical for learning in respect to laying down and/or retrieving memory, especially long-term memory.

The "**O**" in M²OVE stands for **O**lfaction or the sense of smell. Older centers of the limbic system are part of the receptive areas that receive olfactory impulses. This is one of the reasons why olfactory stimuli can cause strong emotional feelings. In the neonate the smell of the mother and her milk is believed to be involved, in part, with infant-mother bonding.

The "**V**" in M²OVE concerns **V**isceral or autonomic responses. The limbic system has direct and indirect connections with the hypothalamus and brain stem reticular formation; hence all behavior, whether overt or convert, has an autonomic (sympathetic or parasympathetic) component. In other words, every action or reaction to internal or external stimuli that is expressed by the somatic system is concurrently expressed by the visceral system. For example, when a normal infant, child, or adult unexpectedly sees a loved one, not only is motorical behavior expressed, but heart rate, temperature, blood pressure, and respiration increases; the pupils dilate as the eyelids open wider; and the eyebrows momentarily elevate.[15-19,33] The reactions are examples of some of the visceral and/or autonomic responses that accompany somatic responses. The reactions above are mild ones in comparison to those that may result from fears, threats, or neglect.[16-18,23,24,27,30,32,34].

The last letter in M²OVE reflects that the limbic system plays a major role in **E**motional tone or **E**motional stability and the way in which one reacts to a situation. There are three subcomponents of emotional tone, "feeding, fighting (or flight), and reproduction." Feeding is not limited to nutritional needs, but of greater importance to emotional needs, or the drive for love. The basic drive to be held, cuddled, talked to, wanted, etc., appears to be an inherent trait of all gregarious animals, and is especially so for humans. Lack of this vital ingredient, especially in the immature or young nervous system, may result in a variety of pathological conditions such as the failure-to-thrive syndrome.[16-18,23,24,27,30,32,34] The word "fighting" is not limited to aggression per se, but also related to retreating (flight) or not reacting at all, as a means of self-preservation. Reproduction, of course, is dependent upon the maturation of the reproductive system, including the hypothalamic-endocrine system.

The other mnemonic associated with limbic function is "FARV," which is used to represent a behavioral sequence or continuum that may result once an emotional pattern is stimulated by some event. The continuum begins with **F**ear (or **F**rustration); if not resolved, **A**nger is triggered. If anger is not repressed or alleviated, it may lead to **R**age, and if rage is not inhibited, **V**iolence may result. The Fear-Anger-Rage-Violence continuum appears to be a behavioral and/or survival trait of the limbic system.[13,14,23,33,35] This is not to say that stimuli that can trigger this reaction must be relayed directly to the limbic system. Rather the limbic system is critically positioned between lower and higher centers of the CNS, and it receives and interacts with all other systems. Also the limbic system appears to be less inhibited, especially early in development when the neo-cortical systems are maturing. With normal maturation, these higher centers begin to inhibit or modify fluctuations in emotional tone of an individual and gradually the FARV continuum is tempered. Lesions of the limbic cortex and/or associated pathways and nuclear centers can release the inhibitory control which the cortical systems have over this system, and the FARV continuum may be remanifested. More commonly, one sees a change in the individual's **M**otivations, **M**emory (learning and/or recall), and **E**motional tone; or these aptitudes may never develop normally if a lesion occurred in the limbic areas either prenatally or perinatally (Figures 3-21 and 3-22).

VI. Neocortical System

The area of the cerebral cortex comprising the neocortical system consists of the parietal and occipital lobes and the posterior parts of the frontal and temporal lobes (Figures 3-14, 3-19, and 3-21). The mnemonic for this area is APES. Most higher primates—i.e., the great APES—have these cortical areas, thus the reason for the mnemonic. Also, $A^2P^2ES^3$ is an abbreviation for the primary functions of these cortical areas: **A**ppreciation and **A**nticipatory behaviors, **P**lanning and **P**rogramming, and then **E**xecuting the behavioral response, which may be either a **S**kill or **S**urvival **S**trategems. A large part of the neocortical sensory areas endow the CNS with the ability to **A**ppreciate various stimuli in the environment, associate previous experiences with new ones, and in so doing, learn how to manipulate or adapt the environment to meet the needs of an individual.

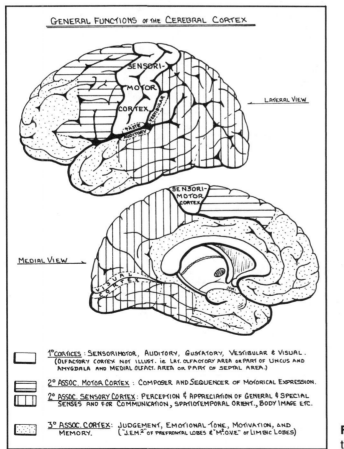

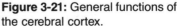

Figure 3-21: General functions of the cerebral cortex.

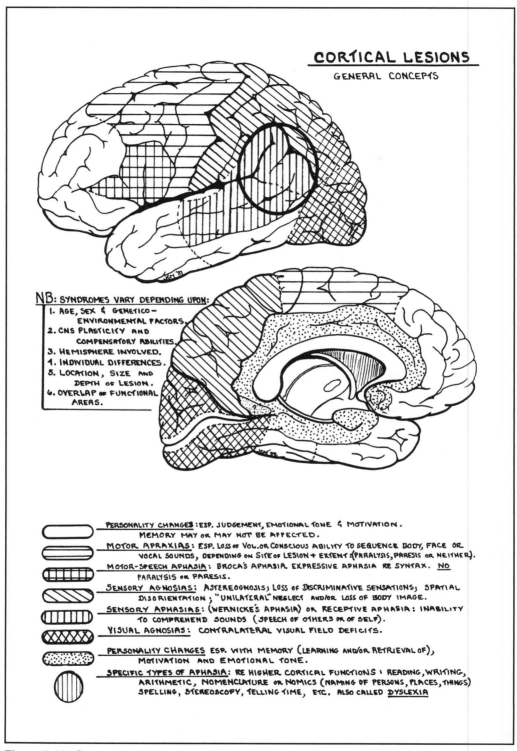

Figure 3-22: Cortical lesions.

The **A**nticipatory cortices (association or secondary motor cortices) endow the CNS with the ability to not only **A**nticipate, but also **P**lan and **P**rogram the moment-to-moment movement or speech patterns that will be most appropriate to environmental events taking place. These planned movement programs are "PASSed" through the kinetic system where the background postural adaptations are added, relayed to thalamic nuclei where synergic (SOS-DEFT^2) are reticular (R^{3}AS + 4 A's), information is integrated, and finally all of these newly integrated impulses are relayed back to the motor cortices. At the same time these reverberating circuits are going through the subcortical (kinetic and synergic) systems, a limbic component is being added to provide "MOVE" (and perhaps some of the "FARV"). Once all of this information has been reassembled in the motor areas of the neocortices, it is ready to be sent over the pyramidal pathways to LMN's (i.e., the corticonuclear tracts to LMN's of cranial nerves and corticospinal tracts to LMN's in the spinal cord) and cause an appropriate behavioral response. All of this anticipatory, planning, and programming activity, and the subcortical circuits involved, occurs prior to the moment when the motor cortices **E**xecute a **S**killed response or a **S**urvival **S**tratagem (ES^3). This circuitry takes approximately 300 to 800 milliseconds to function. In other words, these reverberating circuits are set into motion hundreds of milliseconds before any muscles begin to contract and cause movement (Figure 3-23). In young infants the neocortices have not matured sufficiently, and this intrinsic reverberating circuitry is not believed to be involved until after the cerebral cortices have begun to myelinate and some basic skills begin to develop. Prior to this time, an infant's functional abilities are carried out by utilizing circuitry of the spinal cord, brain stem, archi-cerebellum, and some lower subcortical areas (Figure 3-23). These structures and their circuits are quite capable of endowing an infant with a variety of behavioral patterns, an individual personality, and sufficient abilities to interact with the environment in order to achieve basic needs.

Lesions of these neocortical areas result in a variety of syndromes, each having specific terms, such as apraxia (or dyspraxia), aphasia, agnosia, dyslexia (Figure 3-22). However, the fundamental disability underlying all of these diagnostic terms is an inability of these cortical areas to **A**ppreciate various kinds of stimuli (such as auditory, visual, somatosensory), **A**nticipate events, and then **P**lan and **P**rogram the sequence of correct responses by utilizing appropriate subcortical reverberating circuits so that appropriate behaviors can be **E**xecuted in relation to either **S**killed functions or **S**urvival **S**trategies. Similarly, lesions of the fiber tracts or the reverberating circuits to and from the neocortices not only comprise A^{2}P^{2}ES^3 functions, but may result in pathological conditions—for example, hemiplegia, spastic diplegia, pseudobulbar palsy.

VII. "Neo-Neo" Cortical System of the Cerebral Hemispheres

The prefrontal lobes and the anterior temporal lobes are phylogenetically new (Figures 3-14, 3-19, and 3-21). In growth and development these areas of the brain develop and mature over a very long period. The mnemonic for these areas is JEM, as these cortices are the real "JEM^2" of our nervous system and are believed to separate us from the great APES. These areas endow humans with the ability to have **J**udgment (foresight, hindsight, and insight), especially as judgment related to **E**motional tone, **M**otivation, and **M**emories. These "neo-neo" cortices are intricately related, structurally and functionally, with the rest of the neocortices, limbic system, hypothalamus, and kinetic (basal ganglia) system. These cortices are believed to be the primary areas that

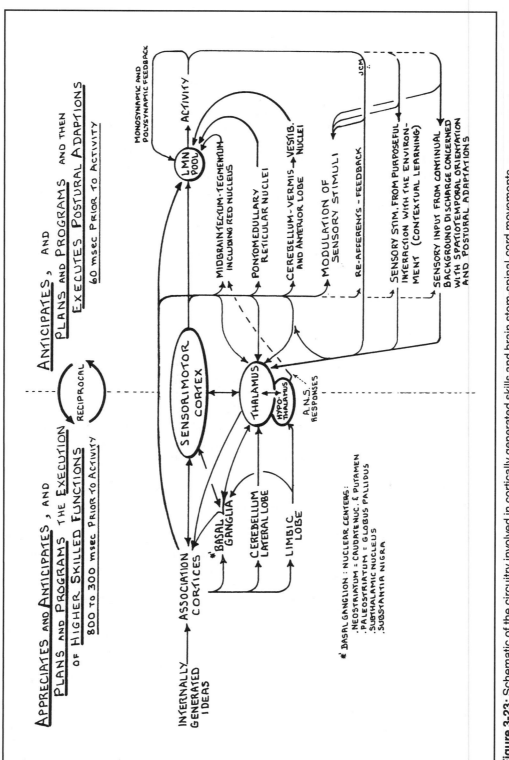

Figure 3-23: Schematic of the circuitry involved in cortically generated skills and brain stem-spinal cord movements.

enable humans to judge the consequences (based upon past experiences) of thought processes or any overt actions that might be taken in response to environmental stimuli. Thus, the "neo-neo" cortices play a major role in influencing neocortical ($A^2P^2ES^3$) functions, by tempering anticipatory reactions and modulating the way in which environmental stimuli are appreciated. These areas also act as a break on the limbic ($MOVE^2 + FARV$) and kinetic (PASS) systems, by modifying emotions and actions in relation to stored memories. Thus JEM^2 cortices enable selection of alternative behaviors or behaviors which would be more appropriate to circumstances of the moment, adapting to those circumstances in which one lives, and modifying short- and long-term goals of an individual in relation to the environment.

Lesions of the prefrontal and anterior temporal lobes may result in a change in an individual's judgment, especially in relation to being able to modify emotional tone, utilizing past memories for coping with new events, and adapting one's motives so that they are more in tune with the demands of the environment (Figure 3-22).

In summary, seven major functional systems have been presented along with mnemonics that are equated with the primary functions and dysfunctions of each system. In growth and development lower systems function first, followed by gradual maturation of higher systems. As these higher systems develop, the degree of functional "overlap" becomes increasingly important, until finally all seven systems are interdependent for normal function. A lesion in one of the systems disrupts this harmony and dysfunction results. The major signs expressed are related to the specific system in which the lesion occurred. However, all of the other systems are affected to varying degrees because of their interdependence.

Neuroplasticity

During the past few decades there has been a revolution in the neurosciences concerning neuroplasticity. Previous concepts considered the CNS to be "hard-wired"; i.e., once all of the nuclei, pathways, and synapses were in place the changes that occurred during growth and maturation were the result of repeated use over time of various circuits, which eventually resulted in the development of different skills. If a lesion occurred in the CNS, it was thought that many of the neurons and pathways involved in a functional circuit would die and permanent deficits would remain. For infants and young children who had CNS lesions, functional improvement was attributed to either "maturation of the NS" or the belief that "the original insult must have spared some functions." In a few cases, especially when there was recovery, it was assumed that an error was made in the diagnosis.

During the 1940's a few neuroscientists began questioning the concept of the "hard-wired" nervous system, and by the 1950's others had joined their ranks. Throughout the last three decades, the older concepts of the "hard-wired" nervous system were modified, and the "soft-wired" or neuroplastic nervous system was recognized, not only in regard to growth and development, but especially in relation to recovery potentials of the CNS following an insult.

A detailed account of the present state of knowledge in the area of neuroplasticity will not be covered in this text. Thousands of research articles and numerous books have been published on this subject and the reader should refer to these for additional information.[5-7,14,20,22,23,28,36-44] Only a brief summary is presented. Table 3-4 concerns microscopic changes that may occur in the CNS following a lesion. Appendix 3-A

Table 3-4
I. NEUROPLASTICITY:
A Summary of Microscopic Changes in the CNS

From Research on Mammals Concerning Enriched vs. Control vs. Deprived Environments, Prenatal, Perinatal and Post-Natal CNS Lesions.

Note: Major research data is based on mice, rats, gerbils, cats and primates. Minor research data is based on humans with few long-term follow-up studies and/or post-mortem data.

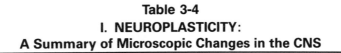

Changes at The Synapse:
Synaptic knobs or spines
Configuration of synapses
Neurotransmitter substances
Speed of conduction across the synapse
Post-synaptic membrane changes

Changes in The Dendrites:
Dendritic sprouting (collateralization or growth)
Dendritic fields

Changes in The Soma or Cell Body:
"Manufactures" cells' chemical energy & transports down axon.
"Induction process": helps to maintain viability of neuron—neuron, neuron—gland, neuron—effectors & neuron—receptors.
Rule: the closer the lesion is to the soma the greater the chances that the neuron will die and vis-a-vis.

Changes in The Axon:
Axonal sprouting at terminals in CNS
Axonal collateralization
Dorsal root sprouting of a peripheral nerve in CNS.
Remodele circuitry (and/or alternate pathways or "aberrant pathways")—anatomical reorganization of circuitry. Found at all levels of CNS and in all areas at these levels and remodeling can occur at all ages following CNS or PNS insult.

Note: In the fetal CNS it appears that neuronal death (due to a lesion) is the "prime initiator" that stimulates the CNS to restore itself.

presents a more detailed annotation of many of the recent research findings, especially as these relate to CNS deficits and neuroplasticity during early development. The important fact is that this relatively new field of knowledge is providing scientific support for many of the rehabilitation techniques that have been and are being used to help individuals maximize their potentials following a CNS lesion.

Individual Differences

Therapists have recognized, from years of observation and treating patients, that every person is different. Individual differences have motivated therapists to tailor their treatment techniques to meet the ever-changing needs of an individual. At the same time, recognition of individual differences has prevented the field of rehabilitation from establishing standardized treatment regimens which, theoretically, could be used to treat all individuals having the same diagnosis. Research in the neurosciences during the past 40 years has substantiated these beliefs and has laid a foundation upon which individual treatment can be justified.

Prior to World War II, it was believed by many that all white male brains were larger and thus more intelligent than the brains of other races and female brains, and that the two hemispheres of a brain were alike in surface configuration, cell types, and functional abilities.[45] Also, it was postulated by some that if offspring had the same parents, they should inherit similar genetic traits. These concepts began to change during and after World War II. Today it is known that no two individuals are morphologically, physiologically, genetically, or biochemically the same—not even identical twins.[11,23] Even the hemispheres of a brain are recognized as being structurally different and have dissimilar functions. Research has verified that female brains are different than male brains, not in relation to intelligence per se, but the way in which the brain develops, matures, and functions. The study of sexual dimorphism in the brains of animals and humans has demonstrated that certain neuronal cell populations are different in the two sexes.[24] These cellular areas not only influence the future behavior of the sexes, but also are influenced by the in utero hormonal environment during gestation.[14] Thus, the in utero environment and the genetic makeup of each embryo/fetus, even though born of the same parents, is different from all other siblings that may be born, just as the perinatal and postnatal environment will be different for each person.

Individual differences are best expressed by the fact that no two fingerprints of an individual are the same; every person's fingerprints are different from everyone else's, including every individual who has ever lived, is living, or will live in the future. In the same way, the soft-wired or neuroplastic nervous system, which is genetically different to begin with, and which is dependent upon environmental stimuli for normal growth and maturation, develops entirely different from every other human on earth. These differences are magnified by the manner in which each human interacts with the environment, modifies these interactions, and learns how to adapt to his/her internal environment. All of these factors, and others noted on Table 3-5, reinforce the concept that everyone is a unique individual. In fact, individual differences and/or uniqueness is enhanced in those who have had a CNS lesion.

Consider all of the variables involved that augment these differences, such as age of insult; degree of CNS maturity; health; sex; environmental and genetic makeup of the individual; the size, location and depth of the lesion (or lesions); how the patient was treated in the hospital, both during and afterwards; and other factors. In other words, all

---

Table 3-5

INDIVIDUAL DIFFERENCES:

* No two people (living today or throughout history) have had the same genetico-environmental endowment and/or exposure; not even identical twins.

* Even though each individual cannot help but be influenced by his/her genetics and environment, the individual, in turn, can modify the way in which these influences mold or shape his/her personality and behavioral patterns.

INDIVIDUAL	FAMILY UNIT
. Sex, race, color, creed, birthplace.	. Caretakers: One, two, or more; age + sex, etc.
. Place in sibling sequence or only child.	. Siblings: Sex, age, place in sibling sequence, multiples and "unexpected".
. Adopted--if so when; previous Hx; genetic endowment.	. Race, color, creed and birthplace.
. Individual drives (motivation) and "need to be".	. Caretaker(s) influence: Strong, moderate, weak.
. Individual talents - recognized or not reinforced or not	. Cultural values and "time of growing up".
. Mental endowment and how this matches expectations of others.	. Standards set (or not) by caretakers and type of standards.
. Body image: physical build; size, wgt; hgt; appearance, et al.	. Economics of family unit - one or both caretakers working, (unemployed), welfare, etc.
. Handicapped or not: Degree of; type of; (mental, physical, visible or not, etc.)	. "SILENT" expectations of family, siblings.
. "Silent" expectations of self vs others at various ages.	. Voiced expectations of family, esp. in relation to handicapped vs. normal family members.
. Educational opportunities utilized or not and why.	. Reality quotient of caretakers.
. Reality quotient.	

INTER-DEPENDENT VARIABLES

GENETICS	ENVIRONMENT
. Sex, race, color, and other physical attributes.	. "Strong (harsh) vs moderate or weak" influences; when, where, how and variability of same.
. Personality factors and affective behavior.	. Cultural standards or values.
. Bonding (types).	. Economic influences.
. "Pre-wired" or genetic "biases" re "that which is strange or different".	. Types of support groups: available or not in the community.
. Circadian rhythms.	. "SILENT" expectations of support groups or personnel in the helping professions.
. "FARV" = Fears, aggression, rage and violence: Allowed or not and/or degree which is tolerated.	. Social or community pressures.
. Territoriality: Personal space and territorial space.	. Peer pressures.
. Genetic diseases and congenital malformations.	. World events and pressures.
. "Traumatic learning".	. Attitudes of the times re research, medicine, and support professions in relation to individual's handicap.

individuals are unique to begin with, and following a CNS insult, they are even more unique in that their brains cannot help but develop, function, and adapt entirely different in comparison to normal individuals.

In summary, the CNS is extremely malleable, or plastic, especially during the developing stages in utero, during infancy, and childhood. Similarly, each individual's nervous system is unique, and especially so if brain-injured. Each must learn from, and react to, environmental stimuli in an individual way. Therapeutic intervention provides these opportunities and enables each individual to maximize his or her potential and adapt to the demands of the environment.

Key Points

1. Postnatal growth and development parallels the hierarchal levels of nervous system development, in that the lower levels mature and function much earlier than the higher levels.
2. The central nervous system is divided into three major areas, or the archi (oldest), paleo (intermediate), and neo (or the newest) components. Major structural units of the CNS can be further subdivided into their respective archi-, paleo-, and neo-components. The archi-, paleo-, and neo-terminology emphasizes the way in which the systems develop and later function together as an integrated whole.
3. Archi-systems are phylogenetically old and are the first to develop and function in humans. Archi-systems are concerned with visceral and endocrine functions, maintenance of homeostasis, postural adaptations, spatiotemporal orientation, sleep-awake, and attending functions.
4. Paleo-areas are intermediate in age and are the next to develop and function. Paleo-systems are primarily concerned with protective responses, patterns of locomotion, and survival mechanisms.
5. Neo-areas are phylogenetically recent, and the last areas to develop and function. Neo-systems enable us to anticipate events, explore and appreciate the environment, and learn from experiences.
6. There is a great deal of overlap between the archi-, paleo-, and neo-systems; however, the neo-areas primarily inhibit or dominate the paleo- and archi-systems.
7. In general, neo-systems are more vulnerable to insult (both prenatally and postnatally) than the paleo-systems, and the paleo- are more vulnerable than the archi-systems.
8. A lesion in one or more areas of the neo-systems may result in a "release phenomenon," which states that the lower or older functional systems are released from "higher" inhibitory control. Lost inhibitory control is usually expressed by abnormal movement patterns, loss of various skills, and/or loss of anticipatory and exploratory capabilities, accompanied by various degrees of retardation, or diminished capacities concerned with sensations, judgment, emotional tone, and learning potentials.
9. The medial longitudinal fasciculus (MLF) is a brain stem-spinal cord archi-pathway of major importance. MLF's function is to coordinate the cranial nerves of the brain stem with the spinal cord and spinal nerves so that all of the peripheral nerves function together in such activities as rooting, sucking, swallowing, visual searching, fixation and tracking, and communication.

10. Paleo-pathways of the spinal cord function as protective systems, relaying information about pain, temperature, touch, and pressure, as well as spatiotemporal adaptation.

11. Neo-pathways of the spinal cord function as exploratory systems, relaying kinesthetic types of sensory information which enable the human to anticipate, appreciate, and explore the environment.

12. The archi-, or oldest, parts of the brain stem function as reflex centers regulating eye movements, sleep-wake cycles, heart rate, respiration, perspiration, etc.

13. Paleo-areas of the brain stem are concerned with integrating sensory stimuli and responding to these stimuli at the protective levels of behavior, as well as spatiotemporal orientation to maintain the body in appropriate postures in relation to the spatial and temporal demands of the environment.

14. Neo-areas of the brain stem are primarily responsible for voluntary control and coordination of skilled functions. These pathways are also important modifiers of incoming sensory stimuli.

15. The archicerebellum develops first and is primarily concerned with balance in relation to antigravity postures and movements.

16. The paleocerebellum is primarily concerned with locomotion, while the neo-areas function in concert with the neocortex and are concerned with circuitry that is involved in learned (or skilled) functions.

17. The cerebellum endows the nervous system with **synergy**, the smooth orderly sequencing of direction, extent, force, timing, and tone involved in all patterns of movement.

18. The diencephalon or thalamus is located in the central depths of the brain and has four main subdivisions: epithalamus, hypothalamus, subthalamus, and dorsal thalamus. The first three are phylogenetically older structures (archi-paleo), while the dorsal is considered a neo-structure.

19. The dorsal thalamus plays a major role in integrating and relaying all kinds of sensory and motor impulses from lower centers to various higher centers of the cerebral cortex.

20. With few exceptions all ascending fibers and collaterals of descending fibers associated with cortical functions must synapse in thalamic nuclei, where they are integrated before new impulses are relayed to their final synaptic destinations.

21. The cerebral hemispheres, or telencephalon, consists of the cerebral cortices, subcortical white fiber tracts, and deep gray nuclei.

22. The cerebral cortex can be subdivided phylogenetically into archi, paleo (insula and limbic cortices), and neo (frontal, parietal, occipital, and temporal). The prefrontal lobes and anterior temporal lobes are phylogenetically recent, thus are referred to as "neo-neo" cortices.

23. During prenatal and postnatal development, the archi-systems of the spinal cord, brain stem, and archicerebellum develop sufficiently to endow the newborn with basic survival reflexes and the visual abilities to fixate upon and track moving objects.

24. The archi-systems of the brain stem, spinal cord, and cerebellum also endow the infant with a predominance of extensor or antigravity tone.

25. There are three kinds of muscle tone recognized in fetal development: passive, active (not gravity dependent), and active (gravity dependent).

26. Development of muscle tone (passive and active) develops in a caudocephalic and distal to proximal sequence. This sequence of muscle tone development prepares

the newborn for basic survival responses, sufficient tone to snuggle for support, or to interact with rhythmical movements to the cadence of the mother's voice.

27. Maturation of functional behaviors, or motor reactions, of the CNS begin in the high cervical levels of the spinal cord and lower brain stem, while protective or primary sensory reflexes of the body develop first in the oral-facial and cervical regions.

28. During growth and development, older systems are not only modified by newer systems, but many of these newer systems are incorporated into and function with the older systems. Eventually, all systems overlap and function together as an integrated whole.

29. Any insult to the seven functional systems of the CNS disrupts their unity and results in various kinds and degrees of dysfunction.

30. Growth and development of an embryo and fetus are governed by genetics and the internal environment in which the organism lives. Postnatally, growth and development, though still regulated by genetics, become more dependent upon stimuli from the external environment.

31. Without environmental interaction, the CNS does not develop normally or reach its optimal potentials.

32. With a viable but abnormal CNS, purposeful stimuli and interactions with the environment are critical for development. Without therapeutic intervention, sensory deprivation is experienced, accompanied by a decrease in neuroplasticity.

33. There are seven functional components of the CNS: sensorimotor-sensory, synergic, kinetic, hypothalamic and reticular, limbic, neocortical, and neo-neocortical. Each of the seven components have specific functions and anatomical areas which provide the human with tone, coordination, movement patterns, autonomic and affective systems, as well as skills and aesthetic systems.

34. The concept of neuroplasticity of the nervous system supports therapeutic intervention and provides scientific support for rehabilitation techniques that enable individuals to maximize their potential following a CNS lesion.

35. The CNS is extremely malleable, or plastic, especially during the developing stages in utero and early childhood.

36. Each individual's nervous system is unique, as no two people have the same genetic and environmental endowment.

Self-study Guidelines

1. List the seven major **structural** divisions of the CNS, the subdivisions, and each of the associated craniospinal nerves and plexuses.

2. Describe myelogenesis of the nervous system.

3. Discuss the archi-, paleo-, and neo-components of the nervous system. Define the terms and relate them to the development of the spinal cord, brain stem, cerebellum, diencephalon, and telencephalon.

4. The archi-areas of the spinal cord, brain stem, and cerebellum endow the infant with what functions?

5. Why does muscle tone develop in a caudocephalic and distal-proximal sequence, as compared to the cephalocaudic sequences of protective reflexes and myelination patterns of the peripheral nervous system?

6. Why is therapeutic intervention critical for the development of an infant with an abnormal CNS?
7. Explain and discuss the importance of neuroplasticity for rehabilitation.
8. Discuss the concept of "individual differences" and its relationship to rehabilitation.
9. Concerning the mnemonics used to understand the seven functional systems of the CNS, list each mnemonic in the appropriate space on the chart and explain what each means in relation to function and dysfunction, and name the major area(s) (structures) of the nervous system concerned with each functional area.

Structural Area(s)	System	Mnemonic	Function/dysfunction Explanations
	Neo-Neo cortic		
	Neo-cortical		
	Limbic		
	Kinetic		
	Hypothalamic-Reticular		
	Craniospinal Nerves		

References

1. Falkner F, Tanner JM: Human Growth. Vol. III. Neurobiology and Nutrition. New York, Plenum Press, 1979.
2. Gilles FH, Leviton A, Dooling EC: The Developing Human Brain: Growth, Epidemiologic, Neuropathology. Boston, John Wrist PSG, 1983.
3. Sarnet HB, Netsky MG: Evolution of the Nervous System. Ed. 2. New York, Oxford Univ. Press, 1981.
4. Yakovlev PI, Lecours, AR: Thee myelogenetic cycles of regional maturation of the brain. In Minkowski A (Ed): Regional Development of the Brain in Early Life. Oxford, Blackwell Scientific Publications, 1967, pp 3-70.
5. Almli CR, Finger S: Early Brain Damage. Vol. I. Research Orientations and Clinical Observations. Vol. II. Neurobiology and Behavior. New York, Academic Press, 1984.
6. Finger S (Ed.): Recovery from Brain Damage: Research and Theory. New York, Plenum Press, 1978.
7. Finger S, Stein DG: Brain Damage and Recovery: Research and Clinical Perspectives. New York, Academic Press, 1982.

8. Leech R, Shuman RM: Neuropathology: A Summary for Students. Philadelphia, Harper & Row, 1982.

9. Rorke LB: Pathology of Perinatal Brain Injury. New York, Raven Press, 1982.

10. Hampden-Turner C: Maps of the Mind. New York, W.W. Norton Co., 1981.

11. Konner M: The Tangled Wing: Biological Constraints on the Human Spirit. New York, Holt, Rinehart & Winston, 1982.

12. Barr M, Kiernan JA: The Human Nervous System: An Anatomical Viewpoint. Ed. 4. Philadelphia, Harper & Row, 1983.

13. Brodal A: Neurological Anatomy in Relation to Clinical Medicine. Ed. 3. New York, Oxford Univ. Press, 1981.

14. Kandel ER, Schwartz JH: Principles of Neural Science. New York, Elsevier/North Holland, 1981.

15. Brown CC (Ed.): The Many Facets of Touch. Pediatric Round Table No. 10. Johnson and Johnson Baby Products Co., 1984.

16. Klaus MH, Kennell JH: Maternal-Infant Bonding. St. Louis, C.V. Mosby Co., 1976.

17. Klaus MH, Robertson MO (Eds): Birth, Interaction and Attachment. Pediatric Round Table No. 6. Johnson and Johnson Baby Products Co., 1982.

18. Klaus MH, Leger T, Trause MA: Maternal Attachment and Mothering Disorders. Pediatric Round Table No. 1. Johnson and Johnson Baby Products Co., 1982.

19. Thomas EB, Trotter S (Eds): Social Responsiveness of Infants. Pediatric Round Table No. 2. Johnson and Johnson Baby Products Co., 1978.

20. Williams PL, Warwick R: Gray's Anatomy. (British) Ed. 36. Philadelphia, W. B. Saunders Co., 1980.

21. Lemire RJ, Loser JD, Leech RW, et al: Normal and Abnormal Development of the Human Nervous System. Hagerstown, MD, Harper & Row Medical Division, 1975.

22. Lund RD: Development and Plasticity of the Brain. New York, Oxford Univ. Press, 1978.

23. Restak R: The Brain. New York, Bantam Books, 1984.

24. Goldberg S, DiVitto BA: Born Too Soon: Preterm Birth and Early Development. San Francisco, W. H. Freeman Co., 1983.

25. Langman J: Medical Embryology. Ed. 4. Baltimore, Williams & Wilkens, 1981.

26. Moore KL: The Developing Human. Ed. 3. Philadelphia, W.B. Saunders Co., 1982.

27. Riesen AH: The Developmental Neuropsychology of Sensory Deprivation. New York, Academic Press, 1975.

28. Bach-y-Rita P (Ed): Recovery of Function: Theoretical Considerations for Brain Injury Rehabilitation. Bern Stuttgart Vienna, Hans Huber Publications, 1980.

29. Suomi SJ: Social development in Rhesus monkeys: Consideration of individual differences. Oliverio A, Zapella M (Eds): The Behavior of Human Infants. New York, Plenum Press, 1983.

30. Suomi SJ, Collins ML, Harlow HF, et al.: Effects of maternal and peer separations on young monkeys. J Child Psychol Psych 17:101-112, 1976.

31. Suomi SJ, Harlow HF: The role and reason of peer friendships in Rhesus monkeys. In Lewis M, Rosenblum LA (Eds): Friendship and Peer Relations. New York, John Wiley & Sons, 1975.

32. Harlow HF: Learning to Love. New York, Jason Aronson, Inc., 1974.

33. Hofer MA: The Roots of Human Behavior. San Francisco, W.H. Freeman Co., 1981.

34. Sasserath VJ, Hoekelman RA (Eds): Minimizing High-risk Parenting. Pediatric Round Table No. 7. Johnson and Johnson Baby Products Co., 1983.

35. Winson J: Brain and Psyche: The biology of the unconscious. New York, Anchor Press/Doubleday, 1985.
36. Andreasen NC: The Broken Brain: The biological revolution in psychiatry. New York, Harper & Row, 1984.
37. Shepard GM: Neurobiology. New York, Oxford Univ. Press, 1983.
38. Stein DG, Rosen JJ, Butters N (Eds): Plasticity and Recovery of Function in the Central Nervous System. New York, Academic Press, 1974.
39. Tsukahara N: Sprouting and the neuronal basis of learning. Trends in Neurosci 4(9):234-237, Sept. 1981.
40. Austin L, Langford CJ: Nerve regeneration: A biochemical view. Trends in Neurosci 3(5):130-132, May 1980.
41. Goldberger ME: Motor recovery after lesions. Trends in Neurosci 3(11):288-291, Nov. 1980.
42. Bliss TVP: Synaptic plasticity in the hippocampus. Trends in Neurosci 2(2):42-45, Feb. 1979.
43. Oakley DA: Neocortex and learning. Trends in Neurosci 2(6):149-152, June 1979.
44. Szekely G: Order and plasticity in the nervous system. Trends in Neurosci 2(10):245-248, Oct. 1979.
45. Gould SJ: The Mismeasure of Man. New York, MacMillan Publishing Co., 1981.

APPENDIX 3-A
NEUROPLASTICITY:
Additional Biological Factors and Pros and Cons

Perinatal Period: 21-22 wks I.U. to 28 Days Postpartum

A: Kennard Principle
The earlier a lesion occurs in development the better the chances are for functional recovery and/or sparing of functional abilities.

B: Genetic Factors Functional recovery following CNS insult:
Susceptibility to CNS insult can be dependent upon "strong" vs "weak" genes (i.e., a "good egg" vs a "bad egg") in relation to one's genetic make-up or dominant and recessive traits.

C: Neurons Pruning and Tuning Concept
Excessive neuronal proliferation during embryogenesis and fetal development parallels one of nature's laws, i.e., the overproduction of progeny, (frogs, fish, sperm, etc). During growth and development in utero excess neurons are "pruned away" as the CNS is "tuned up" to meet the demands of, and interact with, the environment.

D: Neuroglia
While neurogenesis is believed to cease at birth (in humans), neurogliogenesis continues for up to 5 years after birth.
- A severe hypoxic-ischemic episode that affects the basal ganglia can result in too few neurons in relation to "excess" neuroglia. This results in over-myelination of CNS neurons or status marmoratus.
- "Excess" neurons in relation to too few neuroglia result in under-myelination or perinatal telencephalic leukoencephalophy.
- Both conditions result in gross CNS pathology, mental retardation, and functional deficits.

E: Neural Development of the CNS and Behavioral Development
These two processes are time-dependent, i.e., they parallel to one another.
- CNS insult affects (slows down) the rate of both of these developmental processes.
- Training-dependent Recovery (in mice & rats) appears to depend upon CNS fe-organization first. Therefore, training per se may not be coupled to neural or behavioral development and functional recovery, but in primates and humans this may not be the case, i.e., all three processes may be time-dependent.

F: Peripheral Nerve Lesions: sustained at birth
Almost always functional recovery occurs over time; exceptions exist (See Neuroplasticity under Rule changes in the Soma and changes in the Axon Under Dorsal Root Sprouting in Humans).

G: Recovery Potentials Following Perinatal Insult
Statistics include premature, SGA, IUGR, and full-term infants.
- 50-50 chance of "total" recovery vs. all degrees of deficits.
- Thus far medical science is unable to predict who will recover and who won't. Statistics are based on hard signs (not soft signs) in relation to functional abilities.
- Few long-term follow-up studies have been done, especially during the grade school and high school years, except

APPENDIX 3-A continued

- Mental illness and prematurity have been linked (high correlation).
- Teen-age suicides and prematurity have been linked (high correlation).
- Neurological impairment appears to increase as children mature, especially in those originally diagnosed as having mild, moderate, or severe perinatal CNS insult. [Note: Few scientific studies correlate neurological findings with rehabilitation.]

H: Resistance to Hypoxia and/or Circulatory Arrest
- Resistance depends upon the animal's physiological maturity at birth:
  - Precocial animals (calf, fawn, foal, etc) much more vulnerable.
  - Altricial animals (cats, dogs, primates, man, etc.) much less vulnerable.
- Cerebral metabolism in altricial mammals is much lower in the newborn CNS than in the more mature CNS.
- Greater glycogen reserves in newborn altricials can be converted into glucose over a longer period of time and/or during circulatory arrest.

I: Vasculature: Prenatal vs Postnatal Brain: (Humans)
- The prenatal brain has internal and external anastomotic connections between the three cerebral arteries supplying each hemisphere.
- The normal-term neonate and the postnatal brain lacks these internal and external anastomoses. Hence a hypoxic-ischemic episode at birth or shortly thereafter can cause border zone (watershed area) pathology (cell death) in specific and rather critical areas of the brain.

NEUROPLASTICITY:
Miscellaneous Findings in Relation to Recovery Potentials Following CNS Lesions

A: Bonding, Parenting, Motivation, and Learning
If one or more of these parameters is abnormal or missing, non-functional reorganization and hence abnormal development of the CNS usually occurs, and/or there is failure-to-thrive.

B: Dale's Law and Neurotransmitters
This law states that a neuron can produce only one neurotransmitter substance, such as CA (catecholamine), DA (dopamine), NE (norepinephrine).
- Today over 200 (and counting) neurotransmitters have been discovered.
- Neurons are now known to produce a minimum of four (and counting) neurotransmitters per neuron, in varying quantities or mixtures, depending upon the developmental stages and ages of the organism.
- Example: The delicate interplay of CA, DA, and NE in various neural circuits of the CNS are known to play decisive roles in modulating patterns of movement and behaviors. Also they are believed to be implicated in attentional deficit disorders (ADD), hyperactivity, learning and memory problems.
- Experimental replacement of neurotransmitters or their precursors by injection or other means has not, as yet, been successful in the long run.

C: Enriched vs Control vs Deprived Environments
(in relation to "TLC" [bonding & love], nutrition, drugs, kinship & peer relations, security, play and type of environment—stimulating or not.) [See also under Microscopic Changes—Neuroplatsicity and Rehabilitation—Item F. below.]

- In developing organisms an enriched environment is known to cause accelerated growth and development, earlier onset of exploratory behaviors, learning and dexterity, in comparison to controls, and especially in relation to deprived states.
- Brain weight and cortical thickness (especially in certain regions of the cerebral cortex, somatosensory and visual cortices) are enhanced and the neurophil is denser, in enriched state.
- Vis-a-vis in deprived states the cortical thickness (compared to controls) is less, brain weight is less, but body weight may be greater.
- In aged individuals (rats) enriched environments maintain if not increase synaptic density, exploratory behaviors, and an apparent drive to continue learning from the environment; however, in deprived organisms synaptic density, brain weight, cortical thickness, and exploratory behaviors decline rapidly and death comes at a much earlier age (400 to 500 days vs 900 days).
- In elderly humans who are no longer stimulated or self-motivated to learn and explore their environment, and/or poor health makes this impossible, a gradual decline in one's abilities and motivational states appears to parallel neuronal
- depletion, synaptic changes, and actual "shrinkage" of various cortical and sub-cortical structures.
- The age-old dictum "If you don't use it you lose it" has not been disproven to date. Instead, it has been reinforced over and over again during 100 years of intensive research in the neurosciences.

D: Excitatory vs Inhibitory Synapses
Post-lesion Connections and Misconnections

- During reorganization of an organism's nervous system a normal balance must be reestablished between the number of excitatory and inhibitory synapses that influence cell thresholds, and this balance must occur in all of the various nuclear areas that are being re-innervated.
- Excessive loss of excitatory synapses leaves the organism in an inhibitory "floppy to flaccid" state with a depressed affect—i.e., excessive damage to inhibitory centers and circuits leaves an excess of excitatory synapses, thus leading to various degrees of hypertonia, hyperactivity, spasticity, or rigidity.
- The potential for causing changes in the excitatory-inhibitory balance of a re-organizing nervous system is an area of scientific investigation that has been ignored for too long, except perhaps in the field of neuropharmacology and rehabilitation.

E: Maladaptive Circuitry vs Adaptive Circuits

- Until recently (1970s & 1980s) anatomical reorganization of circuits (pathways) following CNS insult was thought to be disadvantageous. This belief was based upon tests of the animals' abilities that were limited to a single specific functional ability such as vision, hearing, touch, reading, writing.
- When tests were changed to include a variety of sensory channels, combined with survival strategies, most anatomical reorganization was found to be adaptive or advantageous to the animal in relation to the demands of its environment.

F: Rehabilitation

- If the rehabilitation techniques are scaled appropriately to developmental environment in the home;
- If the rehabilitation techniques are scaled appropriately to developmental sequences according to each individual's needs and at appropriate ages & growth stages;

APPENDIX 3-A continued

- if the rehabilitation techniques are purposeful (i.e., meaningful to the individual at the time), appropriately inhibiting or stimulating, and repetitive, yet ever changing, to meet the needs of the individual; and
- if the techniques utilize active participation along with goal-oriented behaviors (and not command performances); then
- chances are excellent, based upon our present knowledge of neuroplasticity, that therapists can make effective changes in the CNS which will enable the individual to function on a much higher level in comparison to a matched individual in either a control or a deprived state.

G: A Single Lesion vs Serial Lesions (over time)
- A series of small lesions (with sufficient time between each lesion for healing), usually leaves the experimental animal with minimal or no loss of functional abilities.
- A single large lesion, equivalent in size to all of the serial lesions together, may result in death and/or serious disruption of functional abilities.
- In infants, serial insults may be much less devastating than one large unilateral lesion or two smaller bilateral lesions. [Also see (H.) Territoriality Concept and (I.) Unilateral vs. Bilateral Lesions.]
- In adult humans, multiple small infarcts over time (TIAs) are known to cause little if any overt changes in behavior in comparison to CVAs.

H: Territoriality Concept vs Crossover Re-innervation:
Territoriality Concept: Early in life, if a lesion destroys a vital area of the cerebral cortex of one hemisphere, such as the expressive language cortices of broca, the same or a very similar area in the other hemisphere is believed to take over the functional abilities of the destroyed area. (The young or immature brain is believed to be much more pluripotential, or plastic, in comparison to more mature brains.)
- However, when a given function that has been genetically programmed to function optimally in a certain hemisphere is lost and the other hemisphere takes over that function, the territory which has been taken over cannot develop its own genetic potentials.
- It is only in later stages of neural development (school age and older) that these territorial deficits manifest themselves. These subtle deficits can be devastating both behaviorally and psychologically, especially if help is unavailable and/or the individual is unable to compensate or adapt to the demands of the environment.

Territoriality Concept: In mature brains following a lesion of a cortical area (or its pathways) in one hemisphere, the other hemisphere may not be able to take over the lost function because its functional territories are already committed. If the lost function is regained, this may result from reorganization of the other cortical areas of the same hemisphere which have plurifunctional potentials, i.e., the 2°, 3°, 4°, and 5° association cortices; however,
- mature male brains appear to have less pluripotentiality than do mature female brains (either in one hemisphere or both hemispheres);
- genetic left handers (male and female) appear to have a greater pluripotentiality, and hence functional return, than does the average human brain. (This may hold true for ambidextrous individuals also); and

- right hemisphere lesions (especially in males) usually results in more severe deficits, hence poorer functional recovery, than is seen in left hemisphere lesions.

Cross-over Reinnervation: In experimental animals, a circumscribed lesion in one hemisphere or in a subcortical nuclear area may not result in a territorial takeover of function by the other hemisphere or subcortical area. Instead, the "mirror image" center in the opposite hemisphere may sprout commissural fibers which either

- crossover the midline to re-innervate adjacent areas which have lost their innervation;
- sprout collaterals and new terminals from existing commissural fibers which assist in re-innervating adjacent areas; or
- crossover and re-innervate one or more nuclear centers along the functional pathway and this helps in re-establishing the functional integrity of the system.

<u>Remember</u>: Cell death in the CNS appears to be a primary stimulus for initiating axonal and dendritic sprouting, which helps in reestablishing synapses and maintaining the functional integrity of the system.

I: Unilateral vs Bilateral Lesions: and mirror image vs non-mirror sites

- *Unilateral Lesions:* In developing animals a lesion of the motor cortex, or of the corticospinal tract on one side, can result in the opposite intact hemisphere sending fibers contralaterally as expected but also ipsilaterally to re-innervate LMNs bilaterally. With maturity these animals exhibit mirror image movements. Likewise, the literature records similar cases in which adults exhibit mirror image movements having had a unilateral lesion of the motor cortex when they were very young.
  - A few cases are on record of adults who have had unilateral brain stem lesions of the corticospinal tracts & in several years have regained almost all of their functional abilities.
  - In humans unilateral lesions of the right hemisphere tend to be more handicapping over time than do unilateral left hemisphere lesions, and especially so in males.
- *Bilateral Lesions: Mirror Image Sites vs Non-Mirror Image Sites:*
- *Mirror Image Sites:* These lesions are much more devastating, in that functional takeover by the opposite hemisphere is severely compromised as well as the possibility of reestablishing function by crossover re-innervation; however, this does not imply that nothing can be accomplished by rehabilitation, i.e., the CNS is highly plastic.
- *Non-Mirror Image Sites:* Though usually very handicapping (depending upon size, location, and developmental age of insult), these kinds of lesions offer a greater potential for various degrees of functional abilities in that the intact areas may be able to take over some basic functions and/or assist in re-innervating areas of synaptic loss (either ipsilaterally or contralaterally or both), and thus help to re-establish "alternate," though aberrant, circuitry.

"If centuries of research have told us anything, it is that very rarely if at all is there a tight relationship between the brain and any given behavior"*

* Oswald, S: Lesion-induced Neuroplasticity and the Sparing or Recovering of Function Following Early Brain Damage. In Almli CR, Finger S (Eds): Early Brain Damage. Vol I. New York, Academic Press Inc, 1984, p 76.

CHAPTER 4

Strategies for Developmental and Purposeful Sequences

Objectives

The reader will be able to

1. discuss the nature and developmental course of posture and movement strategies and the adaptation of strategies to sequences;
2. discuss and differentiate postural strategies and movement strategies;
3. define muscle functions and discuss their developmental course and role with posture and movement strategies;
4. define neural functions and discuss their role in development of strategies; and
5. differentiate primitive, transitional, and mature phases as related to sensorimotor development.

Introduction

Movement is an integral part of strategies that constitute developmental and purposeful sequences of adaptation. Growth, maturation, and integration of neuromuscular properties of movement result in development of patterns of movement and postural control, or strategies, that are adapted by a child in performance of developmental and purposeful sequences. Strategies are viewed as component parts of adaptive sequences, since activation and modification of functions occur in response to a child's drive to develop an upright posture and intention to use movements purposefully. Strategies exist for the purpose of activation (movement) and control (posture) of the body or body segments during performance of actions from the simplest act of raising the head in prone to a more complicated act of standing on one foot and hopping. The fact that strategies exist as part of a developmental or purposeful sequence of behavior also means that a child's motivation to meet challenges from the environment and to pursue behaviors beyond current capability serves as a stimulus to facilitate neuromuscular functions required for higher level performance. In this chapter we will examine the nature and developmental course of posture and movement strategies. To study strategies in detail—where they originate, what they do, how they are combined and adapted—is helpful in order to recognize their adaptation in subsequent chapters describing developmental and purposeful sequences.

During the time that structures and functions for movement are being adapted to specific sequential behaviors, they are differentiated according to whether they are suited for performing movement itself or exerting control over movement through postural mechanisms. Functions related to a movement are linked together to form movement strategies, or integrated parts of an action sequence required to create smooth, fast, and directed sequential patterns.[1] Development and use of movement strategies depend on an individual's past experience, present situation, and anticipated outcome. As movement strategies develop, they include both the movement plan itself and the postural adjustments required to support movement.

Functions associated with postural control, such as holding, coactivation of muscle groups, and antagonistic muscle actions, develop along with, and as a part of, the more obvious movement patterns and form postural strategies. Postural strategies are integrated parts of an action sequence required to maintain body position or change position in relation to movement. Development and use of postural strategies also depend upon an individual's past experience, present situation, and anticipated outcome or next required movement. Posture and movement strategies function as a sensorimotor-sensory unit and, although they seem to have entirely different roles in adaptation of movement to developmental and purposeful sequences, they act synchronously; i.e., functions are coordinated to produce integrated action.[2] In developmental and purposeful sequences of behavior, strategies account for a child's ability to move safely in space at whatever level of performance he or she has achieved. Strategies synchronize distribution of postural tone required to secure or change positions, along with movement necessary to initiate action.

Posture and Movement Strategies

Posture and movement strategies create an ability to "move" or "not move" in certain predictable patterns determined by the purpose of moving or ceasing movement. Postural strategies control movement, and movement strategies give rise to purposeful action.[3] Movement tends to displace one body segment with respect to another or to displace the body as a whole with respect to the supporting surface.[2] Movement strategies promote and sequence changes in position of body or body parts. Movement strategies combine muscle actions so that one movement flows into another, and patterns of movement evolve fluently from one another.[4] Action by one group of muscles sequentially enhances or dampens actions by other groups of muscles. Sequence of flow develops from repetition of selected movements, which are simultaneously being adapted to specific developmental or purposeful sequences. With repetition, neural pathways are established so that a particular sequence of movements is associated with a specific outcome or purpose. Once movement strategies are associated with specific outcomes, a strategy can be automatically elicited as soon as an individual anticipates need for that desired outcome. According to Goodgold-Edwards,[5] as children mature their movements are characterized by faster speed, fewer errors, less variability, and therefore more efficient strategies. As a result, greater precision and adaptability are available and better serve the purpose of their intended actions.

Movement strategies that cause displacement of body segments, or the body itself, need to be integrated with mechanisms capable of controlling timing and direction of an action to assure that balance is maintained and movement is purposeful. Postural strategies control both movement of body segments in relation to each other and maintenance of the position of the body in space during movement. Posture is defined as position of body segments at any given time. Postural strategies are considered the means for distributing postural tone needed to maintain positions and for redistributing tone in anticipation or during changes in position due to movement. Postural strategies are similar to that which is termed by Bobath[6] as normal postural mechanism.

Massion[2] states that posture is built on several mechanisms: muscle tone, which gives muscles a type of rigidity and helps maintain joints in defined positions; postural tone, which is added to muscle tone, mainly in extensor muscles that function against gravity; and postural fixation, which acts as a local mechanism to maintain joint position against internal force (such as the weight of other body segments) or external force (such as an object held by one of the segments of a fixated joint). Fixation is obtained by co-contraction of antagonist muscles around joints and will be discussed further with development of muscle functions. Equilibrium as a dynamic component of posture is considered a distinct motion and will be discussed further with development of neural functions.

Development of Strategies

Movement begins in utero. Underlying neurological mechanisms for movement are sufficiently established before birth to transmit stimuli for essentially reflexive movements. Reflexive fetal movements include flexion and extension of an extremity, occasional repositioning of the body, and a few coordinated patterns of movement, such as sucking. When an infant is born, fetal reflexes and movements are adapted to extrauterine life. Neonatal movements provide means by which transactions with the environment are enacted, leading to development of more complex, purposeful movements. Significant factors in the extrauterine environment include gravity, which constitutes a force acting either against or with movement, and surface, which mimics the earth's surface and acts as either a support for posture or a reference point for movement.[3]

A newborn's first movements are generalized and seem to lack control and obvious purpose, although it is clear that the infant enjoys experiencing movement. Only movement around the mouth seems coordinated and purposeful, as an infant adapts sucking and swallowing patterns to survival needs. Generalized movements are confined primarily to the extremities. Even though early movement may seem to the observer to lack purpose, primitive movement serves the purpose of developing muscle functions and establishing neural pathways so that more controlled, directed movements can evolve in the form of posture and movement strategies. In addition, early movements contain incipient patterns of movement, mostly reflexive in nature, but sufficient to give the infant a sense of moving in patterns or rhythms, such as reflexive, reciprocation-type patterns that are seen in the lower extremities. These early movements, or positions assumed momentarily through movement, may give an infant a sense of developmental achievements to come, or a repertoire of past primitive behaviors that can be linked to more mature phenomena as the developmental sequence unfolds.

As a baby matures, generalized movements can be viewed as non-directed, such as repetitive bilateral or reciprocal kicking, or directed, such as swiping at objects (Figure 4-1). Non-directed movements tend to form the basis for the development of automatic

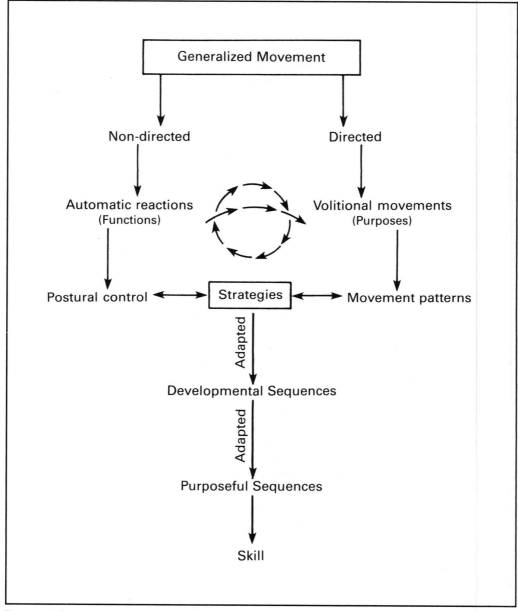

Figure 4-1

reactions, such as righting, protection, or equilibrium. Directed movements tend to develop into volitional movements, such as visually guided reaching or adapting walking to running. As automatic reactions and volitional movements are integrated along the function-to-purpose continuum, a baby starts to use combinations of automatic and volitional movements to form posture and movement strategies and to adapt strategies to developmental and purposeful sequences. A baby's performance with developmental and purposeful activities then takes on a more deliberate quality based on an emerging awareness that movement can be controlled and directed. Deliberateness plays a role in linking the use of automatic reactions as a support for volitional movement, and volitional movement as means for challenging the use of automatic reactions in new situations. For example, after a baby has experienced spontaneous rolling from the influence of righting reactions and wants to make rolling happen deliberately, he may reach across the body with an arm or a leg to start the rolling process, and then let the automatic reactions sequence the rolling pattern. With further adaptation, a baby will not only be able to initiate rolling volitionally, but will also be able to differentiate reaching components and automatic postural control components from the rolling pattern in order to reach for a toy, while maintaining sidelying position.

Development of strategies that support automatic and volitional movement requires structural components for flexion, extension, lateral flexion, and rotation, as well as maturation of mobility and stability, and of combined and blended muscle functions of those components. Movement components and muscle functions develop along with, and because of, nervous system maturation of automatic phasic and tonic reflexes, vertical and rotational righting reactions, support and protective reactions, and equilibrium and midline stability reactions. In each phase of development (primitive, transactional, or mature) movement and combinations of movements facilitated by specific neuronal activity produce specific weight-bearing and weight-shifting patterns of postural control (Figure 4-2).

Posture and Movement Strategies			
Movement Components	**Muscle Function**	**Primitive Reflexes/ Automatic Reactions**	**Postural Control/ Movement Patterns**
Extension		Phasic	
	Mobility	Tonic	
Flexion	Stability	Support	
			Weight bearing
		Righting	
Lateral Flexion	Combined Mobility- Stability		Bilateral Weight Shift/ Movement
		Protective	Unilateral Weight Shift/ Movement
Rotation	Blended Mobility Stability	Equilibrium	Contralateral Weight Shift/Movement

Figure 4-2

Movement Components

At birth, and for a while afterwards, an infant automatically assumes a flexed posture reminiscent of the position experienced in utero. Extension and flexion are the first active movement components to appear first in extremities and specific body segments and then affecting the body as a whole. Extension against gravity is necessary for development of postural tone, especially around the midline and proximal segments of the body. Flexion against gravity is necessary for developing ranges of flexion, which are useful for development of volitional movements. Even though a neonate is often in a flexed posture, flexor muscle groups still need to develop through ranges of movement by moving through the range. Once flexion and extension components have been activated and elongated around a body segment, both components can be used simultaneously to control movement or maintain the position of a particular segment or segments. With further development of movement components and challenges to maintain or move in new ways, activation of flexors and extensors on the same side of the body segment lead to lateral flexion; activation of flexors on one side and extension on the opposite side of the segment, or vice versa, results in rotation patterns of movement. Flexion, extension, lateral flexion, and rotation, with accompanying abduction-adduction, internal rotation-external rotation of the extremities, are the movement components essential to the development of posture and movement strategies. Adaptation of these components to specific strategies depends on maturation of muscle functions associated with each component and maturation of the automatic reactions responsible for developing and directing each component.

Muscle Functions

Stability and mobility muscle functions are dependent upon maturation of CNS reflexes and reactions, and upon physiological development of specific muscles and muscle groups according to their primary function, i.e., stability or mobility.[7,8] All muscles develop mobility first, and many pass through a stability phase before being differentiated into their primary functions. Mobility actions produce "moveability" or change. Mobility actions function as part of movement strategies to carry out a desired sequence of changes in position of the body or body segments. Some muscle groups, especially muscles used for skill activity, function primarily as mobilizers. Mobilizers are characterized by their ability to act with range, speed, and accuracy.[7,8] Mobilizers are usually activated in reciprocal patterns and make use of a wide range of motion.

Stability actions produce "stay-ability," or regulation of change. Stability actions dampen mobility to control movement of the body or body segments during changes in position. Some groups, especially more proximal muscles, function more as stabilizers and produce postural tone. Stabilizers readily respond to constant stimuli from gravity and from the supporting surface.[7,8] Stabilizers maintain contraction in shortened ranges at the midline and around proximal joints for postural stability and control of movement. Stability actions are blended with mobility actions to control posture and movement.

Mobility and stability muscle functions develop sequentially in a cephalocaudal, proximal-to-distal progression. There is overlap between and among the stages, depending on the function-to-purpose adaptation and developmental state of the body segments involved.

Mobility, the first muscle function to develop, is characterized by an activation of muscles and muscle groups in undifferentiated patterns by means of a complete shortening of agonists and lengthening of antagonists. Muscles need to move through a complete range of motion in order to develop an ability to function throughout the range. The concept of elongation of muscles as a prerequisite to developing function is related to the idea of mobility.[9] Muscles, or groups of muscles, to be fully activated and prepared for function, need to be activated in lengthening as well as shortening contractions; e.g., reciprocal kicking or elongation in weight bearing. Development of mobility functions is associated with maturation of phasic reflexes and all righting reactions.

Stability, the second muscle function to develop, is characterized by coactivation, or simultaneous contraction of agonists and antagonists around joints, in order to hold that joint in a particular position to allow the body to maintain postures, even before all the mechanisms for maintaining higher level postures are in place. The concept of coactivation implies that stability is a dynamic quality, which eventually allows holding and moving simultaneously when mobility is blended with stability; e.g., holding head in line with trunk in prone or maintaining hands-knees position. Development of stability is associated with maturation of tonic reflexes and all support reactions.

Combined mobility and stability means that mobility functions are superimposed on stability functions in such a way that a baby can maintain a position and still move within the limited range of that position. Mobility is superimposed around the midline and more proximal joints, while the distal part of the extremities are fixed to a supporting surface. Proximal movement modifies the holding aspect of stability preparing for dynamic stability, and the stability factor modifies the full range of movement preparing for the use of dynamic stability to control movement; e.g., rocking on all fours or bouncing in standing. Combination of mobility and stability is associated with maturation of support and protective reactions and all righting reactions.

Blended mobility and stability means that mobility and stability functions are integrated in such a way that a child can maintain and move freely within positions or move from one position to another while still maintaining desired spatial orientation of head and trunk. When a system has developed blended mobility and stability muscle functions, extremities can move freely in space, since they are no longer needed for protection or support during position changes. Control for position changes and extremity movement comes from dynamic stability functions around the midline and more proximal joints, which controls mobility and adjusts in relation to mobility; e.g., moving from sitting to standing while maintaining vertical orientating of head and trunk or accurate direction of reaching from a sitting position. Blended mobility and stability is associated with maturation of midline stability and equilibrium reactions.

Reflexes and Reactions

Automatic reflexes and reactions are functions of the central nervous system.[6] They are neurological mechanisms that affect predictable patterns of posture or movements. Reflexes and reactions distribute muscle and postural tone in specific posture and movement strategies according to whether the strategies are adapted to purposeful behaviors (e.g., rolling, creeping, walking, reaching) or adapted to purposeful activities (e.g., feeding oneself, cutting a circle from the paper, walking to the store). The terms "reflex" and "reaction" are used to describe specific responses or series of responses to particular sensory input or combinations of sensory stimuli. "Reactions are distinguished from reflexes by their greater complexity and inconstancy of the response."[10, p11] According to this distinction, the term "reflex" is preferred to describe some of the fetal and neonatal responses that are simple, more predictable, and probably result from one or two sources of sensory stimulation, such as tactile and vestibular. The term "reaction" applies to more complex responses that result from integration of simultaneous sensory input, such as tactile, proprioceptive, visual, and auditory. Reactions usually develop from infancy and may be retained with maturity; e.g., the parachute (protective extension) reaction. This text will generally follow the above distinction in terminology.

Reflexes and reactions can be considered in three groupings: primitive reflexes, transitional reactions, and mature reactions. Primitive reflexes include phasic and tonic reflexes and are present at birth. Transitional reactions include righting, support, and protective reactions and develop when the infant is in transition between primitive and mature behavior. Mature reactions include midline stability and equilibrium reactions and are acquired and used throughout life. Detailed descriptions of reflexes and reactions can be found in Appendix 4-A.

Phasic reflexes (Figure 4-3) originate from a variety of exteroceptive, interoceptive, and proprioceptive assimilations. Phasic reflexes usually produce observable movement in response to touch, pressure, movement of the body, or sight or sound received. Some phasic reflexes are part of movement strategies that serve survival functions, such as taking nourishment into the body (e.g., rooting or sucking). Others serve protective purposes, causing withdrawal from unknown sources of stimulation—e.g., avoiding responses—while some relate to strategies that are forerunners of more complex behaviors. For example, reflexes like crossed-extension cause reciprocal limb activity, which prepares for development of higher level reciprocal patterns of movement after postural control has been established.[11]

Phasic reflexes activate muscles and muscle groups through a complete range of motion. Agonist muscles are activated in shortening contractions. Antagonist muscles are dampened and lengthened by reciprocal innervation. Movement through a complete range of motion both by shortening and lengthening is necessary for muscles to develop physiologically through their complete range of motion.[7] Muscle groups with similar function are also aided in developing synergistic action by being activated through complete ranges of motion simultaneously. An outcome of phasic reflexes activating muscles and muscle groups through their complete ranges of motion is the development of mobility and strategies reflecting undifferentiated patterns or full ranges of movement.

Sensory assimilations that initiate primitive mobility also provide feedback from the peripheral to the central nervous system, increasing the infant's awareness of self and environment. Reflexive motor accommodations provide additional exteroceptive, interoceptive, and proprioceptive information about changing positions and motions of body segments. An infant begins to associate certain sensory input with certain predictable responses, such as moving to a touch to obtain the nipple, and can repeat familiar movement patterns to obtain desired results.[12] Spontaneous head turning may indicate hunger, as the infant associates head turning from the rooting reflex with search for the nipple to satisfy hunger. An infant begins to link together a specific outcome or to adapt primitive movement strategies to primitive behaviors and activities.

Tonic reflexes (Figure 4-4) also originate from a variety of exteroceptive, interoceptive, and proprioceptive assimilations. Tonic reflexes are usually seen as postures assumed in response to the position of head and trunk in space or in relation to each other; e.g., tonic labyrinthine reflex or asymmetrical tonic neck reflex.[11-13] Muscle tone is distributed in specific postural patterns, causing cessation of movement or fixation. Tonic reflexes most frequently offset the body's midline and its proximal joints, which are the segments of the body that will eventually provide stabilization to support posture and control movement. Some tonic reflexes distribute tone in opposite patterns on either side of the midline (asymmetrical tonic neck reflex), or above and below the waistline (symmetrical tonic neck reflex). Such differences in distribution may predict types of stabilization patterns that will develop for postural control at higher levels.

Distribution of muscle tone in primitive postural patterns activates muscles and muscle groups in holding contractions at a particular point within the range of motion, frequently at the end of the range of either flexion or extension. Agonist and antagonist muscle groups are prepared for simultaneous partial activation, or coactivation within the range to provide stability.[3,7] Holding strategies produced by tonic reflexes initiate development of stability muscle functions. Stability development is expanded by holding strategies adapted to behaviors requiring action against gravity (e.g., head lift in prone).

As an infant assumes and maintains primitive postures, the system receives feedback from muscle tone distributed in specific holding strategies. Moving from one primitive holding pattern to another, an infant's system receives additional feedback about changes in distribution of tone. Distribution of tone and an infant's awareness of changes

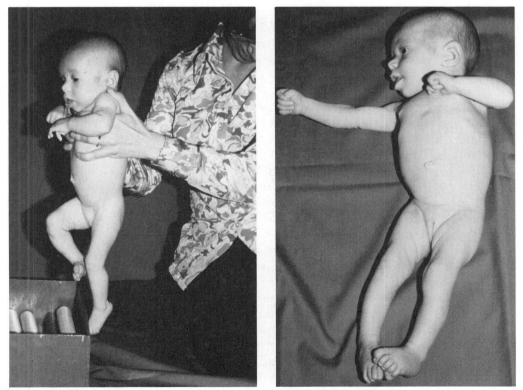

Figure 4-3: Phasic reflex   **Figure 4-4:** Tonic reflex

in distribution prepares for primitive postural strategies to be adapted to higher levels of internal postural control.

Vertical righting reactions (Figure 4-5) activate muscle groups that move the midline of the body into alignment with the center of gravity. Vertcial righting reactions include labyrinthine righting (acting on the head), body righting (acting on the head), and optical righting.[11,14] Reactions are termed according to sensory receptors assumed to be primarily responsible for the reaction. Labyrinthine righting is most likely initiated when an infant moves or is moved in space; labyrinths are stimulated and the infant rights his head. Body righting on head begins when an infant receives asymmetrical or localized pressure to the body from the supporting surface and rights his head toward vertical. Later, development of optical righting comes from visual reception, and the head rights in order to orient visually to the world. Different sensory assimilations result in the same accommodation of vertical righting; when assimilations are received simultaneously, they are integrated so that a single source of input as a stimulus for vertical righting is no longer identifiable.

Vertical righting reactions are not present at birth, but develop with central nervous system maturation and environmental contact. Reactions are adapted from primitive behaviors of head lift and head alignment. Vertical righting begins with the head moving against gravity, righting itself vertically in prone, supine, and lateral positions. Neck muscles are activated and develop extension, flexion, and lateral flexion. With further maturation, movement of the head elicits a vertical chain reaction. Stimulus for righting is transferred from neck to trunk muscle groups, and trunk muscles are activated in synergy with neck muscles through a complete range of motion. As the trunk follows the head, the baby assumes a prone extension posture, participates in pull to sit, or raises the head and trunk in sidelying. Vertical righting reactions are used during transition to maintain head and trunk alignment as well as to develop higher level stability reactions. As neck and trunk muscle groups develop toward midline, they are prepared for coactivation around the midline in order to maintain vertical alignment with the center of gravity.

Vertical righting reactions also activate extremity musculature by chain reactions in patterns corresponding to activated neck-trunk synergy. As extension develops in the neck and trunk, the upper and then lower extremities develop full extension; as the head and neck flex, flexion spreads to affect the extremities; when lateral flexion develops, the corresponding upper, then lower, extremities extend and abduct. The extremity patterns activated by vertical chain reactions are undifferentiated; however, musculature is activated, which will be adapted to protective and balance reactions after extremity support reactions are developed.

Rotational righting reactions (Figure 4-6) include neck righting and body righting on the body.[11,14] Rotational righting reactions are not present at birth, but are adapted from primitive turning behaviors. Reactions are termed according to whether rotation is initiated by turning the head or by turning a trunk segment. Rotational righting reactions activate muscles, which cause the head and trunk to rotate around the central axis of the body. Primary sensory assimilations needed to initiate neck righting are tactile input, stimulating head turning, and proprioceptive input from neck muscles activated in turning. However, visual and auditory receptions are rapidly integrated as sources of stimuli for rotational righting. A baby may turn his head toward a sound or to look at a toy. If sufficient rotation is placed upon the central axis of the body, other body segments will automatically follow in the same direction to maintain alignment.

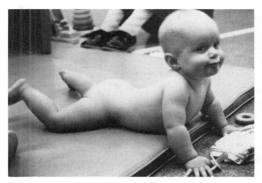

Figure 4-5: Vertical righting

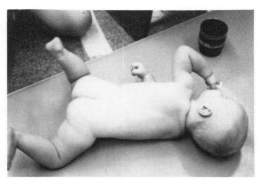

Figure 4-6: Rotational righting

Neck righting is initiated by independent head turning. Rotation of the neck stimulates neck proprioceptors and labyrinths and rotates vertebral segments. Combined stimuli from neck rotation is transmitted to the trunk by a chain reaction, and the trunk follows to align itself with the head in sidelying. Neck righting moves the trunk and limbs as a unit because differentiation of body segments has developed only between the head and trunk, and not between the upper trunk and pelvis.

However, the trunk elongates as a baby rolls from supine to sidelying. Elongation of the trunk stimulates proprioceptors and activates trunk muscles to move from sidelying to prone. Elongation, increased tactile pressure in sidelying, and assistance from extremities pushing and pulling stimulate trunk muscles and facilitate a body righting on body reaction, or rotation between trunk segments during turning. Repetition of body righting on body reaction facilitates rotation between upper trunk and pelvis, and differentiates body segments. Differentiation of trunk segments is necessary for deliberate rolling from sidelying to prone. Rotation between body segments also means that a baby can initiate rolling by rotating either head or upper or lower trunk, significantly modifying his rolling pattern.

Differentiation of body segments by maturation of rotational righting reactions brings about development of counterrotation. Since body segments can move independently of each other, and muscle groups have developed to rotate segments in either direction, the child can rotate one segment in one direction and interrupt the pattern by rotating another segment in an opposite direction. The effect of rotation-counterrotation is to begin to balance rotation around the midline and modify the complete rotation pattern. When rotation-counterrotation strategies are being used to control posture, the shoulder and hip on the same side are observed to move in opposite directions. Rotation-counterrotation patterns of movement achieve more significance as they are adapted to the development of equilibrium reactions.[9]

Both vertical and rotational righting reactions activate muscle groups that move the body as a whole in space. Righting reactions control movement in a particular sequence so that transitory equilibrium is not lost during movement.[13] New positions achieved by means of righting reactions are stabilized and maintained by development of support reactions. Later, using support reactions and combinations of vertical and rotational righting reactions to change positions prepares for maturation of equilibrium reactions. Vertical and rotational righting reactions are first integrated when an infant turns the head and simultaneously rights the head toward vertical. Combined vertical-rotational

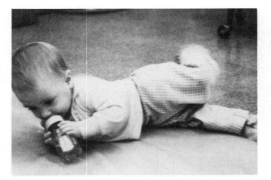

Figure 4-7: Rolling supine to prone

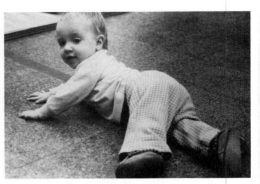

Figure 4-8: Pushing toward sitting

righting reactions are often seen as an infant rolls from supine to prone, or pushes up into sitting from rolling or sidelying (Figures 4-7 and 4-8). The combination of rotation within the body axis, while assuming or maintaining a vertical posture with support, develops into the same components that are used for equilibrium without support from the extremities.

Support reactions (Figure 4-9) develop from adaptation of primitive holding strategies. Support reactions are elicited when supporting areas of the body (e.g., palm of hand, sole of foot, buttocks) contact the supporting surface.[14] Exteroceptive stimulation from touch to the surface, and proprioceptive stimulation from pressure and stretch of distal musculature, produce sensory assimilations for support reactions. Motor accommodation is accomplished by coactivation of muscle groups of the appropriate extremity or about the midline. Tactile-presssure input causes an initial movement away from the source. An infant essentially pushes away from the source of stimulation (supporting surface) while maintaining contact with supporting surface. Following the chain of movements away from a contact point, muscle groups are coactivated with antagonists to stabilize around joints and bear weight or support posture in that position. When palms of the hands contact the supporting surface, an infant extends arms to push up to support in an on-hands position. When sensory assimilations are localized on the buttocks, the infant straightens his neck and trunk to sit in a vertical posture. Similarly, as soles of the feet contact the surface, lower extremities and then neck-trunk muscles are coactivated for standing.

Support receptors are a major source of input to alert the system to any changes in posture. As an individual moves, or is moved in space, pressure from the supporting surface to the body surface is altered. Pressure may be increased, localized, moved, or completely changed to another area of the body. Alterations in tactile-pressure input received cause automatic changes in distribution of supporting responses in order to adjust a position in space. Support functions may be transferred from one extremity to another, from one side of the body to the other, or from upper to lower body segments and reverse.

Support for posture is trunk-centered before the infant develops support reactions. At every level of development, the extremities support new postures before any purposeful movement in the posture develops. Once the limbs are freed from total support, they can protect the body by extending, reversing the chain effect from support reactions to protective reactions.

Protective reactions (Figure 4-10) of the extremities allow one to seek out, or return to, a support base to sequence movement flow or to protect the body when environment demands exceed the child's capacity to adapt.[3,11] Protective reactions are elicited as accommodations to vestibular assimilations from moving in space, to tactile-pressure alterations from supporting surfaces, and to sensory awareness of impending change. These assimilations are integrated and available to initiate extension of extremities toward the supporting surface whenever protection from falling or use of support for moving is required. Following initial input for a limb extension synergy, the pattern is completed by chain reactions. Development of protective reactions contributes to activation of limb extensors through a complete range of motion.

Once protective reactions are developed, they are always available for use in their original form; i.e., given appropriate input, extremities automatically extend in any plane of the body to protect by seeking support. In addition, protective reactions are adapted to alternate with support reactions in performance of such reciprocal behaviors as walking. Protective reactions are also adapted to purposeful sequences, such as seeking out pivot points on the supporting surface in order to turn cartwheels or to hop.

Midline stability reactions (Figure 4-11) are adapted primarily from vertical-rotational righting and support reactions. Midline stability reactions are defined as invisible, or barely discernible, adjustments in posture around the midline and proximal joints. Dynamic stability muscle functions are facilitated by influence from gravity on stretch receptors of postural muscles and from alteration in touch-pressure reception from supporting surfaces. A child responds with constant, but barely observable, changes in distribution of postural tone, which keeps the midline of the body aligned with the center of gravity. A child uses midline stability reactions to maintain vertical postures, even before equilibrium reactions have developed. After equilibrium reactions develop, they are blended with midline stability so that the two types of reactions function on a continuum. Midline reactions control postural adjustments within a confined area related to the center of gravity. As soon as a child moves away from the center significantly, equilibrium reactions are elicited for balance.

Equilibrium reactions (Figure 4-12) are compensatory movements used to regain midline stability when alignment of midline with gravity is significantly disturbed.[14]

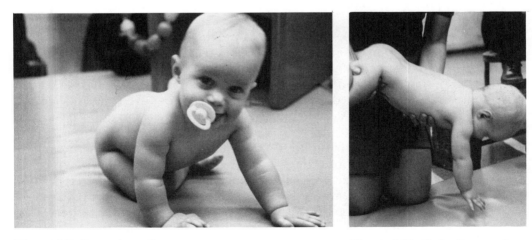

Figure 4-9: Support reaction   **Figure 4-10:** Protective reaction

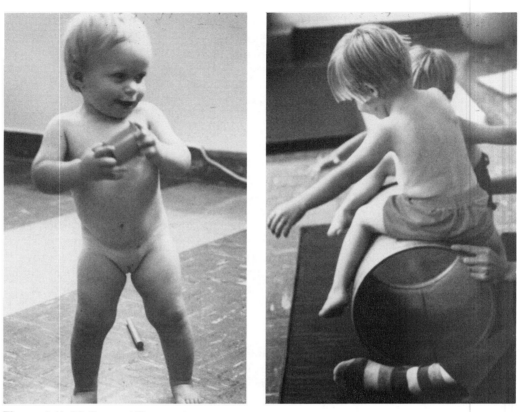

Figure 4-11: Midline stability reaction   **Figure 4-12:** Equilibrium reaction

Equilibrium reactions adapt vertical-<u>rotational</u> righting, particularly neck and trunk rotation with flexion, in order to move toward realignment with the center of gravity. Protective reactions are available in case the equilibrium response is not sufficient for regaining balance. Tactile-pressure, vestibular, and sensory assimilations are integrated to produce equilibrium reactions. Equilibrium reactions encompass several observable sequential movements:

1. Movements away from the center of gravity to the extent that balance may be lost elicits rotation and flexion of neck and upper trunk back toward the center.
2. Lower trunk segments may counterrotate to balance the rotational effect of the upper portions and control the degree of rotation. As upper portions of the body come back to midline, there is barely observable reverse in the rotation and counterrotation patterns of the upper and lower segments in order to stop the adjustment at midline.
3. Extremities on one side of the body moving back toward midline may extend and abduct to pull the body back toward center alignment.
4. Opposite extremities may also assist in bringing head and trunk back toward the midline but, in addition, are prepared to protect and support the body if balance is lost. When support-protective reactions are used, the extremity responses are accompanied by rotation and extension of the neck and trunk.

Postural Control and Movement Patterns

Movement components, with their inherent muscle functions and neural mechanisms responsible for reflexes and reactions, are combined into continuous actions as they develop in utero and after birth. Neural mechanisms activate muscle responses in patterns that we have come to recognize as reflexes or reactions, as well as patterns of volitional movement. An infant begins to respond to gravity by using combinations of righting reactions, which control the position of the body in space, and muscle functions that create support reactions for maintaining new positions in space. An ability to maintain positions by bearing weight on specific segments of one's body and the ability to change position by shifting weight from one segment, or combinations of segments, to another provides some of the postural stability required to control movement. Posture and movement strategies make use of four increasingly complex weight-bearing, weight-shifting patterns.

1. Weight bearing (Figure 4-13) means an infant can maintain a position in space supported by bearing weight on a specific aspect of trunk or extremities. An infant assumes and maintains a position by weight bearing before being able to move within that position.

2. Bilateral weight-shift/movement pattern (Figure 4-14) means an infant can move forward and back, or up and down, using upper or lower extremities bilaterally and shifting weight from upper to lower parts of the body, and vice versa. Flexion and extension are primary components in bilateral patterns.

3. Unilateral weight shift/movement pattern (Figure 4-15) means an infant can shift weight to one side of the midline, supported by either the trunk or extremities on that side, and then move the extremities on the opposite side of the body. When used for forward progression, the pattern for movement resembles a two-step process of shifting weight and moving with a side-to-side movement, such as seen in early walking.

4. Contralateral weight-shift/movement pattern (Figure 4-16) means that rotation within the body axis allows one body segment to rotate in one direction while the adjacent segment rotates in the opposite direction. Weight can then be shifted to one upper extremity and the opposite lower extremity while the other upper and lower extremities move. Contralateral weight shifting makes it possible for a child to shift weight and move forward simultaneously. With a one-step process for forward progression, movement patterns are smoothed out. Reciprocal patterns of the upper extremities can be adapted to nonweight-bearing situations as well, with control for reciprocal arm swing coming from rotation and counterrotation of trunk segments.

During development of primitive strategies, movement components of flexion and extension are developing, along with accompanying functions of mobility and stability. Primitive mobility and phasic reflexes produce undifferentiated patterns of movement through a complete range of flexion or extension. Primitive stability and tonic reflexes produce holding or fixing postures in either flexor- or extensor-dominated positions. Primitive postures and movements generally affect movement and positioning of the extremities or positioning of the body as a whole. Support for posture is trunk-centered and comes more from external sources (such as the crib, floor, or someone's arms) than from within the body itself.

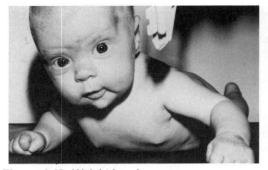

Figure 4-13: Weight bearing

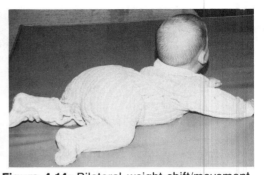

Figure 4-14: Bilateral weight-shift/movement pattern

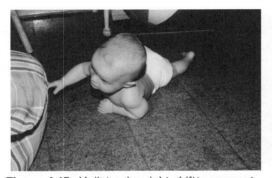

Figure 4-15: Unilateral weight-shift/movement pattern

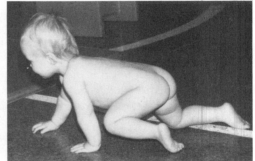

Figure 4-16: Contralateral weight-shift/movement pattern

Development of transitional strategies begins several months after birth and continues until mature postural control and movement patterns have developed. For transition to higher level postures, primitive reflexes are adapted to righting, support, and protective reactions. Muscle functions are stabilized around neck, trunk, and proximal joints to support new positions in space. Proximal stability is combined with mobility functions to allow movement within postures and between positions. Weight bearing on extremities signifies that support for posture is extremity-centered, meaning that control for posture is developing in the neck, trunk, and more proximal joints. Weight-bearing support reactions, combined with vertical righting reactions, lead to bilateral weight-shift patterns of control for movement in space. Weight is transferred to lower portions of the body so that upper portions can move and vice versa. Bilateral weight-shift patterns, combined with vertical-rotational righting reactions, lateral flexion of neck and trunk, and support and protective reactions, lead to unilateral weight-shift patterns for control of movement. Weight is transferred to one side of the body and/or upper and lower extremities on the same side of the body, while extremities on the opposite side of the body move. Lateral flexion of the trunk produces elongation on the opposite, weight-bearing side of the body, which prepares for development of trunk rotation patterns.

Development of mature strategies implies that muscle functions are blended in such a way that posture is controlled by stability and mobility within the body axis and is not dependent upon the extremities for support of positions in space. The extremities move freely in space, controlled by countermovements with the trunk or more proximal joints. Midline stability reactions and equilibrium control the balance between postural control and movement, and provide automatic responses that allow a child to maintain a position, to move within a position, and change position without changing his/her general orientation in space. Dynamic postural control, based on equilibrium and movement-countermovement model, assumes that an equilibrium point for the body in space or the extremities in relation to the body is a position where the torques around a joint, generated by antagonist muscles and external forces, are equal and opposite. A given level of activation is directed toward opposing muscle groups, and there is a gradual shift in the equilibrium point until balanced position is achieved.[14] Dynamic stability means that movement is controlled by movement.

Summary

Posture and movement strategies are composed of movement components, muscle functions, and reflexes and reactions that are integrated into postural control and movement patterns. Strategies develop from generalized movements that are present at birth. Strategies depend upon nervous system maturation and environmental interaction for their development. Strategies are adapted to developmental and purposeful sequences as they develop through primitive, transitional, and mature phases of development.

Key Points

1. Strategies are viewed as component parts of adaptive sequences.
2. Strategies exist for the purpose of activation and control of the body or body segments during performance.
3. A child's motivation to interact with environmental events serves as a stimulus to facilitate neuromuscular functions.
4. During development, structures and functions for movement are adapted to specific behaviors and differentiated according to whether they are suited best for movement or control.
5. Postural strategies control movement, and movement strategies give rise to action.
6. Movement strategies promote and sequence changes in position of body or body parts.
7. Postural strategies both control movement of body segments in relation to each other and maintain body position in space during movement.
8. Non-directed movements of an infant form the basis for development of automatic reactions, while directed movements of the infant develop into volitional movements.
9. Muscles and muscle groups have stability and mobility functions dependent upon maturation of reflexes and reactions.
10. There is overlap among the developmental stages of mobility and stability muscle functions, depending upon the function-to-purpose adaptation.

11. Neural functions (reflexes and reactions) distribute muscle tone in specific posture and movement strategies according to whether strategies are adapted to purposeful behavior or activities.

12. Reflexes and reactions can be considered in three groupings: primitive reflexes, transitional reactions, and mature reactions.

13. Phasic reflexes activate muscles and muscle groups through a complete range of motion. Tonic reflexes are viewed as postures assumed in response to head and trunk position in space or in relation to each other.

14. Vertical righting reactions activate muscle groups that move the midline of the body into alignment with the center of gravity. Rotational righting reactions activate muscles that cause head and trunk to rotate around the central axis of the body.

15. Support reactions are elicited when supporting areas of the body contact the supporting surface and function to alert the system to changes in posture. Protective reactions are elicited as accommodations to movement through space, and function to allow a person to seek out or return to a support base.

16. Midline stability reactions function to maintain vertical postures and control postural adjustments within a confined area. Equilibrium reactions are compensatory movements used to regain midline stability when the person's alignment of midline with gravity is significantly disturbed.

17. Weight-bearing and weight-shift/movement patterns develop through transitional and mature phases to provide ability to move within a position and change positions.

18. Strategies develop through primitive, transitional, and mature phases. The primitive phase is characterized by generalized movement patterns, phasic and tonic reflexes, mobility muscle functions, and the need for external sources of postural control. The transitional phase is characterized by stability and combined mobility/stability muscle actions, by the emergence of righting reactions, and by weight-bearing, bilateral, and unilateral weight-shift patterns. The mature phase continues the maturation of reactions for the emergence of automatic balance reactions, blended mobility/stability functions, and contralateral weight-shift/movement patterns.

Self-study Guidelines

1. Explain postural strategies as they relate to movement.
2. Describe movement strategies and compare/contrast with postural strategies.
3. What are the stages of muscle functions? Describe each stage.
4. Compare and contrast reflexes and reactions.
5. Differentiate phasic and tonic reflexes.
6. What are the functions of vertical and rotational righting reactions?
7. Differentiate support and protective reactions and describe the function of each.
8. Define midline stability reactions.
9. Match reflexes, reactions, and muscle functions to primitive, transitional, or mature phases.
10. Explain purposes of primitive, transitional, and mature phases.

References

1. Brooks V: Motor control: How posture and movements are governed. Phys Ther 63(5):664-673, 1983.
2. Massion J: Postural changes accompanying voluntary movements: Normal and pathological aspects. Human Neurobiology 2:261-267, 1984.
3. Holt K: Movement and child development. Clinics in Developmental Medicine. No. 55. Philadelphia, J.B. Lippincott Co., 1975, p 2.
4. Shaffer LH: Rhythm and timing in skill. Psych Rev 89:109-122, 1982.
5. Goodgold-Edwards S: Motor learning as it relates to the development of skilled motor behavior: A review of the literature.Phys Occup Ther in Peds 4:5-16, 1985.
6. Bobath K: A neurophysiological basis for the treatment of cerebral palsy. Clinics in Developmental Medicine. No. 75. Ed 2. Philadelphia, J.B. Lippincott Co., 1980.
7. Stockmeyer S: Sensorimotor approach to treatment. In Pearson P, Williams C (Eds): Physical Therapy Services in the Developmental Disabilities. Springfield, IL, Charles C. Thomas Pubs., 1972, pp 186-222.
8. Coogler E: Differentiation of human skeletal muscle. A self-instructional package. HEW Grant # 5-DOI-AH-50524-02, Georgia State University, 1973.
9. Bly L: The Components of Normal Movement During the First Year of Life and Abnormal Motor Development. Neurodevelopmental Treatment Association, Birmingham, AL, Pathway Press, 1983.
10. Andre-Thomas: The neurological examination of the infant. Clinics in Developmental Medicine. No. 1. Philadelphia, J.B. Lippincott Co., 1964, p 11.
11. Fiorentino MR: Reflex Testing Methods for Evaluating CNS Development. Springfield, IL, Charles C. Thomas Pubs., 1965.
12. Touwen B: Neurological development in infancy. Clinics in Developmental Medicine. No. 58. Philadelphia, J.B. Lippincott Co., 1976.
13. Peiper A: Cerebral Function in Infancy and Childhood. New York, Consultants Bureau, 1963.
14. Carter MC, Shapiro DC: Control of sequential movements: Evidence for generalized motor programs. J Neurophysiology 52:787-796h, 1984.

Appendix 4-A
Reflexes and Reactions[11-14]

Reflex/Reaction	Description	Phase	Related Muscle Functions
1. Phasic Reflexes			
Rooting	Touch to corner of mouth elicits head turning towards stimulated side	Primitive	Mobility
Moro	Gentle head drop in supported supine posture elicits abduction-extension of arms, followed by arms coming together in arc over body	Primitive	Mobility
Flexor withdrawal	Touch-pressure to sole of foot of extended leg elicits flexion and withdrawal of stimulated leg	Primitive	Mobility
Crossed extension	Touch-pressure to sole of foot of leg held in extension elicits flexion, followed by extension of opposite leg; or flexion of one leg elicits extension of opposite leg	Primitive	Mobility
Bauer's	Sufficient leg flexion-foot dorsiflexion in prone for sole to touch surface elicits extension of leg and flexion of opposite, or crawling movements	Primitive	Mobility
Stepping	Held in upright position so feet touch surface elicits alternating flexion-extension stepping movements, especially if trunk is bent forward	Primitive	Mobility
Placing legs	Held in upright position and dorsum of foot touched by table edge elicits flexion followed by extension of leg so foot is placed on table	Primitive	Mobility, Stability
Placing arms	Touch to dorsum of hand from table elicits arm flexion followed by placing hand on table	Primitive	Mobility
Avoiding	Light touch on the palm or dorsum of the flexed hand elicits finger extension	Primitive	Mobility

Appendix 4-A—Reflexes and Reactions (continued)

2. Tonic Reflexes

Tonic labyrinthine	Positioning in supine elicits general extension pattern throughout body; positioning in prone elicits general flexion pattern	Primitive	Mobility
Asymmetrical tonic neck	Head turning elicits extension of face-side arm and leg and flexion of skull-side	Primitive	Mobility, Stability
Symmetrical tonic neck	Head dorsiflexion elicits arm extension and leg flexion; head ventroflexion elicits arm flexion and leg extension	Primitive	Mobility, Stability
Magnet	Touch-pressure to sole of foot with leg flexed elicits extension of leg touched	Primitive	Mobility, Stability
Primary standing	Held in upright position so feet touch surface elicits extension of legs to "stand"	Primitive	Stability
Plantar grasp	Touch-pressure to ball of foot elicits flexion of toes	Primitive	Mobility, Stability
Traction	Pressure on the palm of hand elicits finger flexion followed by flexion of arm	Primitive	Mobility, Stability
Grasp reflex	Pressure on the palm of hand and stretch to finger flexors elicits finger flexion	Primitive	Mobility

3. Vertical Righting Reactions

Labyrinthine righting acting on head	Movement in space causes head and trunk to move toward a vertical orientation in space	Transitional	Mobility
Body righting acting on body	Asymmetrical or changing touch-pressure on the body surface from the supporting surface causes head and trunk to move toward a vertical orientation in space	Transitional	Mobility
Optical righting	Visual awareness causes head and trunk to move toward a vertical orientation in space	Transitional	Mobility

Appendix 4-A—Reflexes and Reactions (continued)

4. Rotational Righting Reactions			
Neck righting	Neck rotation causes the rest of the body to turn as a whole in same direction to align head and trunk with each other	Transitional	Mobility
Body righting acting on body	Rotation of one body segment causes adjacent body segments to rotate in sequence in the same direction to align head and trunk with each other	Transitional	Mobility
5. Supporting reactions	Touch-pressure from supporting surface to body support receptors causes maintained extension of trunk, arms, or legs to hold position		Stability Combined mobility and stability actions
6. Protective reactions	Moving in space and changing touch-pressure information from supporting surface causes arms or legs to extend and protect the body from losing balance.	Transitional	Mobility Combined mobility and stability actions
7. Midline stability reactions All positions	Vertical alignment with gravity is maintained by constant adjustment in response to gravity and supporting surface	Mature	Blended mobility and stability functions
8. Equilibrium All positions	Compensatory movements used to regain midline stability if alignment with gravity is significantly disturbed	Mature	Blended mobility and stability functions

CHAPTER 5

Developmental Sequences

Objectives

The reader will be able to

1. list key behaviors for each of the five basic developmental sequences according to their primitive, transitional, and mature phases of development;
2. identify and describe key behaviors for each of the five basic developmental sequences;
3. identify movement components, muscle functions, reflexes/reactions, and postural control/movement patterns for each of the key behaviors;
4. analyze key behaviors according to their antecedents, purpose, and contribution to development of higher levels of behavior; and
5. apply specific aspects of developmental sequences to understanding of deviations from normal development.

Introduction

Achievement and use of upright posture, such as standing and walking, and an associated ability to explore and manipulate the environment, are underlying innate goals of a child's developmental quest. Developmental behaviors that lead to upright functioning, such as creeping, provide not only early forms of movement for exploration, but also facilitate lower extremity components required for walking. Behaviors like creeping also contribute to development of upper extremity components required for reaching and grasping. Once a child is upright, walking becomes a major means for exploration and frees upper extremities from their support role, thereby creating possibilities for upper extremity exploratory and manipulative abilities to develop.

Literature concerned with central nervous system maturation identifies "hard-wired" and "soft-wired" systems (Figure 5-1). The hard-wired aspect of the human nervous system is thought to be comprised of certain genetic endowments that are "pre-programmed" with specific behavioral drives (e.g., getting up and walking on two feet). However,

Hard-wired System		Soft-wired System
Developmental Sequences	Intentionality	Purposeful Sequences
Upright Posture		Gross Motor Skills
Reach/Grasp		Fine Motor Skills

Figure 5-1

genetic potential for walking, and all developmental steps leading to walking, is realized when a child "learns" developmental sequences. As the nervous system matures, a child learns by experimenting with potential behaviors, by repetition of essential components, by adding variety to the ways in which steps to upright functioning can be accomplished and, in general, by actively engaging in the process of adapting nervous system functions required for upright posture. Neuromuscular functions, which were identified as part of posture and movement strategies, are adapted to each predictable developmental step along the continuum. Genetic endowment provides both potential to achieve an upright position and a drive to deliberately pursue the potential. The combination of potential and drive to achieve make up a child's intrinsic motivation to experiment and learn by actively doing.

Actively doing something takes on more significance with the concept of a soft-wired system. The soft-wired system contributes to ways in which a child can smooth out and time movements in purposeful sequences of adaptation and, eventually, in skill performance. Behaviors that develop sequentially for upright functioning can be differentiated from their developmental sequences and directed toward accomplishment of purposeful sequences. With purposeful sequences, a child can intentionally use a developmental pattern, or part of a pattern, to respond to an environmental event. Intentionality changes the way a movement pattern is being directed. The change reflects new combinations of movements that were initially intrinsically motivated and now include the extrinsic motivation that comes from an environmental challenge.

Responding to goals outside of self brings about purposeful sequences of movement. As movement is used more purposefully and directed away from self, coordination and direction of movement in relation to objects and persons in the environment become more critical. In general, strategies used for developmental sequences leading to upright are adapted to purposeful sequences used for gross motor skills. Strategies used for reach and grasp are adapted to purposeful sequences used for fine motor skills.

Ability to perform skillfully is considered part of genetic potential, but development of skills requires special practice and varies according to individual genetic makeup. We all have potential functions available to play the piano. In order to play skillfully, an individual needs to develop purposeful sequences of movement required for piano-playing and practice. Some players will succeed more than others, based on greater genetic potential, motivation, and more practice.

This chapter will explore progressive development of five basic developmental behaviors. Information about behaviors and relationships among behaviors has been gleaned from observations of normal development and synthesis of information found in the literature (see Bibliography). The five behaviors are discussed according to the primitive, transitional, and mature phases of development. The behaviors include the child's achievement of creeping, sitting, rolling, standing/walking, and reaching/grasping. Adaptation of developmental sequential behavior to development of purposeful sequential behavior is discussed in Chapter 7.

Each developmental progression is described according to its key behaviors. Key behaviors are like snapshots taken at certain points along the progression and signify an identifiable point at which a child is adapting previously acquired behaviors to achieve a new behavior, or modifying a previously acquired behavior because of a new experience. By learning the sequential development of key behaviors, the reader can analyze behaviors according to their antecedents, purpose for present level of functioning, and contribution to development of higher level behaviors. This knowledge is particularly significant when applying concepts from normal development to ideas about analyzing and treating dysfunctional behaviors.

The primitive phase of each developmental behavior has some behaviors that can be viewed as forerunners, or primitive versions of the outcome for that progression. The baby may momentarily maintain or assume a posture with support, such as primary sitting or primary standing, or put together primitive forms of limb movement, such as primary crawling or walking. Primitive versions are seen only in the first few days or weeks after birth and are not evident in later months when the baby is developing mature strategies for these behaviors. Perhaps primitive forerunners give the baby's system a sense of a behavior to be pursued and contribute to baby's drive to achieve a behavior.

Posture and movement strategies that are used during primitive development are also important to consider in relation to intervention programs for dysfunctional behavior. Primitive patterns of undifferentiated movement, fixation patterns of postural control, and primitive reflexes are often part of abnormal behavior that accompanies central nervous system dysfunction. Strategies used during transitional phases of development, such as righting reactions, protective-support reactions, or combined mobility/ stability patterns, modify primitive behavior in normal development. Aspects of these transitional strategies are often replicated in intervention programs designed to remediate abnormal development. Mature strategies represent goals of intervention programs. Whether or not a child with dysfunction acquires mature strategies depends on the nature and cause of dysfunction, a child's potential, and the intervention program. Aspects of dysfunction and intervention will be discussed in Chapters 8, 9, and 10.

Creeping

Creeping provides a means for locomotion before movement in upright posture has been achieved. During the progressive development from prone to creeping, a baby develops neck and trunk <u>extension</u> against gravity, combines extension with flexion for neck and trunk postural tone, and moves to an extremity-supported rather than trunk-supported posture. During the process, the baby also gains lateral flexion and rotation in trunk in order to use flexion and extension together for shifting weight and moving forward or changing position, adapts reciprocal limb movement to trunk stability in order to initiate reciprocal movement patterns, and develops blended mobility and stability components in the upper extremities that can be adapted to reach and grasp. In a child's quest for upright functioning, posture and movement strategies developed with creeping are differentiated for use in upright locomotion (e.g., midline postural tone, lower limb reciprocation) and upper extremity functions (e.g., upper extremity reciprocation, proximal control).

Development in prone and creeping provides a particularly clear example of changes in weight-bearing and weight-shifting patterns. Emergence of weight bearing in the cephalocaudal direction is evident; first weight bearing occurs around head and upper chest, then progresses to weight on-elbows and mid-trunk, to mid-trunk in prone extension, to hands and pelvis, hands and knees, knees, and finally feet. Bilateral weight bearing and weight shifting in the upper and lower extremities accompany the cephalocaudal changes in weight distribution through the trunk. After bilateral patterns have been established in upper extremities and upper trunk, and lower extremities and lower trunk, then unilateral and contralateral weight-shift patterns appear, first in upper body segments and then in lower body segments. Unilateral and contralateral weight shift patterns support both crawling on tummy and creeping on hands and knees.

Key behaviors (Figure 5-2) associated with development of creeping include .

Primitive Phase
Protective Head Turning
Primary Crawling
Head Lift-Primitive Support

Transitional Phase
Head Control-On Elbows
On Hands
Prone Extension
Pivoting
Crawling

Mature Phase
Creeping

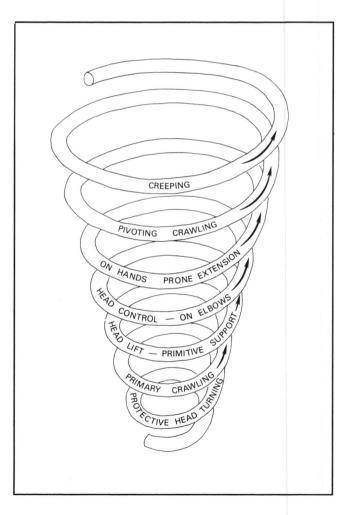

Figure 5-2: Key behaviors of creeping

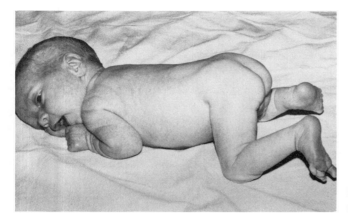

Figure 5-3: Flexed posture in prone

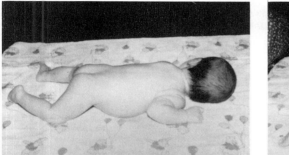

Figure 5-4: Head turned to one side

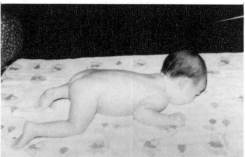

Figure 5-5: Head lift while turning

Protective Head Turning

Description and purpose. At birth, a flexed body posture predominates, especially when a baby is placed in a prone position. Upper extremities are flexed and adducted with shoulders internally rotated and elbows positioned behind the shoulders. Lower extremities are flexed under the pelvis. Weight is therefore forward and baby's face is pressed down on the supporting surface. The baby's flexed posture is adapted from fetal flexion and influenced by the tonic labyrinthine reflex in prone (Figure 5-3).

A baby tends to turn her head to one side or the other when placed face down on a supporting surface in order to assure airway clearance for breathing. Head turning is a protective response. Once in prone, a baby will tend to turn her head from one side to another periodically, altering her flexed posture momentarily. Each time she turns her head she must lift it slightly at midline in order to clear the surface and protect her access to air. Each slight lift activates neck extensors against gravity, modifies flexed posture, prepares for prone head raising, and, eventually, development of righting reactions (Figures 5-4 and 5-5).

Movement Components: Neck extension

Muscle Functions: Mobility

Reflex Reactions: Tonic labyrinthine reflex

Postural Control/Movement Patterns: Weight bearing more on face and upper portions of body

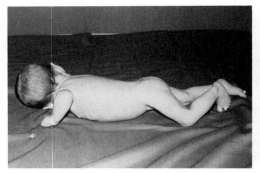

Figure 5-6: Primary crawling

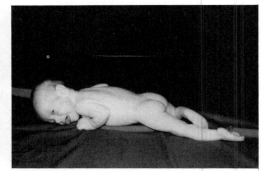

Figure 5-7: Primary crawling

Primary Crawling (Figures 5-6 and 5-7)

<u>Description and purpose</u>. Flexed posture of the neonate is also altered by primary crawling (Bauer's reflex). Full range of flexion of the lower extremities sometimes increases dorsiflexion of the foot to the extent that the sole of the foot contacts the supporting surface. Tactile pressure on the sole of one foot can cause complete extension of that lower extremity and increased flexion of the opposite extremity. The result is a rhythmical, reciprocal-like pattern of lower extremity movement. Movement of the extremities may be sufficient to move the body along the supporting surface, even though upper portions of the body are not part of the primitive pattern. However, elements of lower extremity flexion-extension and reciprocal nature of the pattern will be adapted to crawling and creeping when higher level posture and movement strategies are available for trunk and extremity control and coordination. Primary crawling is one of the forerunner behaviors for prone/creeping.

<u>Movement Components</u>: Lower extremity flexion/extension in a reciprocal pattern

<u>Muscle Functions</u>: Mobility through complete ranges of lower extremity flexion/extension

<u>Reflex/Reactions</u>: Bauer's reflex

<u>Postural Control/Movement Patterns</u>: Weight bearing more on face and upper portions of body; movement in lower portions of body

Head Lift - Primitive Support (Figure 5-8)

<u>Description and purpose</u>. By about 2 months of age, a baby adapts neck extension, which was initiated with head turning in prone, to head raising, and deliberately lifts her head momentarily from the supporting surface. Initial head lift is accompanied by head movement downward toward the shoulders to retract and fix the head on shoulders. Neck retraction is utilized by the infant to stabilize the head on shoulders prior to the time when sustained neck extension and upper extremity support are available for holding the head up in space. Neck retraction is accompanied by shoulder elevation as another means for holding head in space. Neck retraction allows primitive holding of head in space so that the upper extremities can begin to move forward into weight-bearing positions. Although shoulders are still internally rotated and elbows are still behind shoulders, more abduction of shoulders appears and will eventually contribute to bringing elbows in line with shoulders.

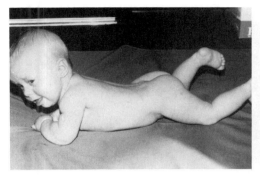

Figure 5-8: Head lift - primitive support

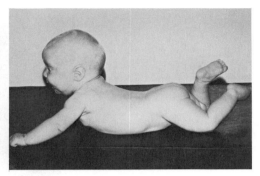

Figure 5-9: Symmetrical posture

<u>Movement Components</u>: Neck extension accompanied by retraction
<u>Muscle Functions</u>: Mobility for head raising; primitive stability for holding
<u>Reflex/Reactions</u>: Beginning vertical righting reaction
<u>Postural Control/Movement Patterns</u>: Weight bearing more on upper trunk and flexed upper extremities

Head lift and primitive support prepare for symmetrical postures and bilateral extremity weight bearing in prone. Emergence of symmetrical tonic neck posture influences prone adaptations, particularly extremity postures. Neck extension facilitates symmetrical tonic neck posture of upper extremity extension and lower extremity flexion (Figure 5-9). Arms come forward in full range of primitive extension with abduction and assume a primitive weight-bearing posture on fisted hands. Besides reversing the upper extremity flexion pattern, primitive support on extended arms lifts chest farther from the supporting surface. Extension developing in the neck has an opportunity to begin moving down to upper back, while neck flexion, developing in supine, begins to modify neck retraction and makes it possible for extension to expand in a caudal direction. Neck and trunk extension will be further developed and expanded when more stable weight bearing on-elbows and on-hands emerges during transition.

Symmetry and head control in space are characteristic of behaviors that mark initiation of the transitional phase for prone. During transition, primitive head-neck and upper extremity responses are modified and adapted to vertical righting and support/protective reactions. These reactions influence development of creeping since extension expands to include the trunk and extremities. Muscles that extend the body are activated against gravity to develop stability components for postural control. Extension of the neck and trunk also moves the body away from a supporting surface and into a position which facilitates support, first on upper extremities and then on all-fours. During transition, a baby develops an ability to move forward and backward through space supported by four extremities.

Head Control-On Elbows (Figure 5-10)

<u>Description and purpose</u>. Between 3 and 4 months of age more mature aspects of head raising in prone and support on arms become evident. A baby can raise head in midline from 45° to 90° off the supporting surface. Neck extension, facilitated by vertical righting reactions, in turn facilitates upper trunk extension in a chain-reaction

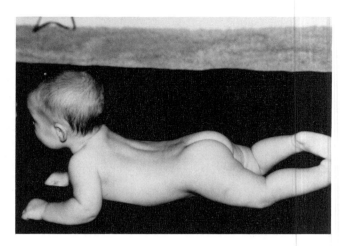

Figure 5-10: Head control on elbows

effect. Neck retraction is modified by integration of neck flexion, which has developed in supine, with neck extension. Activation of flexors with extensors elongates extensors and allows development of extension to expand to upper trunk. Addition of upper trunk extension provides more control along the midline and begins to facilitate muscle groups which stabilize scapulae in relation to trunk. Upper trunk and scapular stability provide control for changes in upper extremity support patterns.

Upper extremity patterns change from primitive extension for support to elbow flexion, with weight on forearms and elbows, aligned slightly in front of shoulders. As flexion develops around shoulders and upper trunk, combinations of flexion and extension create the shoulder stability that supports forearm weight bearing. As flexion expands to upper trunk, elbows move slightly in front of shoulders, signifying that head, upper trunk control, and shoulder stability have developed. With more proximal stability to control posture, upper extremity abduction decreases and shoulders come into more neutral rotation. Hands may remain fisted if additional stability is needed. Weight bearing is localized essentially on forearms and mid-trunk. Head control in space is possible because neck extensors and flexors are coactivated and supported by stability in adjacent body segments. The baby can use flexion in combination with extension and look down at toys without losing control over head position in space. Baby can also turn head from side to side and still keep head raised in space. Head turning differentiates head from other body segments and prepares for weight shifting, and ultimately rolling, at higher levels of development. As extension moves down over the pelvis, primitive lower extremity flexion is modified. Pelvis assumes more of an anteriorly tilted posture and lower extremities are less flexed but remain abducted and externally rotated. The position of lower portions of the body provides stability or point of fixation for movement emerging in upper body.

Movement Components: Neck, upper trunk, and shoulder extension; neck, upper chest, and shoulder flexion; neck rotation

Muscle Functions: Mobility—head raising; stability—head in space, on-elbows; combined mobility/stability—head turning

Reflex/Reactions: Vertical righting reactions; upper extremity support reactions

Postural Control/Movement Patterns: Bilateral weight bearing on forearms; mid-trunk weight bearing on supporting surface

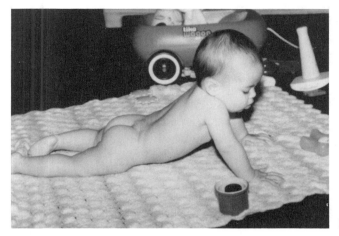

Figure 5-11: On hands

On Hands (Figure 5-11).

<u>Description and purpose</u>. By 5 months, extension expands down through the upper extremities as well as trunk. A baby can assume an on-hands posture in prone. Increased upper extremity extension allows the baby to push up from on-elbows to on-hands. Increased pressure from concentration of weight bearing on hands facilitates support reactions and further increases extension, especially through the elbows, in order to hold upper trunk further from the supporting surface. At first, hands may be fisted as a means of increasing extensor stability through the extremities and shoulders. When more proximal shoulder stability increases and is adapted to on-hands posture, hands will be open, allowing more stimulation from supporting surface to palms of hands. Open hands promote more pressure on support reaction receptors and therefore more facilitation of extension, as well as more inhibition of hand grasp reactions.

On-hands posture means that the upper trunk moves farther away from the supporting surface. Extension moves down over the hips, and the pelvis and hips assume more weight bearing, acting as an anchor for upper body development of mobility and stability functions. With more extension through the hips, lower extremities move out of flexed, abducted postures into more extended, neutrally rotated positions. Changes in lower extremity postures pave the way for unilateral weight shifting when upper body control is sufficiently developed for weight shift.

Upper body movement and control increase because baby is responding to a challenge to achieve higher level behaviors. With upper trunk off the supporting surface, the baby can align head and trunk in much the same way as head and trunk will be aligned in an upright posture. Flexor groups are further activated, while extensor groups are elongated and activated with flexors against gravity. Head control and shoulder-scapulae stability increase significantly as baby pushes farther away from supporting surface and confines upper body weight bearing to hands. Coactivation and combined mobility and stability of neck and shoulder muscle groups expand to include flexors and extensors of upper trunk. Baby has enough stability to rock forward and back and from side to side on extended arms within limited range. Rocking begins to bring in lateral trunk flexion, which will support unilateral weight shifting. Stability around the pelvis and hips, as well as support on hands, provides distal fixation, and allows rocking, facilitating mobility and stability combinations at the shoulders and within the trunk.

<u>Movement Components</u>: Upper extremity, upper and lower trunk and hip extension

<u>Muscle Functions</u>: Mobility—trunk extension; stability and combined mobility/stability—neck and trunk

<u>Reflex/Reactions</u>: Vertical righting reactions; upper extremity support reactions

<u>Postural Control/Movement Patterns</u>: Bilateral weight bearing on upper extremities and hips

A baby's experience in on-hands posture modifies functioning in the on-elbows posture. Being in an on-hands position contributes to an increase in shoulder stability and expansion of extension coactivated with flexion down through the upper trunk. Increase in shoulder stability supports shifting weight onto one upper extremity instead of two extremities. Expansion of extension and combinations of flexion and extension through the trunk support lateral trunk flexion—and eventually rotation—required for shifting weight onto one upper extremity. In addition, expansion of extension over the hips means that the hips assume weight bearing and provide a point of stability for upper body weight shifting. Initially, unilateral weight-shift components are not well enough developed to allow weight shifting in the on-hands position. But if a baby resumes a more secure, previously acquired on-elbows posture, the components described above can be used by the baby to shift weight onto one forearm and free the other arm for reaching, and eventually for crawling and creeping.

According to the adaptation theory, new behaviors, such as asssuming and maintaining on-hands posture, develop as modifications of previously acquired behaviors, such as on-elbows. In addition, previously acquired behaviors are modified by new behaviors; e.g., maintaining on-elbows posture is modified to shifting weight and reaching in on-elbows posture after on-hands posture has been attained (Figure 5-12).

Unilateral weight shift onto one arm affects the rest of the body posture as well. Weight shift to one side of the trunk causes elongation of weight-bearing side and shortening, or lateral flexion, of opposite side. Besides affecting the trunk, unilateral weight shift increases separation between humerus and scapula on weight-bearing side, results in more weight bearing on one hip, and more neutral rotation of lower extremity on weight-bearing side. Shifting weight back toward midline in prone occurs when baby reaches forward with arm and trunk rotates to follow. Components of equilibrium in prone emerge with weight shifting in and out of sidelying.

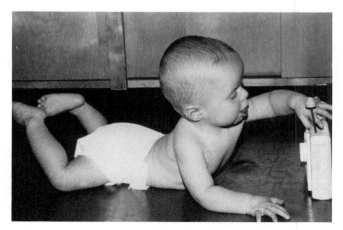

Figure 5-12: On-elbows reaching

Prone Extension (Figures 5-13 and 5-14)

<u>Description and purpose</u>. Between 4 and 6 months of age, the baby lifts head more frequently and farther from the surface. Extension of the neck and upper trunk facilitates extension over the hips and into the lower extremities. The baby assumes a position of full extension in relation to maximum effect of gravity and maintains extension without support from the extremities. Maintaining midline extension against gravity will be adapted along with midline flexion to develop postural tone in the neck and trunk. Meanwhile, with prone extension, the baby activates extensor muscle groups through a full range of motion, while simultaneously elongating and preparing antagonistic flexor muscles to act with the extensors. Extension of the upper trunk is assisted by upper extremity flexion and scapular adduction, which act with upper trunk extensors to help lift the trunk off the supporting surface. Scapular adductors are activated, while neck, upper trunk, and shoulder flexors are elongated in preparation for increased scapular-shoulder stability in upper extremity weight bearing. Use of upper extremity flexion and scapular adduction to facilitate spinal extension is repeated by the child in early sitting, standing, and walking. The posture forms the basis for the "high guard" position in upright. Unfortunately, in cases of dysfunction, the prone extension pattern can develop without appropriate balance from flexor muscle group development, and the child tends to use the posture abnormally for postural control. Therefore, facilitation of full extension with upper extremity flexion and scapular adduction is not used in therapy for facilitation, but is instead modified so only necessary components are facilitated, along with appropriate flexor patterns.

A normal baby moves in and out of prone extension easily, practicing both extension and combinations of flexion and extension. Baby will move from full extension posture to rest in on-elbows position, or on-hands posture, or amphibian position, and then resume full prone extension. Baby can also rock back and forth in full extension, increasing facilitation of extensors against gravity, and may move arms and legs in swimming-like movements. The baby is beginning to play with movement of body or extremities, superimposed on postural control of the body in relation to gravity.

<u>Movement Components</u>: Neck, trunk, hip, and lower extremity extension; scapular adduction

    <u>Muscle Functions</u>: Mobility-extension; stability-scapular adduction

    <u>Reflex Reactions</u>: Vertical righting reactions

    <u>Postural Control/Movement Patterns</u>: Weight bearing—mid-trunk

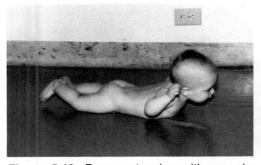

Figure 5-13: Prone extension with scapular adduction

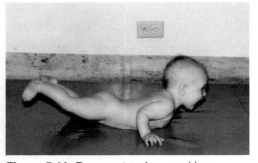

Figure 5-14: Prone extension - rocking

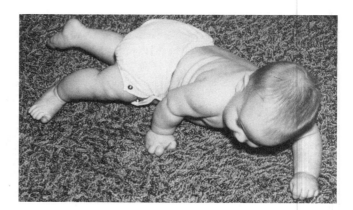

Figure 5-15: Pivot in circle

Pivoting (Fig. 5-15)

<u>Description and purpose</u>. Between 5 and 6 months of age, babies begin to pivot in a circle in the prone position in order to experiment with movement in space and begin to reach for objects that are slightly out of reach. Pivoting adapts neck, trunk, and hip extension from prone extension patterns, and combines midline extension with all components of extremity movement: flexion, extension, abduction, adduction, internal rotation, and external rotation. Pivoting is one way in which the child activates, co-activates, and combines components of movement in prone before and during use of the components for moving forward in space.

Pivoting begins with neck and trunk extension, followed by unilateral weight shift onto one side of the body, using a combination of vertical and rotational righting as well as support reactions to control weight shift. With weight shift, the weight-bearing side is elongated and the non-weight-bearing side is shortened by lateral flexion. Elongation and extension on the weight-bearing side facilitates hip extension and more neutral rotation of lower extremity on that side and more hip flexion and external rotation on the opposite side. Separation of functions between sides of the body begins in prone with pivoting, and is further developed with crawling and creeping. Initial pivoting is accomplished more by pushing and pulling with upper extremities, but as neuromuscular functions mature, both upper and lower portions of the body are involved in pivoting.

Usually, a baby starts to move by reaching with the arm on non-weight-bearing side, followed by pushing with the arm on weight-bearing side. The lower extremity on the non-weight-bearing side acts as a stability point for upper body movement by flexing and abducting at the hip and extending at the knee and ankle. The foot as a stabilizing point allows more rotation to develop between upper and lower segments of the trunk, which increases the freedom and range of upper body movement. Meanwhile, with rotation, the lower portions of the body can become involved in pivoting. Instead of using lower extremities for stabilization, the extremities begin to move in opposition to the upper extremities, increasing rotation between body segments, and bringing forth a contralateral weight-shift pattern of postural control. The lower extremity on the non-weight-bearing side pushes with the upper extremity on the weight-bearing side and weight is shifted contralaterally so that the opposite extremities can push and pull together. Introduction of contralateral patterns is significant at this point, but children will not be able to adapt contralateral weight shifting to forward movement in space until contralateral movement patterns develop with crawling and creeping.

<u>Movement Components</u>: Extremity abduction/adduction; trunk lateral flexion and rotation

<u>Muscle Functions</u>: Mobility and combined mobility/stability—extremities

<u>Reflex/Reactions</u>: Vertical righting reactions

<u>Postural Control/Movement Patterns</u>: Unilateral weight shift; beginning contralateral weight shift

Crawling

<u>Description and purpose</u>. Crawling describes the way a baby moves on tummy, either using extremity movement or weight-shift patterns. Trunk-centered support on tummy provides stability for adaptation of extremity movements to bilateral, unilateral, or reciprocal patterns of movement as trunk and extremity weight bearing is shifted bilaterally, unilaterally, and contralaterally. Crawling begins bilaterally around 6 months of age, usually after some prone extension or pivoting have been observed. Bilateral crawling patterns become unilateral, and by 8 months are usually reciprocal.

Bilateral crawling (Figures 5-16 and 5-17) is initiated from the on-hands posture. With trunk supported by the surface and distal aspect of upper extremities fixed to the supporting surface, the baby pushes back or pulls forward through space. Both upper extremities push or pull together, creating a bilateral pattern of postural control/movement. With hands fixed to the supporting surface, movement occurs at the more proximal joints, especially around the shoulder-scapular region. Proximal movement of extremities with distal fixation for control develops combined mobility-stability muscle functions around proximal joints and prepares for free extremity movement in space. Pushing back also transfers weight back toward wrist and facilitates finger extension in weight bearing as part of the total upper extremity extension pattern. Although many babies begin to move with bilateral postural control/movement strategies, bilateral movement patterns are not replicated in treatment. Babies at risk for developmental delay or abnormal tone often retain bilateral patterns of control and need to develop separation between sides of body and unilateral-contralateral weight-shift patterns.

<u>Movement Components</u>: Upper extremity and upper trunk flexion/extension

<u>Muscle Functions</u>: Combined mobility/stability

<u>Reflex/Reactions</u>: Vertical righting reaction; upper extremity support reactions

<u>Postural Control/Movement Patterns</u>: Bilateral weight shift from the upper extremities to lower extremities or lower extremities to upper extremities

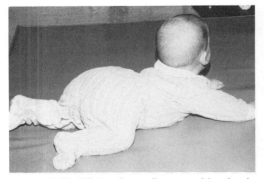

Figure 5-16: Bilateral crawling - pushing back

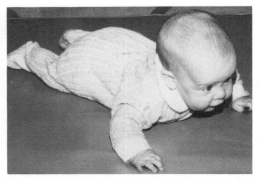

Figure 5-17: Bilateral crawling - pulling forward

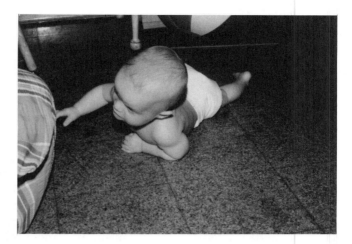

Figure 5-18: Unilateral crawling

Unilateral crawling (Figure 5-18) appears when unilateral weight-shift patterns, which originally developed with on-elbows reaching and were enhanced by pivoting, are adapted to bilateral crawling patterns. Child shifts weight to one side of body, but instead of reaching sideways to move in a circle, reaches forward with upper extremity while flexing and abducting lower extremity on the same side. The baby moves forward with a unilateral pattern of control/movement consisting of weight supported on one side of the body and movement executed by arm and leg on the opposite side of the body.

Unilateral weight-shift pattern in crawling is supported by lateral trunk flexion on the mobile side of the body and elongation on the weight-bearing side of body. Unilateral weight shift promotes a combination of side-to-side and forward movements. Reaching out with the upper extremity introduces blended mobility-stability functions to crawling, but actual movement of body in space is still controlled by combined mobility-stability. Beginning adaptation of vertical-rotational righting to equilibrium reactions in prone is seen again as child shifts weight to one side without activating rotational righting, but instead pulls back toward midline with beginning trunk rotation.

<u>Movement Components</u>: Upper extremity extension/flexion; lower extremity flexion/abduction-extension/adduction; trunk lateral flexion/rotation

<u>Muscle Functions</u>: Combined mobility/stability; beginning blended mobility/stability in shoulder

<u>Reflex/Reactions</u>: Vertical/rotational righting reactions: beginning equilibrium reactions

<u>Postural Control/Movement Patterns</u>: Unilateral weight shift

Reciprocal crawling (Figure 5-19) usually develops after the child has assumed hands-and-knees posture and expanded coactivation of trunk flexors and extensors in an extremity-supported posture. When a child resumes trunk supported posture, reaching from on-hands emerges, which facilitates rotation of upper trunk (Figure 5-20). In addition, expansion of combined flexion-extension to lower trunk while in hand-knee position prepares for development of rotation in the lower trunk as well. With upper and lower trunk segments capable of rotation in opposite directions, contralateral weight-shift patterns can emerge and facilitate reciprocal forward progression. The child's initial experience with contralateral weight shift in pivoting, combined with increased trunk control and experience with unilateral crawling, are adapted to contralateral or

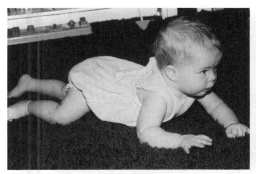 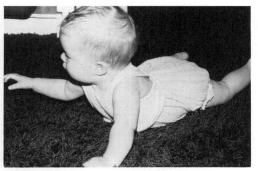

Figure 5-19: Reciprocal crawling   **Figure 5-20:** On-hands reaching

reciprocal crawling. Weight is shifted to one upper extremity and the opposite lower extremity, while the contralateral extremities reach out to move forward through space. The rotation-counterrotation between upper and lower trunk segments facilitates contralateral weight shift and makes simultaneous moving forward possible while shifting weight.

    <u>Movement Components</u>: Upper extremity extension/flexion; lower extremity flexion/abduction-extension/adduction; trunk rotation

    <u>Muscle Functions</u>: Combined mobility/stability; blended mobility/stability-upper extremities

    <u>Reflex/Reactions</u>: Vertical rotational righting reactions; equilibrium reactions

    <u>Postural Control/Movement Patterns</u>: Contralateral weight shift

Creeping (Figures 5-21 and 5-22)

    <u>Description and purpose</u>. Creeping describes the way a child moves around on hands and knees. In order to creep, a child needs enough trunk control to maintain the trunk in a position horizontal to gravity and without support from a supporting surface. The extremities remain in contact with the supporting surface as the main source of stability in a creeping position. To get into a creeping position, a child often combines upper extremity pushing back from bilateral crawling with hip flexion from unilateral crawling, and pushes back onto hands and knees. Once in hand-knee position, a child rocks back and forth, combining mobility and stability around shoulders and hips, as well as through the trunk. Rocking back and forth repeats bilateral weight-shift patterns and prepares for adaptation of unilateral and contralateral patterns required for reciprocal creeping.

    Before creeping, a child often moves between hands-knees rocking and reciprocal crawling, and occasionally assumes hands-feet posture. Hands-feet is an adaptation of prone extension and gives the child an opportunity to again activate extensors against gravity, but with extremity-centered support rather than trunk-centered support (Figure 5-21). By moving between posture requiring higher levels of control, like hands-knees, and back to already established postures, which have been combined with movement such as reciprocal crawling, movement already integrated with established posture is associated with a higher level posture. Eventually, the movement pattern is adapted to the higher level posture. For example, reciprocal movement of extremities from crawling is adapted to hands-knees posture in order for creeping patterns to develop. First unilateral and then contralateral weight shifting is adapted to hands-knees posture so

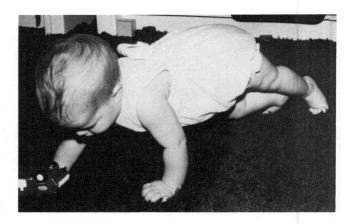

Figure 5-21: Hands-feet support

that child creeps with first unilateral and then contralateral postural control/movement strategy. Blended mobility-stability muscle functions control extremity movement in space, with both unilateral and contralateral patterns.

When the unilateral weight-shift pattern is adapted for creeping, the pattern to assume hands-knees posture from prone changes. Rather than pushing back onto all fours, a child shifts weight onto one side, extends upper extremity, laterally flexes trunk on the same side, flexes lower extremity, and gets up onto hands and knees. As contralateral weight shift affects reciprocal creeping, getting up into creeping changes also. A child gets up onto one upper extremity and the opposite lower extremity, reinforcing contralateral patterns and smoothing out the pattern of simultaneously getting up and moving forward in creeping. Between 8 and 10 months of age, most children are creeping reciprocally. Maturation of contralateral reciprocal patterns in creeping is enhanced by the child's activity in standing. Pulling up into standing facilitates co-activation of flexors and extensors in lower trunk and hips, and leads to expansion of rotation through lower trunk, thereby improving contralateral weight shifts affecting lower extremities.

Rotation and accompanying rotational righting reactions also influence a child's ability to assume sitting from creeping. With rotation developed in the lower trunk, a baby can stabilize with upper extremities and rotate into sitting and back to creeping. Rotating from creeping into sitting facilitates rotation with flexion of trunk in preparation for developing equilibrium in sitting.

    <u>Movement Components</u>: Neck, trunk, and extremity components working together
    <u>Muscle Functions</u>: Blended mobility/stability patterns
    <u>Reflex/Reactions</u>: Vertical/rotational righting reactions; equilibrium reactions
    <u>Postural Control/Movement Patterns</u>: Unilateral, then contralateral, weight-shift patterns

Sitting

Sitting provides a means for assuming and maintaining a vertical, antigravity posture of head and trunk before standing in an upright posture is possible. Sitting ability is retained throughout life as a position of rest, or to provide postural control required for school, work, leisure, or socialization. During progressive development from supine to

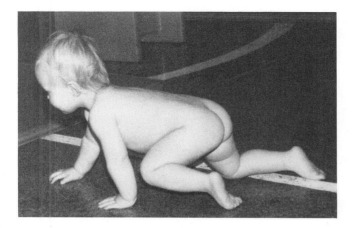

Figure 5-22: Creeping

sitting, the baby develops head, trunk, and extremity <u>flexion</u> against gravity, combines flexion with extension in preparation for developing postural tone along the midline of the body and stability around proximal joints, maintains sitting posture with upper extremity support, frees upper extremities from support role and sits unsupported, adapts lateral flexion and rotation components to move from sitting into creeping and creeping back to sitting using complete rotation patterns, assumes sitting using partial rotation pattern, and eventually assumes sitting using symmetrical pattern. Complete rotation, partial rotation, and symmetrical patterns to assume sitting are further elaborated in Chapter 6.

Sitting, and getting to sit, is particularly illustrative of integration of righting, support, protective, midline, and equilibrium reactions as mechanisms of upright functioning. Getting to sit from prone is initially controlled by an interplay between vertical righting combined with rotational righting and appropriate placement of extremities for support. Maintaining sitting with support from upper extremities allows a child to experiment with letting go of support, align midline of body with center of gravity, and rely on combinations of vestibular and visual perceptions of position in space and assimilations of pressure on the buttocks to maintain vertical posture. Getting to sitting facilitates patterns of movement that are adapted to equilibrium reactions. Maintaining sitting facilitates patterns of movement which are adapted to midline stability reactions. Both equilibrium and midline reactions enhance freedom of movement and use of upper extremities in sitting posture and are adapted to assuming and maintaining standing/walking as well.

Sitting not only frees upper extremities from the support role assumed in prone/creeping and early sitting, but well-established sitting posture provides the background tone needed for upper extremity movement in space. Mobility-stability functions and separation of extremity movement from trunk movement begins in both prone and supine, using supporting surface to help control the extremity movement. Once stability is established in upright posture, trunk and scapular-shoulder stability is blended with extremity mobility to control free movement. Upper extremities can be used to transfer objects, manipulate objects bilaterally, and cross the midline to obtain objects. Lower extremities can be used to assist with changes in position while the child continues to maintain an upright orientation with head and trunk.

Key behaviors (Figure 5-23) associated with development of sitting include

<u>Primitive Phase</u>
Primary Sitting
Head Lag
Head Align

<u>Transitional Phase</u>
Pull to Sit
Hands to Feet/Feet to Mouth
Supported Sitting

<u>Mature Phase</u>
Sitting.

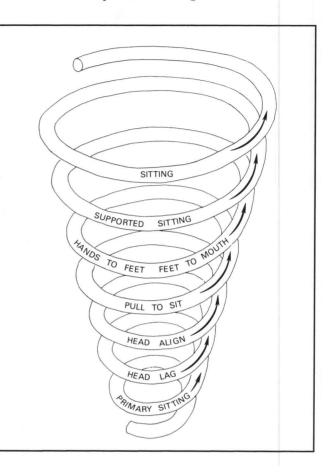

Figure 5-23: Key behaviors of sitting

Primary Sitting (Figure 5-24)

<u>Description and purpose</u>. Primary sitting is one of the early behaviors that seems to be a forerunner to sitting behaviors that follow. If a newborn baby is placed and held in a sitting position, the baby will momentarily try to right herself and maintain head and upper trunk in the upright posture. Attempts to straighten head and trunk are brief and uncoordinated, but may give the baby a sense of sitting. The baby is probably responding to touch pressure assimilations on the buttocks that become more localized in supported sitting than in supine lying. Being upright may also influence the vestibular system and bring forth some primitive attempts to right head. Both pressure on buttocks and vertical head righting are significant sources of stimulation for sitting balance at higher levels of development.

<u>Movement Components</u>: Extension
<u>Muscle Functions</u>: Mobility
<u>Reflex/Reactions</u>: Early attempts—vertical righting reaction
<u>Postural Control/Movement Patterns</u>: Weight bearing

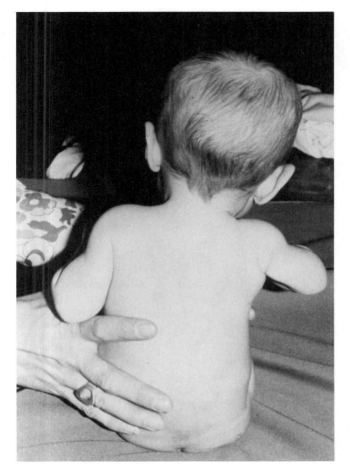

Figure 5-24: Primary sitting

Head Lag (Figure 5-25)

<u>Description and purpose</u>. Whenever a baby is lifted from a supporting surface, the person lifting always takes care to support the baby's head, realizing that the baby does not have sufficient control over own head in space. If a baby is pulled up from supine, using only the arms for holding, the extent of newborn head lag is evident. Head lag results from lack of head righting reactions to counteract the effect of gravity on head and neck musculature and effect of the tonic labyrinthine reflex, which facilitates supine extension in newborn babies. Movement through space may also activate a Moro reflex, which also initially facilitates extension of head and neck in supine. It is difficult for a baby to activate flexor muscle groups against gravity or in conjunction with extensor action. However, stretch on the flexor muscles and effect of gravity on vestibular receptors eventually act to facilitate flexion and bring about head alignment and control in supine and pull to sit.

<u>Movement Components</u>: Extension
<u>Muscle Functions</u>: Mobility
<u>Reflex/Reactions</u>: Tonic labyrinthine: Moro reflex
<u>Postural Control/Movement Patterns</u>: Weight bearing

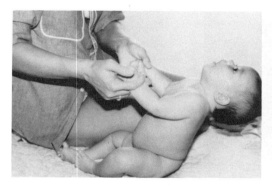

Figure 5-25: Head lag

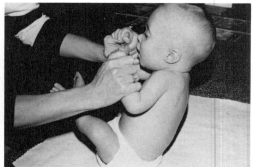

Figure 5-26: Head align

Head Align (Figure 5-26)

Description and purpose. A baby's response to being pulled to sit, or lifted up from supine, changes with activation of neck flexors against gravity. First evidence of flexor activation in supine is noted around 2-3 months of age, when a baby attempts to keep head aligned during pull to sit. Effect of flexor development is also noted when the baby can hold head in midline more consistently in supine. Head alignment in midline, either in supine or in pull to sit, contributes to development of symmetry and decreased asymmetry in supine. During pull to sit, activation of neck flexors is facilitated by pressure on palm of baby's hands as well as traction on arms. Pressure on palms of a newborn or very young infant often stimulates a sucking response and general increase of flexor tone in neck and upper trunk. With increased flexor tone, the baby can keep head aligned with body while being pulled up. Flexor tone in the upper extremities increases with grasp and also facilitates pulling up. Even with assistance from general activation of flexion, it is difficult for baby to keep head aligned while moving against gravity. To assist with head alignment, the baby elevates shoulders in an attempt to stabilize head on shoulders. Although shoulder elevation is an adequate substitute for neck coactivation in a normally developing baby, elevation can become part of an abnormal fixation pattern if continued as an adaptation at higher levels of development. Instead, righting reactions and activation of a full range of neck flexion need to develop in order to integrate head lag.

 Movement Components: Flexion
 Muscle Functions: Mobility
 Reflex/Reactions: Sucking
 Postural Control/Movement Patterns: Weight bearing

Pull to Sit (Figure 5-27)

Description and purpose. By 4 months of age, symmetry in supine is apparent with flexion well enough developed to allow the baby to hold head in midline, bring hands together easily, and initiate head righting when pulled to sit. Between 4 and 5 months there is a significant change in pull-to-sit behavior, with the emergence of vertical head righting. As a baby is pulled up, the head rights toward vertical and comes forward slightly ahead of the body. Neck and upper trunk flexors are activated through a full range of motion and are prepared to act with extensors for coactivation functions of postural control. With repeated experience in pull to sit, flexors through the lower trunk

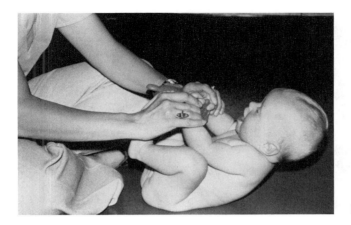

Figure 5-27: Pull to sit

are activated and prepared to act against gravity or with extensors. Upper body adaptations are modified with repeated experience as well. As baby pulls into flexion with arms and combines upper extremity flexion with scapular adduction, upper trunk extension is coactivated with rapidly developing upper trunk flexion. Upper trunk extension, facilitated by scapular adduction, is adapted from prone extension behavior. Baby aligns head and trunk when held in an upright sitting posture. Lower extremities remain flexed and abducted to provide a wide base of support.

Movement Components: Neck and trunk flexion

Muscle Functions: Mobility

Reflex/Reactions: Vertical head righting

Postural Control/Movement Patterns: Weight bearing

Hands to Feet/Feet to Mouth (Figures 5-28 and 5-29)

Description and purpose. Once midline head control in supine and supine head righting appear, supine flexion patterns develop rapidly. Baby is able to reach into space with first upper and then lower extremities. At first, holding extremities in space is often reinforced by bringing hands or feet together at midline. Later, with more control, baby can reach and hold objects, reach for knees or feet, and bring feet to mouth. Reaching freely with upper extremities contributes significantly to development of range and control over upper extremity movement. Reaching against gravity helps develop and blend upper extremity movement components while also facilitating separation between humeral and scapular components of upper extremity. Baby's supine position, along with newly developing scapular adduction, holds scapulae against the upper trunk so that scapular mobility is differentiated from humeral mobility. Scapulae begin to develop stability functions, which support further separation and control over upper extremity movement. Between 4 and 5 months, the baby not only reaches more accurately for objects in space, but also begins to direct reaching toward knees, and then to feet.

Reaching for knees and feet not only expands upper extremity movement patterns, but also encourages development of lower trunk and lower extremity function. Baby brings knees up to meet hands by activating lower abdominal muscles, along with hip and knee flexor muscle groups. Activating abdominal muscles and lifting hips off supporting surface facilitates posterior pelvic tilt. Posterior tilt is combined with anterior pelvic tilt, which is developing with extension in prone, in order to mobilize the pelvis

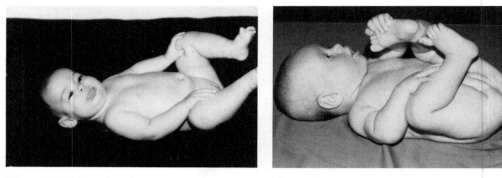

Figure 5-28: Hands to knees   **Figure 5-29:** Feet to mouth

and separate pelvic movement from upper trunk movement. Pelvic mobility and separation is necessary for positioning pelvis for stability in sitting, as well as developing pelvic rotation in creeping, rolling, walking, and moving in and out of most positions. Flexion and posterior tilt are further enhanced as baby reaches and plays with feet. In addition, hands to feet requires hip flexion with knee extension, and therefore differentiates full lower extremity flexion patterns. With hip flexion and knee extension, baby can hold legs up against gravity and prepare for sitting posture—i.e., trunk extended, hips flexed, and knees extended.

Between 5 and 6 months, baby increases range of lower body movement by bringing feet to mouth. Baby's perception of self is greatly enhanced by hands to knees to feet, and especially feet to mouth. Baby is accustomed to exploring hands and objects with mouth, so exploring feet not only adds to baby's information about self but also contributes to baby's oral-motor development.

Baby plays with the variety of postures and movements available in supine, using posterior and anterior pelvic tilt to move in and out of "bridging" (lifting hips in extension with feet flat on supporting surface) postures, or bridging on one side and rotating pelvis toward other side, or holding feet with hands and rolling to side. Generally, baby's activities in supine contribute significantly to differentiation of body segments; i.e. separation of extremity movement from trunk movement, separation of one extremity from another, and separation between upper and lower trunk segments.

Movement Components: Flexion—neck, trunk, extremities

Muscle Functions: Combined mobility/stability; blended mobility/stability

Reflex/Reactions: Vertical righting reaction

Postural Control/Movement Patterns: Weight bearing; bilateral and unilateral weight shift

Supported Sitting (Figure 5-30)

Between 5 and 6 months of age, a baby who is placed in a sitting position will lean forward with rounded back and support on bilaterally extended arms. Supporting on extended arms is adapted from protective-support reactions which are developing in prone. Lower extremities are flexed, abducted, and externally rotated to provide a wide, stable base of support. With a stable base and distal support on upper extremities, mobility is combined with trunk stability whenever the baby turns her head and shifts weight from one upper extremity to the other. Shifting weight changes pressure on the buttocks, while facilitating head righting with upper trunk rotation, and these combinations of assimilations and accommodations prepare for equilibrium and independence in sitting.

Movement Components: Neck and trunk flexion/extension; rotation

Muscle Functions: Stability; combined mobility/stability

Reflex/Reactions: Vertical righting reactions; upper extremity and buttock support reactions

Postural Control/Movement Patterns: Weight bearing

By 7 to 8 months of age, a baby is no longer interested in staying in supine, and rolls quickly into prone. From prone, baby is able to assume sitting, using a variety of patterns. As soon as the baby can get into hand-knee position, she may push back between legs to assume supported sitting, or shift weight to one hip and push up, using arms for support. When a baby can sit unsupported, getting into sitting with more rotation of trunk and less push from arms is possible, as noted in description of creep-to-sit sequence of movement.

Sitting (Figure 5-31)

Attempts to get into sitting using upper extremity support combine mobility with stability through lower trunk and hip region and facilitate hip control for sitting without support from upper extremities. The baby lets go of support and aligns head and trunk over hips. Activation of extensors for postural tone may be reinforced by recalling scapular adduction with upper extremity flexion. Posture may also be secured by fixing

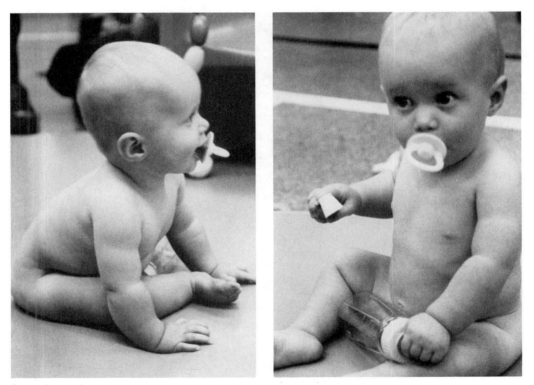

Figure 5-30: Supported sitting   **Figure 5-31:** Sitting

the pelvis in anterior tilt position. Lower extremities remain flexed, abducted, and externally rotated. As flexion, extension, and rotation are blended in unsupported sitting, and midline stability develops, the baby's arms come down from full flexion into readiness to protect in either forward or sideward protective responses. The baby adapts pelvic mobility, which was originally practiced in supine, and experiments shifting weight slightly in anterior, posterior, or lateral planes, responding to touch-pressure on the buttocks.

With more lower trunk stability, the baby can use hands freely for two-handed activity, or rotate away from midline and back to reach objects (Figure 5-32). Occasionally, the baby may lose balance while reaching and can recall protective reactions to return to upper extremity support for sitting, or may position one upper extremity in flexion and scapular adduction in order to fix the upper trunk for balance, while reaching with opposite upper extremity. However, balance based on equilibrium and midline stability becomes more consistent after the baby has pulled to stand, as well as after the baby has rotated between creeping and independent sitting and back to creeping. Both higher level achievements enhance pelvis-hip control in sitting. Evidence of increased midline

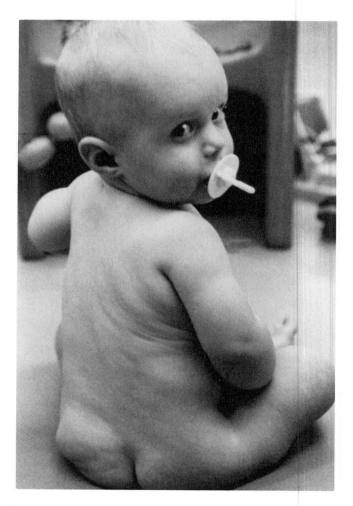

Figure 5-32: Sitting with rotation

and hip control is apparent when baby can sit with one leg extended with more adduction and neutral rotation, even though the other leg may remain flexed and abducted in a more fixed position. When both lower extremities extend into a long sitting position, control around the hips is even more established, although a threat to balance may cause one lower extremity to return to flexion-abduction to fix for balance (Figure 5-33). With more lower trunk stability and lower extremity extension, child can begin to pivot in sitting by abducting and adducting lower extremities. Pivoting in sitting is similar to pivoting in prone and allows child to reach object more easily. Lower extremity abduction-adduction is also enhanced.

Initial position shifts between creeping and sitting and back to creeping are controlled more by upper extremity support reactions combined with rotation along the midline of the body (Figure 5-34). Gradually, upper extremity participation decreases and one lower extremity serves as a pivot point for moving between positions. Using the lower extremity to initiate and control movement around the midline enhances rotation-counterrotation between upper and lower body segments. With mature midline stability, baby can maintain upright alignment of neck and trunk while lower extremities change

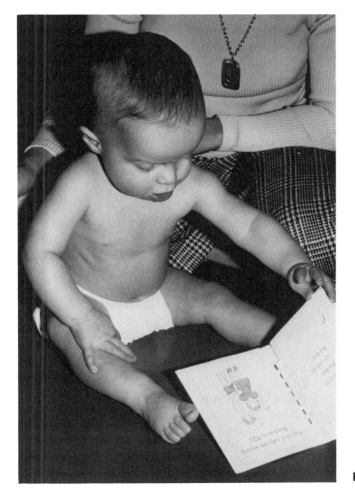

Figure 5-33: Long sit

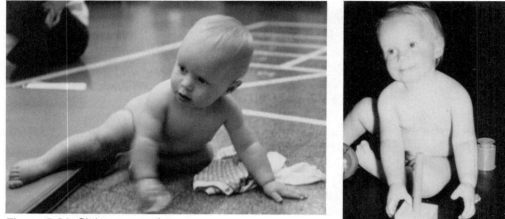

Figure 5-34: Sitting to creeping

Figure 5-35: Mature sitting

position (side sit, long sit, tailor sit). Or, baby can change from sitting to standing without disturbing vertical alignment in space (Figure 5-35).

Movement Components: Neck, trunk, and extremity components working together

Muscle Functions: Blended mobility/stability

Reflex/Reactions: Midline stability; equilibrium reactions

Postural Control/Movement Patterns: Contralateral weight shift for moving in and out of sitting and reaching from sitting

Rolling

Rolling (Figure 5-36) provides a means for changing position in space, or moving through space before forward progression develops in prone posture. Rolling also leads to a baby's ability to maintain sidelying positions and use upper extremities for two-handed play in sidelying. During the progressive development of rolling, a baby develops rotation between body segments, e.g., between head and the rest of the body, or between head and upper trunk segment, upper and lower trunk segments. Rotation emerges from combinations of extensor and flexor patterns of movement. In early rolling, the influences of flexion and extension of neck and trunk segments are obvious. For example, in supine, a baby may initiate rolling from a flexed posture, like supine hands-to-feet position. Upon reaching sidelying in flexion, the baby lifts and turns her head toward prone, facilitating extension throughout the body. Early evidence of rotation between segments is seen first in the neck when the head is turned to initiate or complete the pattern. A similar series of events occurs in prone when a baby in on-hands position increases the amount of extension in the neck and trunk, turns head, elicits asymmetrical changes in extremity tone, and "falls" into supine. In both incidences of early rolling from supine and prone, association between some head turning and patterns of complete flexion and extension through the rest of the body provides the foundation for more discrete combinations of flexion and extension to emerge and support development of rotation between midline body segments.

As a baby uses either flexion or extension to initiate rolling with either extension or flexion to complete the rolling pattern, aspects of total flexion or extension patterns are differentiated and combined for smoother, more efficient rolling. At the same time head turning, accompanied by neck rotation, facilitates rotational righting reactions between head and trunk and between trunk segments. The righting reactions are mainly responsible for facilitation, sequencing, and controlling the movement between segments. Facilitating specific muscle groups to act in sequence for a particular movement pattern, such as rotation, is part of the differentiation process. In rolling, flexor-extensor actions are differentiated so that flexors on one side of the body can be activated to initiate the roll, followed sequentially by activation of extensors on the opposite side of the body to complete the roll. Rotation and diagonal patterns of movement across the midline of the body develop, and separation between body segments is facilitated.

Separation between body segments in rolling can be described as the ability to move one segment prior to moving its adjacent segment, or the ability to hold one segment stable while moving adjacent segment, or moving segment in the opposite direction than its adjacent segment. Rotational patterns of movement, separation between segments, and rotational righting reactions are linked together through maturation and development of neuromuscular functions in rolling. Together they produce chain reactions of movement through space so that movement of one segment facilitates movement of its adjacent segment, or opposite movement of an adjacent segment can control movement of the lead segment. The process of control of movement by movement is adapted to equilibrium reactions for postural control and sequential movement patterns at higher levels of development and adaptation.

Key behaviors (Figure 5-36) associated with development of rolling include

Primitive Phase
Primary Turning

Transition Phase
Spontaneous Rolling
Deliberate Roll to Prone
Deliberate Roll to Supine

Mature Phase
Rolling

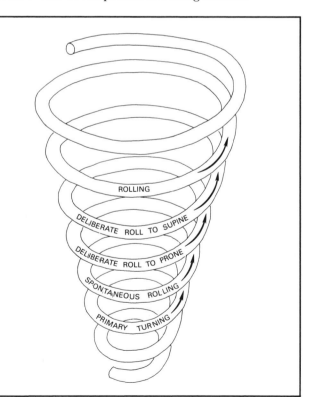

Figure 5-36: Key behaviors of rolling

Primary Turning (Figures 5-37 and 5-38)

<u>Description and purpose.</u> Rolling depends on rotation between body segments. Rooting during the newborn period is a forerunner to development of neck rotation and rolling. The rooting reflex begins in utero and is available to the newborn as a means of seeking nourishment. Touch on the side of the face of a newborn causes baby's head to turn toward the touch in search of a nipple and to start sucking. A baby may associate head turning with satisfying hunger and tend to repeat head turning in response to hunger or in search of hand to satisfy need to suck. In addition, visual functions and auditory responses develop rapidly after birth. Baby's efforts to visually follow moving objects or persons, as well as frequent experiences turning toward voices and other sounds, mean that turning head from side to side in supine is enhanced by stimulation from the environment as well (Figure 5-39). Protective head turning in prone, which was previously described as a primitive key behavior of creeping, also contributes to early development of neck rotation patterns. Right after birth there is limited range of movement between head and rest of the body. Head and body often move together, especially if the baby is under stress from crying or attempting movement. With specifically directed neck movement, elicited by touch, visual, or auditory assimilations, range of neck movement increases and separation between head and rest of the body increases. With neck movement, proprioceptors located in the neck musculature and vertebral segments are facilitated and accommodate first with asymmetrical postures, and later with righting reactions.

Primary head turning begins to influence distributions of muscle tone in the trunk and extremities. Asymmetrical tonic neck reflex posture is elicited from stimulation of neck proprioceptors during head turning (Figure 5-40). Extension of extremities on the face side of the body and flexion of extremities on the head side of the body are accompanied by arching of the trunk. Tendency to arch by extending body is also influenced by tonic labyrinthine reflex in supine. Arching with head turned increases pressure on the face side of the body and creates a source of stimulation for automatic trunk turning toward sources of pressure (Figure 5-41). Asymmetrical postures are not obligatory for normally developing infants, but may become a frequent position of rest, thus providing stimulation for primary trunk turning. A baby may play with head turning and trunk turning in preparation for rolling from supine to prone. Vigorous repetition of asymmetrical extension can bring the baby toward sidelying and may elicit some flexion in sidelying. Trunk extension followed by flexion, or flexion followed by

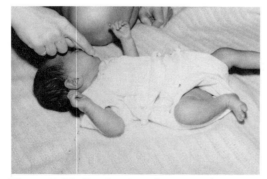

Figure 5-37: Rooting for primary turning

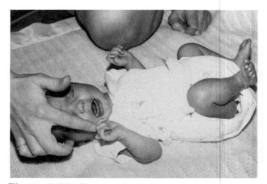

Figure 5-38: Rooting for primary turning

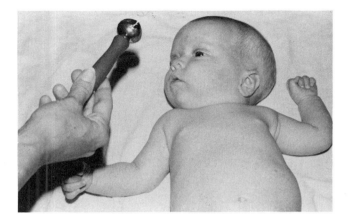

Figure 5-39: Visual following

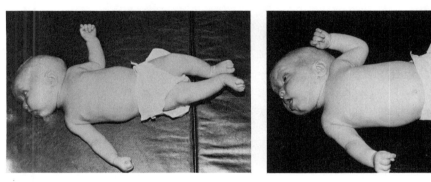

Figure 5-40: Asymmetrical posture   **Figure 5-41:** Arching

extension, is sometimes used to facilitate early rolling and combine flexion and extension into rotation patterns.

Movement Components: Neck rotation

Muscle Functions: Mobility

Reflex/Reactions: Rooting; asymmetrical tonic reflex

Postural Control/Movement Patterns: Weight bearing

Spontaneous Rolling (Figures 5-42 to 5-47)

Description and purpose. Spontaneous rolling promotes some of a baby's first changes of position in space from prone to supine, or supine to prone. Spontaneous rolling may be initiated from different positions, and seems to begin when baby loses postural control in a position, or uses primitive patterns of movement in combinations that result in early rolling. Baby does not seem to intend to change position at first, and is often surprised by the change. The experience of spontaneously changing position probably influences emergence of deliberate rolling at higher levels of development.

Around 4 months of age, if a baby is in prone position with head raised, resting on-elbows or on-hands, head turning may elicit an asymmetrical tonic neck response and affect the baby's arm posture. The imbalance that occurs from flexion in one supporting arm and extension in the other supporting arm allows baby to push with extended arm and fall over the flexed arm into sidelying. If the baby's arm movement is vigorous

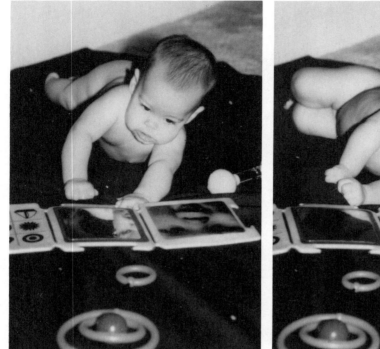

Figure 5-42: Spontaneous rolling from prone

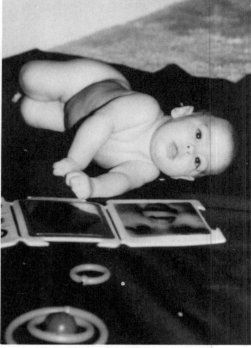

Figure 5-43: Spontaneous rolling from prone

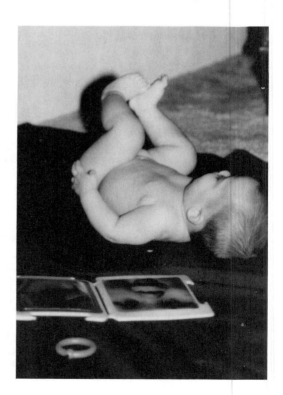

Figure 5-44: Spontaneous rolling from prone

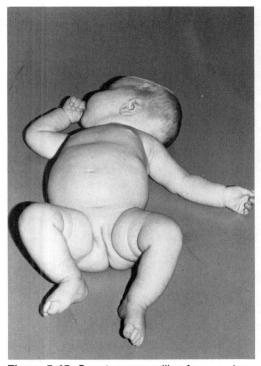

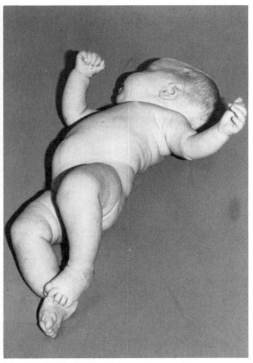

Figure 5-45: Spontaneous rolling from supine

Figure 5-46: Spontaneous rolling from supine

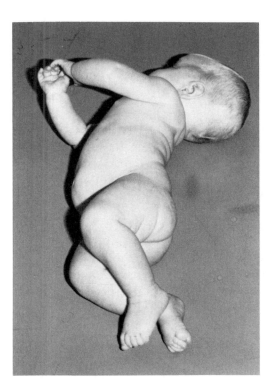

Figure 5-47: Spontaneous rolling from supine

enough, or if the baby assists with trunk extension, she may fall all the way from prone into supine.

Also at 4 months, neck righting reactions begin to appear in supine. Neck righting is a rotational righting reaction and introduces rotation components to rolling patterns. When a baby turns her head to the side in supine, rotation between head and body segments activates proprioceptors in muscle components and vertebral segments, which cause the body to follow rotation of head, and the baby rolls spontaneously to sidelying. Activation of neck proprioceptors began with primary head turning and previously facilitated asymmetrical postures in supine. With maturation of higher level righting reactions, head turning affects the trunk as well, so that trunk turns as a whole to realign with head. Use of righting reactions to align and realign body segments will be expanded as righting reactions continue to mature and serve as a control for movement in space. Once in sidelying, baby attempts to move into prone by extending trunk and pushing with foot. Although occasionally successful, further development of components is necessary for rolling supine to prone.

For some babies, spontaneous rolling supine to prone is enhanced between 5 and 6 months of age with appearance of hand-to-feet behavior in supine. As baby experiments with holding feet in hands and shifting weight slightly from side to side, lack of midline stability and equilibrium in supine make it difficult for baby to shift weight back toward midline, and gravity and neck righting assist baby to roll toward sidelying. Meanwhile, in sidelying, pressure from supporting surface is localized from baby's back to baby's side. Pressure facilitates lateral vertical head righting, which is combined with rotational neck righting so that baby can continue head turning toward prone and trunk can follow to assume prone position. Rotation is still essentially between head and trunk until rotational righting reactions mature further.

> Movement Components: Neck rotation
> Muscle Functions: Mobility
> Reflex/Reactions: Rotational/vertical righting
> Postural Control/Movement Patterns: Weight bearing

Deliberate Rolling (Figures 5-48 to 5-50)

Description and purpose. Deliberate rolling is evident when a baby appears to participate more in initiating and carrying through with a rolling pattern. Deliberate rolling not only makes it possible for the baby to complete a spontaneously initiated roll more consistently, but also contributes to separation between trunk segments and further maturation of rotational righting reactions. A baby participates more in rolling by pulling upper trunk segment with arm, or pulling lower trunk segment with leg, or pushing lower trunk segment with foot.

Between 6 and 7 months, baby in prone may use one foot to rotate pelvis on trunk. Rotation between lower and upper trunk segments facilitates upper trunk to follow lower trunk until baby assumes sidelying posture. Once in sidelying, lateral head righting is facilitated which, in turn, facilitates lateral trunk flexion and elongation on the weight-bearing side of the trunk. From sidelying, baby can continue to roll by combining head turning and reaching with upper extremity, which encourages upper trunk to rotate on lower trunk, and complete the roll to supine. Upper trunk rotating on lower trunk separates trunk segments and, along with maturation of nervous system, facilitates rotational righting between trunk segments. Or, the lower extremity may lead baby to roll from sidelying to supine, encouraging lower trunk to rotate on upper trunk and further facilitating rotational righting reactions.

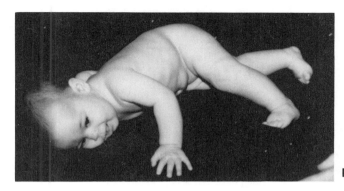

Figure 5-48: Deliberate rolling from prone

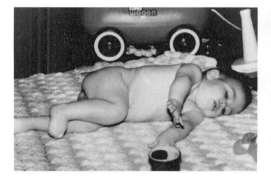

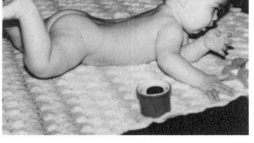

Figure 5-49: Deliberate rolling from supine   **Figure 5-50:** Deliberate rolling from supine

By 7 months, deliberate rolling from supine is observed. After baby turns head and initiates neck righting, assistance from upper extremity pulls upper trunk into rotation slightly ahead of the lower trunk. Separation between upper and lower trunk segments facilitates muscle proprioceptors and vertebral segments, and, along with maturation of the nervous system, also encourages expansion of rotational righting.

Deliberate rolling from supine is also enhanced by baby's use of lower extremities. Bridging and half-bridging in supine develops separation between upper and lower trunk segments. In addition, ability to flex hips and hold legs extended in supine allows baby to develop control to direct movement of lower extremities. When baby either bridges and rotates lower extremities to one side, or raises one or both legs in supine and rotates them to one side, rotation between trunk segments facilitates rotational righting so that upper body follows lower trunk rotation and baby can roll deliberately from supine to prone. Although deliberate rolling appears in many forms, there are some commonalities among the patterns. Deliberate rolling is an interaction between developing rotational righting reactions and separation between body segments, facilitated by use of extremities to lead movement of segments and source of further facilitation of righting reactions within the central axis of body. Rotational righting reactions that develop with deliberate rolling are adapted to automatic rolling as well as patterns for assuming sitting from prone at higher levels of development.

<u>Movement Components</u>: Neck and trunk rotation
<u>Muscle Functions</u>: Mobility
<u>Reflex/Reactions</u>: Rotational righting reactions
<u>Postural Control/Movement Patterns</u>: Unilateral weight shift

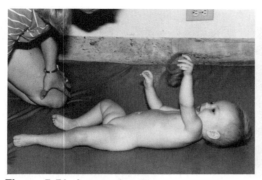 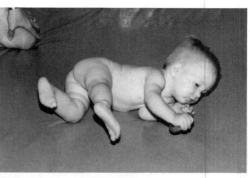

Figure 5-51: Automatic rolling   **Figure 5-52:** Automatic rolling

Automatic Rolling (Figures 5-51 and 5-52)

<u>Description and purpose</u>. Automatic rolling is evident by 8 or 9 months of age. With automatic rolling, rotational and vertical righting reactions are fully developed and integrated with each other. Baby can initiate rolling from any body segment, and other body segments will automatically follow to complete the pattern from supine to prone, or prone to supine. Rotation occurs around the central axis of the body without assistance from extremities. In fact, baby can roll while holding objects in hands. Baby also can begin to roll in one direction and change to opposite direction by activating opposite segments.

Activating body segments in sequence and in opposition to each other increases baby's control of movement by opposite movement that is used to maintain sidelying positions, and can be adapted to development of equilibrium reactions. In order for a baby to maintain sidelying, rotation between body segments is balanced so that if lower segments are rotated slightly forward from sidelying, upper segments are rotated slightly backward and baby maintains sidelying with minimal support from extremities.

<u>Movement Components</u>: Neck and trunk rotation working together
<u>Muscle Functions</u>: Mobility
<u>Reflex/Reactions</u>: Rotational/vertical righting reactions; equilibrium reactions
<u>Postural Control/Movement Patterns</u>: Contralateral weight shift

Standing/Walking

Standing and walking provide a means for locomotion in an upright posture, utilizing lower extremities for support and freeing upper extremities for carrying objects and further development of skill capability. Upright locomotion also leads to such skills as running, hopping, skipping, and participation in numerous games, sports, shopping and recreational activities. A child develops an ability to stand and walk by associating, differentiating, and adapting essential elements of flexion, extension, and rotation accompanied by righting, midline stability, and equilibrium reactions with extremity support, protection, separation, and reciprocation that were developed during creeping, sitting, and rolling. A baby first pulls up into standing by holding onto persons or objects; stands by holding on or supporting with upper extremities or trunk, climbs, walks, or cruises around objects while holding on, squats, stands unsupported, walks unsupported and runs, skips, and jumps. Observing a child's first attempts at standing and walking independently underscores the intrinsic motivation associated with the child's innate drive to walk. The child is delighted with the accomplishment and seems to pursue the activity for its own sake. The child gets up, stands, takes some steps, falls, and gets up again without much regard for walking to something, but more for the joy of walking itself.

Standing and walking behaviors provide a particularly excellent opportunity to observe adaptation of previously acquired behaviors to development of new behaviors. Although adaptation of old-to-new and new-to-old behaviors has appeared throughout the developmental progressions, the fact that standing and walking are comprised almost entirely of differentiated aspects of creeping, sitting, and rolling, and performed under potentially more stressful spatiotemporal conditions, means that spiraling effects of adaptation and stress will be more obvious to the observer.

Key behaviors (Figure 5-53) associated with development of standing and walking include

Primitive Phase
Primary Standing
Primary Walking

Transitional Phase
Pull to Stand
Supported Standing
Supported Walking

Mature Phase
Squatting
Standing
Walking

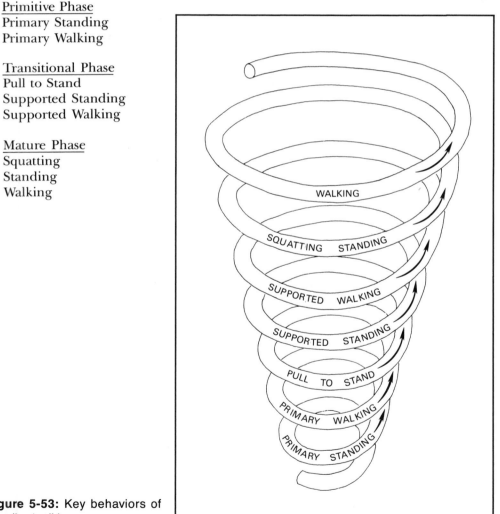

Figure 5-53: Key behaviors of standing/walking

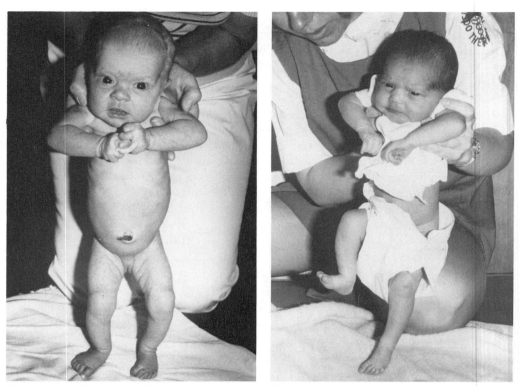

Figure 5-54: Primary standing   **Figure 5-55:** Primary stepping

Primary Standing (Figure 5-54)

Description and purpose. If a baby is held in a standing position right after birth, the baby will momentarily bear weight on feet and seem to stand with support. The response is similar to primary sitting, but pressure is on soles of feet instead of buttocks, and the extension elicited affects both the lower extremities and the trunk. Primary standing is a forerunner to standing behavior that will develop after a baby has acquired the necessary mobility and stability to support independent standing. After the first few weeks or first month after birth, primary standing can no longer be elicited. A baby may even pull lower extremities into flexion if placed in standing, and will not usually bear weight consistently until more postural tone is present in the rest of the body.

Movement Components: Extension of lower extremities
Muscle Functions: Mobility
Reflex/Reactions: Primitive support
Postural Control/Movement Patterns: Weight bearing

Primary Walking (Figure 5-55)

Description and purpose. Like primary standing, primary walking is a forerunner to later functions. If a baby is held in supported standing and moved slightly forward, baby will take steps in a primitive reciprocal pattern. Primary walking is similar in pattern to primary crawling. Increased stimulation on the bottom of one foot causes extension of that lower extremity and flexion of opposite extremity, followed by extension of flexed extremity and flexion of opposite extremity, etc. The flexion-extension pattern of lower extremities is activated through full ranges of motion, which contributes to activation of these muscle groups in reciprocal patterns. Primary walking can only be elicited for a few weeks to a month or so after birth. Only after baby has developed enough postural tone for supported standing, combined with reciprocal patterns from crawling and creeping, will stepping movements emerge again as part of upright locomotion.

Movement Components: Flexion/extension—lower extremities

Muscle Functions: Mobility

Reflex/Reactions: Crossed extension reflex

Postural Control/Movement Patterns: Weight bearing

Pull to Stand (Figures 5-56 and 5-57)

Description and Purpose. Pulling up to a standing position precedes supported and unsupported standing and walking. Both pull to sit in supine and crawling/creeping weight-shift patterns in prone are adapted to pull-to-stand patterns. Progressively more refined pull-to-stand patterns influence higher developmental levels of standing and walking. Motivation to pull up to stand is linked to a drive for upright locomotion and early attempts at pulling up may be seen at 7 months of age, even though postural tone for standing is still in the process of developing.

In order for a baby to begin to pull to stand, lower extremities must be prepared to bear weight. Around 5 to 6 months, appearance of a positive supporting reaction in the

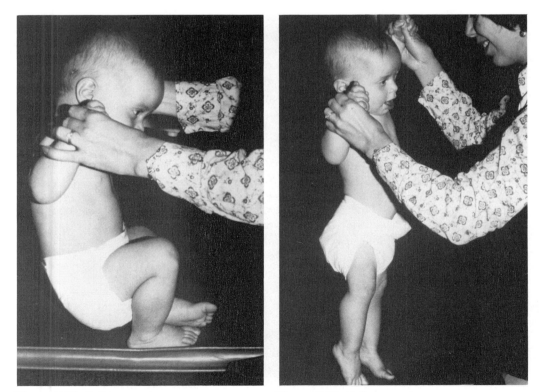

Figure 5-56: Pull to stand   **Figure 5-57:** Pull to stand

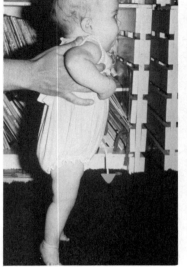

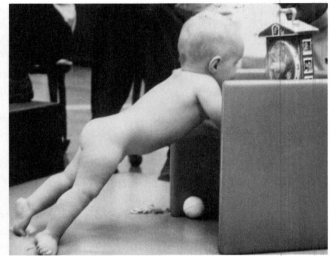

Figure 5-59: Bilateral pull to stand

Figure 5-58: Positive support

lower extremities provides initial weight-bearing capability (Figure 5-58). As a baby is held and lowered down toward the floor in an upright posture so that the balls of the feet contact the supporting surface, there is a general increase in extensor tone up through the lower extremities and trunk. The baby "stands" on toes and maintains trunk and head in upright posture with support. Positive supporting is one of the extremity support reactions. Once present, the reaction is combined with lower extremity protective (parachute) reaction so that a baby anticipates need for extension and weight bearing, and extends and abducts lower extremities before touching supporting surface. The parachute reaction retains the extension component of hips and knees, but modifies plantar flexion and the tendency to stand on toes. However, extensor tone is so necessary for upright functioning, and so strong when elicited by positive support, that modification and blending with flexion will continue for several years.

Appearance of positive support modifies pull-to-sit responses. As a baby is pulled up from supine and anticipates possibility of standing, instead of coming only to sit, the baby can now adjust lower extremities in anticipation of weight bearing and be pulled up to stand, as soon as soles of feet are stimulated by supporting surface. Full extension may be elicited due to activity of the positive support reaction. Despite the fact that extension is not yet blended with flexion for independent standing, the child has discovered the possibility of pulling self to standing, a behavior to pursue. Most babies are pulling up between 8 and 9 months, and can usually lower self down by 10 months.

Bilateral pull to stand is adapted from being pulled to stand (Figure 5-59). As soon as a child can crawl or creep over to an object, the object can be used to pull self to stand. Baby uses upper extremities to stabilize upper part of body while moving lower extremities into a position for standing. Baby tends to push back onto lower extremities and straighten knees and hips in a bilateral pattern of movement, rather than pull legs under trunk in preparation for standing. Bilateral weight-shift pattern is similar to the pattern used for pushing back into the creeping position from prone, and serves to combine mobility and stability functions in preparation for more mature patterns of assuming standing.

Getting down from standing is more difficult than getting up. At first the baby will cry to be helped down, or sit down abruptly. With more experience getting up, baby will develop ability to combine mobility and stability in order to lower self into squat, while continuing to hold on to an object.

Movement Components: Extension—trunk and lower extremities

Muscle Functions: Combined mobility/stability

Reflex/Reactions: Positive supporting reaction; vertical righting reaction

Postural Control/Movement Patterns: Bilateral weight shift.

Unilateral pull to stand (Figure 5-60) is adapted from bilateral pull to stand and unilateral crawling patterns. Once the child has combined mobility and stability in lower portions of the body by getting into and out of an upright posture, and has developed ability to shift weight to one side of the body without losing balance, unilateral pull-to-stand patterns emerge. Child shifts weight to one knee while holding on to an object with both hands and brings opposite foot into plantigrade position, shifts weight onto plantigrade foot, and rises to stand. Emphasis is on moving forward over foot to extend leg rather than pushing back to stand.

Movement Components: Extension—trunk and lower extremity; lateral flexion—trunk; flexion/abduction—lower extremity

Muscle Functions: Combined mobility/stability; blended mobility/stability

Reflex/Reactions: Vertical righting reaction

Postural Control/Movement Patterns: Unilateral weight shift

Contralateral pull to stand (Figure 5-61) is adapted from unilateral pull to stand and contralateral creeping patterns. Once the child has refined lower trunk rotation by creeping, and experienced weight shift to one side to pull to stand, then the unilateral weight-shift pattern can be modified to include trunk rotation and counterrotation as a means for shifting weight and moving up into standing simultaneously. By adapting rotation-counterrotation to unilateral weight shift, contralateral weight-shift patterns in pull to stand emerge. With contralateral weight shift, the child gains more control over lower extremity movement and placement, so that eventually getting to standing can be accomplished without holding on for balance. In order to use contralateral weight shift for pull to stand, the child shifts weight onto one knee while holding on with the opposite upper extremity to maintain balance. Holding on with one upper extremity includes reaching forward with upper trunk rotation. In order to free non-weight-bearing lower extremity, bring extremity forward, and place foot in plantigrade position, the child rotates lower trunk segment backward. As child rises to standing, lower trunk on the lower extremity weight-bearing side rotates forward to neutral, while upper trunk segment rotates back to neutral. By using rotation and counterrotation to support contralateral pull-to-stand position, child is able to simultaneously maintain upright alignment while moving forward and upward into standing.

Movement Components: Trunk rotation and all components in unilateral pattern

Muscle Functions: Combined mobility/stability; blended mobility/stability

Reflex/Reactions: Vertical/rotation righting reactions; midline stability reaction

Postural Control/Movement Patterns: Contralateral weight shift.

Supported Standing (Figure 5-62)

Description and purpose. Once a child can pull to stand, supported standing is possible, using postural tone which is developing around midline, as well as support from holding or leaning against objects in the environment. Being in standing, even with support, gives the child more opportunities to develop or refine components for

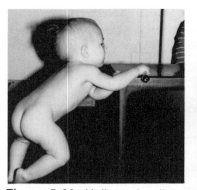

Figure 5-60: Unilateral pull to stand

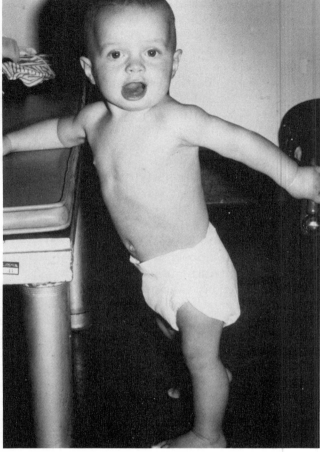

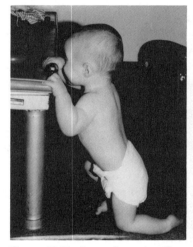

Figure 5-61: Contralateral pull to stand

Figure 5-62: Supported standing.

unsupported standing and walking. Although the child may pull to stand on toes, especially in early standing, once up and well supported, the child will usually come down into a plantigrade foot position. Supported standing also allows the child to use bilateral weight-shift patterns to combine flexion with extension of lower extremities. At first, the child holds on and bounces up and down in standing to combine flexion and extension in lower extremities, trunk, and shoulders. As the child gains ability to lower self into squat, muscle components are combined through full range of motion to assist with integration of lower extremity extension patterns. As extension with stability increases in supported standing, child will experiment with rotating upper trunk on lower trunk while holding on in standing, or shifting weight in squat by rocking in different directions while holding on. Rotating and shifting weight slightly away from and back toward midline facilitates development of midline stability equilibrium for independent standing.

<u>Movement Components</u>: Extension with flexion
<u>Muscle Functions</u>: Combined mobility/stability—lower extremities
<u>Reflex/Reactions</u>: Lower extremity support reactions
<u>Postural Control/Movement Patterns</u>: Weight bearing; bilateral weight shift

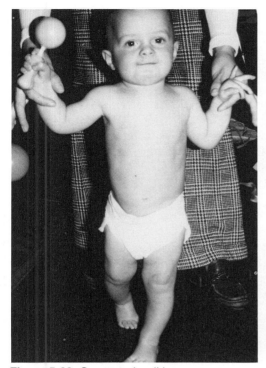

Figure 5-63: Supported walking

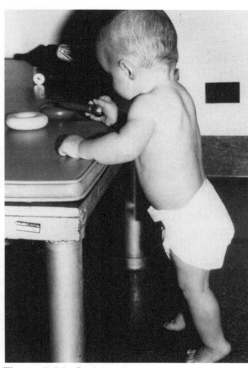

Figure 5-64: Cruising

Supported Walking (Figure 5-63)

Description and purpose. With stability in supported standing, a child can adapt lower extremity reciprocal patterns from creeping and weight-shift patterns from getting to stand in order to take steps in supported walking. Initially a child shifts weight unilaterally to one lower extremity and abducts the other extremity to step sideways, shift weight onto the abducted extremity, and adduct opposite extremity sideways. A child abducts and adducts upper extremities in coordination with lower extremity movements. Supported walking sideways around objects, such as furniture, appears between 10 and 11 months and is often called cruising (Figure 5-64). The pattern for cruising is probably adapted from pivoting in prone or sitting since the weight-shift, abduction/adduction patterns of the extremities are similar.

As balance in supported standing improves and the baby can maintain standing with a light hand hold, cruising patterns change as well. Instead of stepping sideways, the baby can hold with one hand and turn away from the supporting objects and toward the direction of movement. As a result, the baby begins supported walking forward. Walking forward with support encourages the baby to narrow the base of support by bringing lower extremities into more neutral rotation and stepping forward instead of sideways. Stepping forward with lower extremities in more neutral rotation is adapted from mature creeping. In creeping, stimulation on the dorsum of the foot during forward movement encouraged ankle dorsiflexion. In supported walking, forward lower extremity movement, accompanied by dorsiflexion of foot, leads to heel-toe pattern of upright locomotion.

Supported walking is further facilitated when the baby begins walking with first both hands and then one hand held. At first, lack of trunk control and lower extremity crossing pattern are evidence of need for further stability for walking. Often, with both hands held, a baby flexes upper extremities and adducts scapulae in order to increase extension and stability in upper trunk. Using scapular adduction to increase trunk extension is adapted from similar behaviors noted in prone extension and unsupported sitting. In supported standing, the baby uses the pattern to prepare for unsupported standing and walking. By about 12 months of age, when child is walking with trunk and lower extremity control, as long as one hand is held or holding on, a child is prepared to walk independently.

    Movement Components: Lower extremity components working together
    Muscle Functions: Blended mobility/stability—lower extremities
    Reflex/Reactions: Midline stability reactions
    Postural Control/Movement Patterns: Unilateral weight shift

Squatting (Figure 5-65)

Description and Purpose. Squatting is a behavior that begins during the transitional phase of development. A baby lowers body down from supported standing, using a bilateral movement strategy, and moves into supported squatting. Squatting without holding on requires maturation of midline stability reactions and appears with mature phase of standing/walking. As a child moves down into full flexion of lower extremities with trunk and head in upright orientation, the child can shift weight slightly away from and back toward midline without losing balance. The child relies significantly on changes in pressure on soles of feet as means for making postural adjustments of head and trunk in relation to gravity. Information from pressure receptors is combined with the vestibular response to movement in squat. The child has an opportunity to practice adjusting head and trunk to an upright orientation, while using the security of lower extremity flexion as part of a base of support rather than less controllable lower extremity extension and narrow base of foot support.

Squatting becomes a common play position for children for many years. Squat position brings a child close to the ground for numerous floor games, and is a posture from which change of position is easy. From a squat position, the child can get to standing easily, or rotate around into sitting. Squat also plays a role in blending muscle functions and smoothing out patterns of getting to stand. As noted in the information related to the positive supporting reaction, undifferentiated lower extremity and trunk extension, initially facilitated by being placed in an upright posture with stimulation on balls of feet from supporting surface, is a strong reaction. In order to decrease repeated full extension response to foot stimulation, the baby spends time in squat, which allows pressure stimulation on foot and full flexion to be combined.

    Movement Components: Flexion—lower extremities
    Muscle Functions: Blended mobility/stability
    Reflex/Reactions: Midline stability reactions
    Postural Control/Movement Patterns: Weight bearing

Standing (Figure 5-66)

Description and purpose. A child's experience with supported standing, supported walking, and getting up and down from standing facilitates development of midline stability required for independent standing. Once a child has experience holding onto support in an upright position, she can begin to experiment with letting go and balancing self momentarily. Early attempts at independent standing are characterized by wide base of lower extremity support and full range of toe flexion in an attempt to hold onto the supporting surface. Additional characteristics include upper extremity flexion with scapular adduction (high guard), either continuously or whenever balance is threatened as well as a tendency to move slightly away and back to center of gravity as a means for further development of midline stability without support in standing. As the child gains stability in standing, toe flexion decreases. Toe extension, and perhaps even ankle dorsiflexion, appear whenever a child begins to lose balance backwards. Foot dorsiflexion in response to displacement of body in space is considered part of equilibrium reactions.

Upper extremity patterns change as well. Arms come down from high guard into readiness-to-protect position, which is a position somewhere between full elbow flexion and full elbow extension. Readiness to protect implies that use of arms in high guard is not required as a means for increasing upper trunk stability. Instead, stability around the midline alone is sufficient for maintaining upper trunk in upright alignment in standing. Child begins to rely more on midline reactions and proprioceptive information from soles of feet to facilitate appropriate degree and distribution of stability in order to maintain and move in an independent standing position.

Additional means for maintaining independent standing appear after a child has had some experience with independent walking. Protective reactions in the form of stepping appear as a means for maintaining balance whenever a child moves away from the center of gravity beyond range of midline stability reactions. Falling forward produces forward walking steps. Falling sideways results in crossover steps to the side. Falling

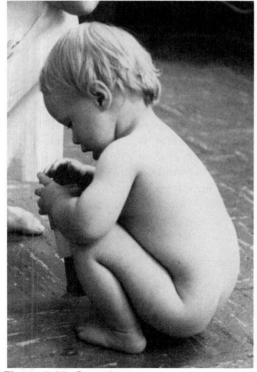

Figure 5-65: Squatting

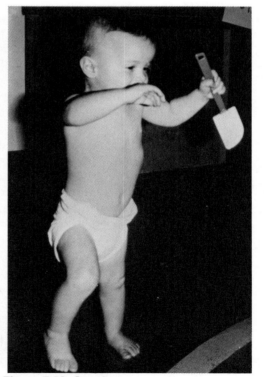

Figure 5-66: Standing

backward facilitates steps backward. When equilibrium reactions in upright are well-developed, forward loss of balance is countered by extension of neck, upper trunk, and hyperextension of shoulders and plantar flexion of feet before lower extremity protective stepping reactions are elicited. Backward loss of balance is counteracted by flexion of neck and upper trunk, forward flexion of shoulder, foot dorsiflexion, and toe extension before stepping back is used to maintain upright. Movement toward the side brings forth more classic equilibrium reactions, including neck and trunk rotation back toward center of gravity, abduction of extremities toward center of gravity, and either horizontal adduction of the opposite upper extremity to assist or abduction of that extremity in readiness to protect. If an equilibrium reaction is insufficient for maintaining balance, crossover stepping may be used for catching balance. Generally, loss of balance in any direction elicits protective reactions from upper extremities when all other recovery or lower extremity protective reactions have been unsuccessful. But once equilibrium is well established and combined with patterns of movement developed with walking, coordinated movement in standing can be adapted to skilled activities or games requiring movement in standing, such as batting a ball or dancing in place.

Movement Components: All movement components working together

Muscle Functions: Blended mobility/stability

Reflex/Reactions: Midline stability; equilibrium reactions

Postural Control/Movement Patterns: Contralateral weight shift

Walking (Figure 5-67)

Description and purpose. By the time a child begins walking, most of the components for walking have already developed, along with creeping, sitting, rolling, and independent standing; for example, control over vertical alignment of head and trunk in space, weight shift/movement patterns of trunk and extremities, and reciprocal movement of extremities. The average age for walking is usually 13 months, although many children walk earlier and others may not walk until 15 months or more. First signs of independent walking appear when a child takes a few steps from object to object, after pulling up or being placed in standing. If the child falls, or wants to move rapidly or greater distances, more established creeping patterns are called forth for locomotion.

Development of consistent independent walking includes enough control to rise to standing from middle of floor independently (Figure 5-68), start and stop walking with support, and catch self when falling. Early walking depends on protective reactions, both upper extremity protective extension and lower extremity stepping, as a means for child to lean forward in standing and take steps. During early walking, a child delights in propelling self forward, falling down, getting up, and trying again. Walking is such a joy for children that once experienced it becomes a child's preferred mode of locomotion, even for covering short distances. Intrinsic motivation previously termed "walking for the sake of walking" is quickly adapted to extrinsic motivation of walking from place to place and object to object.

Initially, a child uses upper body stabilization as a means for controlling upright posture while simultaneously shifting weight to one lower extremity and stepping forward with opposite lower extremity. Upper body posture of scapular adduction and upper extremity flexion is adapted from a pattern developed with pivot prone and used to facilitate spinal extension in prone and again in sitting and standing. The pattern is even more obvious and more likely to recur in independent walking because stress associated with maintaining and moving in an upright posture requires reinforcement

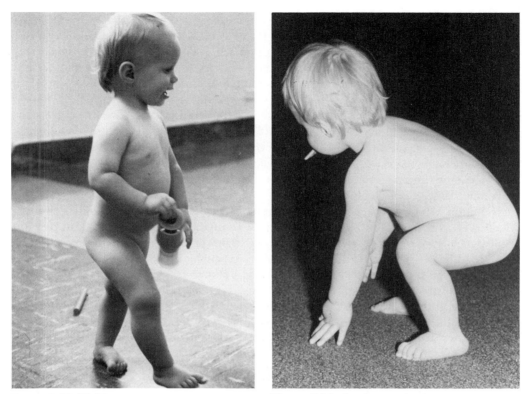

Figure 5-67: Walking   **Figure 5-68:** Getting to stand

of extension. Stabilization is also reinforced if the child walks while holding small objects in hands. Holding objects for stability is adapted from supported walking with hand held, and probably gives a child a sense of support for walking independently.

When the child is using upper body stabilization for upright postural control, walking is characterized by unilateral weight shift from side to side with lateral trunk flexion. Early walking is a two-step process of shifting weight to one lower extremity and stepping forward with opposite lower extremity, using combined hip and knee flexion and contact with foot flat on surface. Walking is with a waddling type of gait characterized by side-to-side weight shift. Once the child has experienced early walking, posture and movement strategies from previous developmental progressions are adapted to walking and modify both postural control and movement patterns in upright. Adaptation of midline stability and equilibrium reactions modify postural control in walking and facilitate changes in weight-shift and extremity patterns of movement. Midline stability and equilibrium reactions promote blending of flexion and extension along midline of neck and trunk, and adaptation of rotation to the child's ability to shift weight and move forward at the same time. At first, midline stability is evident when upper extremities assume a readiness-to-protect position part way between full flexion and full extension. In a readiness position, upper extremities can either resume flexion to reinforce trunk extension as needed, or extend to protect if balance is lost.

With rotation, the child begins to develop contralateral weight-shift patterns and use arms and legs in reciprocal patterns of movement. Contralateral weight shift allows upper part of body to rotate in an opposite direction from the lower part of body so that the arm on one side swings forward while leg on opposite side swings forward for heel strike. The other arm swings back while other leg engages in push-off for next step. Pelvic rotation becomes a major source of control over lower extremity movement from push-off to heel strike. Rotation-counterrotation between shoulders and pelvis results in reciprocal extremity movement patterns. Observation of reciprocal upper and lower extremity patterns, as well as narrower base of support in walking, are indications that blended muscle functions, facilitated by midline stability and equilibrium reactions, are supporting contralateral weight-shift patterns of control.

A child's experience with walking, and later running, smooths out the pattern so that shifting weight and stepping forward occur simultaneously as a one-step process. Lower extremity components include pelvic rotation, hip flexion, knee extension, and ankle dorsiflexion. Heel strike and push-off modify the flat-footed gait of early walking. Moving from heel strike to push-off changes stimulation on soles of feet and provides information about position in space and speed of movement. Information from stimulation to soles of feet, along with visual and vestibular information, enhances rapid adjustments in posture and movement during walking.

By 22 months, children seldom fall while walking, can walk fast, and attempt stairs by holding on and taking one step at a time. As running begins, walking becomes even more coordinated. By 24 months, children may walk down stairs holding on; by 30 months, they can alternate feet going up stairs; and by 36 months, they can alternate feet going down stairs.

> Movement Components: All movement components working together
> Muscle Functions: Blended mobility/stability
> Reflex/Reactions: Midline stability; equilibrium reactions
> Postural Control/Movement Patterns: Contralateral weight shift

Manipulative Prehension

Manipulative prehension develops from a baby's innate motivation to explore and manipulate the environment, combined with stimulation from persons and objects in the environment. Reach for exploration and grasp for manipulation are, therefore, both intrinsically and extrinsically motivated. Reaching develops along with behaviors previously described in this chapter; i.e., prone-creeping, supine-sitting, and rolling. Grasp and accompanying release begin with reflex activity and are integrated when higher level functions develop in the hand itself, as well as the rest of the body. For example, early attempts at grasping objects are influenced by a grasp reflex. As soon as an object touches the palm of a baby's hand, all the fingers flex fully on the object. But, after palm of the hand has been desensitized with weight bearing, and baby develops more isolated finger motions with maturation, baby can respond to touch of objects with appropriate amount and type of flexion required for grasping the object. Objects, as well as neuro-muscular functions, shape the direction and type of grasp required for hand adaptation to objects. Once grasp patterns are developed and adapted to holding objects, further maturation of hand functions supports manipulation of objects grasped by the hand.

Upper extremities functions can be considered either automatic or volitional. Automatic functions include weight bearing, weight shifting, protecting, and balancing. Development of these automatic functions have already been described in this chapter. Volitional functions include reaching, grasping, releasing, and manipulation, and develop in a sequence from controlled reach to controlled grasp to controlled release to controlled manipulation. Control over volitional functions depends on development and adaptation of automatic functions to volitional functions. For example, weight bearing on upper extremities, which develops stability, precedes reaching into space with upper extremity. Weight shifting onto upper extremity, which develops combined mobility-stability, precedes accurate, graded reaching into space, which depends on blended mobility-stability. In addition to adaptation of mobility and stability developed during weight bearing and weight shifting, separation between humerus and scapula, also gained during developmental sequences, frees the upper extremity from general body movement, so that movement away from and toward body is both possible and controlled.

Reaching includes both movement and direction of movement of the baby's arm and hand in space. Reaching places the hand in contact with the environment so that grasp responses can develop and be adapted to specific functions. Reaching requires separation of the upper extremity from the rest of the body, as well as upper extremity proximal control over movement in order to accommodate to spatial and temporal dimensions of moving in space. Activation of upper extremity function through various planes of movement with varying degrees of support from body and environment facilitates both separation and control. In supine, reaching begins with swiping at objects, first to the side and later at midline. Swiping, and later reaching in supine, contributes to development of flexion and flexion-extension of upper extremity against gravity, as well as first separation between scapula and humerus. The supine position promotes scapular stability since pressure on scapulae from supporting surface holds scapulae against trunk, even before musculature for scapular stability has developed (Figure 5-69). As baby reaches out to the side or up toward objects at midline, scapulae are basically held against upper trunk, while arms move away from and back toward trunk. Bringing hands to midline also is enhanced in supine, since baby can bring hands together across chest before developing ability to bring hands together and hold against gravity at the same time. Hands to midline eventually supports transfer of objects and crossing the midline functions.

In prone, reaching begins with achievement of on-elbows and on-hands postures (Figure 5-70). Once a baby in on-elbows position can maintain and bear weight on one upper extremity, the other upper extremity is free to reach forward in order to move body forward, or to obtain a toy. Reaching from prone facilitates extension of upper

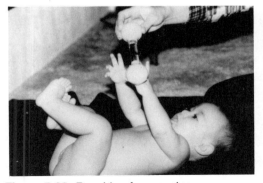

Figure 5-69: Reaching from supine

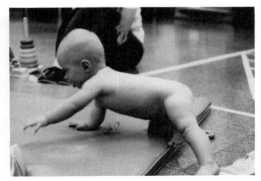

Figure 5-70: Reaching from prone

extremity against gravity. When upper trunk-scapular stability is well enough established to hold scapulae close to the trunk, separation between scapula and humerus also is enhanced. Reaching from prone to move body forward is repeated with each mode of crawling and creeping. In order for baby to adapt reaching to move to reaching for an object, the reaching pattern is differentiated from full crawling or creeping pattern. The baby maintains posture on tummy or on hands-knees and reaches forward just with arm to contact object.

In rolling, reaching begins with deliberate rolling as baby uses upper extremity to assist movement of body in space (Figure 5-71). A baby develops reaching in a pattern of horizontal adduction, which enhances ability to bring hands to midline and to cross midline with upper extremity. Once automatic rolling patterns and sidelying postures are established, the baby can differentiate reaching to roll from complete rolling pattern. Reaching in a horizontal plane across body can then be used to obtain objects on opposite side of body. Crossing midline with extremities and simultaneous maintenance of stable posture usually implies that equilibrium reactions are present. In fact, once reaching is differentiated from the supine, prone, or rolling sequence, which facilitated reach, equilibrium and midline stability patterns make it possible for a person to use reaching purposefully in all planes of movement.

Release of objects held in hand develops along with grasp. Early grasping patterns are stimulated by touch on the palm of the hand. The reflexive nature of early grasp often produces strong, ungraded flexion of fingers, which is difficult to blend with finger extension. As a result, a baby may grasp an object easily, but have difficulty releasing the object. Release can be facilitated by child's use of environment, or own body, before extension is well enough developed for voluntary release.

Before 4 months of age, objects may be placed in baby's hand and be retained momentarily. Release is usually involuntary as a result of general movement of the upper extremity, or touch on the hand itself. Once a baby can voluntarily reach and grasp objects, and bring hands to midline in supine, mouthing objects is possible. Mouthing assists with early release because if a child can stabilize an object in the mouth, pulling the hand off the object is much easier (Figure 5-72). By 6 or 7 months of age, transferring object from one hand to another serves a similar purpose; i.e., child stabilizes object with receiving hand and releases hold with other hand. Initially, object is pulled from the holding hand, but with more control over extension of fingers, pulling and releasing occur simultaneously. Baby needs stability of receiving hand becoming holding hand in order to activate finger extension.

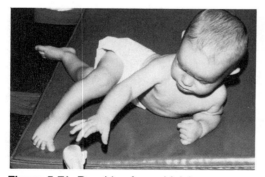

Figure 5-71: Reaching from sidelying

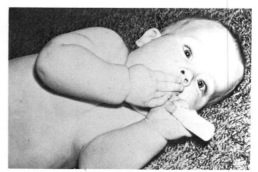

Figure 5-72: Object mouthing

By 7 months of age extension of upper extremities, including fingers, is developing rapidly along with protective and support reactions. Baby begins to drop objects down from a height, like the highchair. Dropping objects requires a full extension pattern of the extremity, and represents the beginning of voluntary release of a supporting object. Baby watches objects dropped and seems to enjoy control over movement of objects. Cause-effect relationships and object permanence are enhanced by dropping, and later throwing, objects.

By 10 to 11 months, a child is picking up smaller objects between thumb and fingers and release is also refined. In order to execute extension of fingers without using extension of rest of extremity, child returns to support by resting ulnar side of hand on supporting surface or another object. With support, more controlled extension of thumb and fingers for release is possible. By about 1 year of age or so, voluntary release without support is developing, although a child will work for many months, even years, to control the range of finger extension required to release certain objects, as well as timing release for accurate completion of some tasks.

Grasp and manipulation support a child's drive to obtain and explore objects in the environment. Grasp and manipulation develop along with developmental sequences described in this chapter. Primitive, transitional, and mature grasp patterns will be described, along with some significant oral motor and visual-motor behaviors that accompany development of grasp and manipulation. Key behaviors associated with development of manipulative prehension (Figure 5-73) include

Primitive Phase
Primary Grasp
Primary Release
Swiping

Transitional Phase
Scratching
Crude Palmar Grasp
Reach and Pat
Palmar Grasp
Index Probing
Instinctive Grasp

Mature Phase
Visual Orientation
Inferior Pinch
Superior Pinch
Prehension
Manipulative Prehension

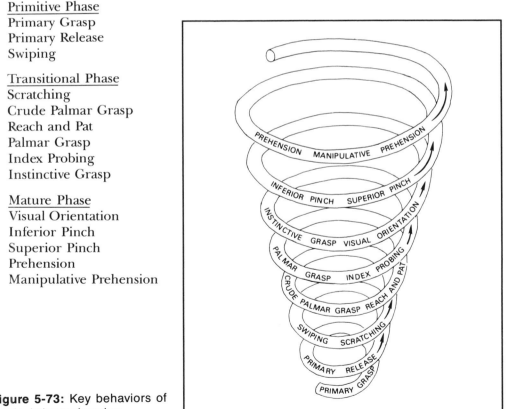

Figure 5-73: Key behaviors of manipulative prehension

Primary Grasp (Figures 5-74 and 5-75)

<u>Description and purpose</u>. Primary grasp activates flexor components of the hand and upper extremity. Pressure on the palm of the hand during the newborn period elicits flexion of fingers, followed by palmar flexion of the wrist and flexion of the elbow. Total flexion of the extremity in response to pressure on palm activates flexor components through full range of motion and is known as the traction response. If traction response is strong, it would be possible (although not desirable) to lift the baby off a supporting surface by applying pressure to palms and holding hands. Traction may be a forerunner to behaviors that develop with pull to sit at higher levels of development. If traction persists under dysfunctional conditions, objects placed in a child's hand will be grasped and pulled toward a child's body, greatly interfering with visual inspection and manipulation of objects.

<u>Movement Components</u>: Flexion
<u>Muscle Functions</u>: Mobility
<u>Reflex/Reactions</u>: Traction
<u>Postural Control/Movement Patterns</u>: None

Between 1 and 2 months, traction response of primary grasp is modified to a grasp reflex (Figure 5-73). With the grasp reflex, pressure on palm elicits flexion of fingers, but not the rest of the extremity. Flexion is usually stronger on ulnar side of hand. Thumb may be adducted to radial side of hand or in palm. Ability to flex fingers without eliciting a pattern of total extremity flexion is significant for development of reach and grasp, since a child must be able to maintain extension for reach while simultaneously manipulating objects away from the body, using finger flexion. Modification of traction to grasp

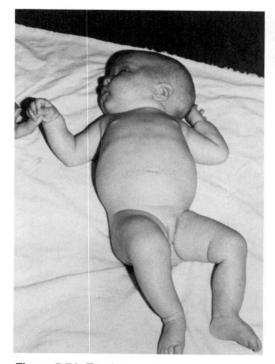

Figure 5-74: Traction response

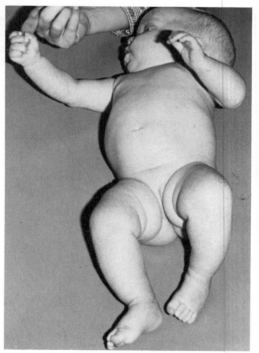

Figure 5-75: Grasp reflex

reflex is due in part to appearance of increased neck rotation and accompanying asymmetrical tonic neck reflex. When the baby perceives touch on palm and turns head toward source of stimulation, the ATNR facilitates extension in upper extremity on face side, modifying tendency to flex due to traction.

If dysfunction is present, grasp reflex may continue to cause the child to flex fingers when an object is placed in hand. Sustained grasp reflex interferes with development of release. If ATNR continues to influence postural tone, it will be difficult to flex the extremity and bring objects to mouth or transfer them to other hand.

Movement Components: Flexion—fingers; extension—upper extremity

Muscle Functions: Mobility—fingers; stability—upper extremity

Reflex/Reactions: Grasp reflex; asymmetrical atonic neck reflex

Postural Control/Movement Patterns: Weight bearing

Primary Release (Figure 5-76)

Description and purpose. In order for a baby to release as well as grasp objects, extension needs to develop in the hand, along with flexion. During the newborn period, the avoiding response facilitates extension of fingers. Later, posture and movement strategies that promote extension throughout the upper extremity will also influence development of more mature release. Avoiding response elicits extension in fingers in response to a light touch on the hand, especially dorsum of the hand. Fingers extend momentarily and return to partially flexed or flexed posture. Touch on the hand may come from a person, or from the baby contacting objects, like blankets, in the environment. Extension of fingers elicited by touch and other assimilations may be forerunners to voluntary finger extension, which appears at higher levels of development. Other sources for stimulation of extension during the primitive phase of development include Moro reflex and ATNR, which facilitate finger extension as part of upper extremity extension patterns.

Movement Components: Extension

Muscle Functions: Mobility

Reflex/Reactions: Avoiding, Moro, ATNR

Postural Control/Movement Patterns: Weight bearing

Two other factors significantly influence development of reach and grasp, and will be noted as appropriate in description of key behaviors of grasp. One is a baby's ability to bring hand and objects to mouth (Figures 5-72, 5-77), and the other is baby's ability to visually track objects, own hand, objects and hand together, and use vision to direct hand movement (Figure 5-78). Only minimal information on vision considered essential to discussing development of reach and grasp is presented here. There is extensive literature available regarding development of vision and visual perception in infants.

Getting hand into mouth allows a baby to explore hand through tactile reception before visual inspection is possible. Tactile receptors around the mouth are more mature and discriminating at birth because of their survival functions. Hand to mouth also allows baby to explore mouth with hand, adding to development of oral-motor functions. Later, a child will bring objects to mouth for manipulation of the object and facilitation of some upper extremity movement components.

Infants' ability to use vision for "grasping" the environment is more advanced than hand grasp functions. As a result, a baby has many opportunities to view hand, hand in motion, objects, and objects in motion before actually adapting hand to grasp objects in space. During primitive phase of development, a newborn can visually fix on objects or

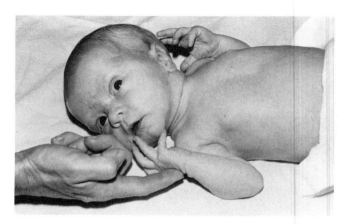

Figure 5-76: Primary release

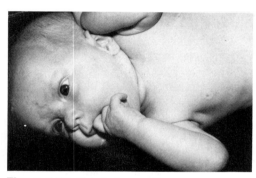

Figure 5-77: Hands-to-mouth

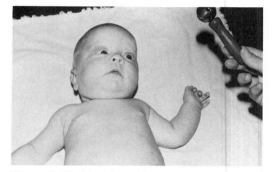

Figure 5-78: Visual tracking

faces, move eyes with head, and soon differentiate eye movement from hand movement. By 1 month, baby fixes longer on objects and may track moving objects to midline; by 2 months, focus increases, may track past midline with hesitation, and may demonstrate some vertical tracking; by 3 months, convergence at midline, midline regard for objects, especially shifting gaze from object to object, tracking 180° horizontally across midline, and vertical tracking, which is more upward than downward, appear.

Swiping (Figure 5-79)

<u>Description and purpose</u>. By about 3 months of age, baby has increased opportunities to view hand in space and begins to swipe at objects. The ATNR brings the hand into baby's visual field on one side. Baby has an opportunity to view own hand for longer periods of time due to the primitive postural stability provided by an ATNR. At 3 months there also is an increase in baby's ability to focus on objects in space (Figure 5-80). If an object such as a rattle comes into view, a baby can glance from hand to rattle and attempt to contact the rattle by swiping at it. Movement from the shoulder is activated against gravity. Fingers will often flex in either primitive anticipation of grasp or means to control shoulder movement, or both. Baby usually cannot maintain visual gaze on an object while moving hand toward it, thus, looks away after initiating movement. Swiping represents early reaching for objects, perhaps visually initiated, but not yet visually guided or posturally controlled. If dysfunction is present, difficulty initiating and

controlling swiping-type movement is frequently observed, even at later ages. Maintaining visual contact with object during reaching may also be difficult, perhaps because integrating movement and visual information is not developing.

Movement Components: Neck rotation; upper extremity flexion/extension
Muscle Functions: Mobility
Reflex/Reactions: Asymmetrical tonic neck reflex
Postural Control/Movement Patterns: Weight bearing

By the end of the primitive phase, baby is weight bearing on fisted hands in prone, able to change weight bearing from radial to ulnar or ulnar to radial side of hand by turning head, and is beginning to bring hand to mouth in supine. Weight bearing on fisted hands increases stretch of finger extensors and helps facilitate active finger extension in weight-bearing and non-weight-bearing postures (Figure 5-81). Turning head in prone weight bearing elicits an asymmetrical tonic neck posture in baby's arms and shifts weight bearing between ulnar and radial sides of hands (Figure 5-82). Early weight shifting prepares for ulnar side to provide stability for radial mobility, either playing with toys in weight bearing, or cutting with scissors in non-weight bearing. In supine, baby's experience with swiping facilitates more flexion in upper extremity and allows baby to bring hand to mouth as long as head is turned toward one side, eliminating some effect of gravity on flexion. Hand to mouth control allows baby to choose hand mouthing at any time. As baby keeps head more in midline and hand follows, flexor patterns develop which can act against gravity.

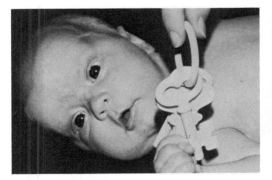

Figure 5-79: Swiping

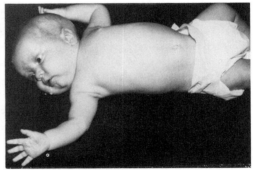

Figure 5-80: Hand regard

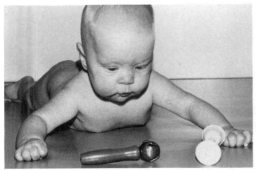

Figure 5-81: Weight bearing on fisted hands

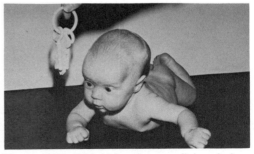

Figure 5-82: Weight-bearing—radial and ulnar sides

Scratching (Figure 5-83)

<u>Description and purpose</u>. By 4 months, baby can support on elbows with weight distributed between hands, forearms, and elbows, and can bring hands together across chest in supine position. When hands are in contact with supporting surfaces or own body, babies seem to enjoy scratching the surface, using alternating flexion and extension of all fingers together. Scratching provides an opportunity for a baby to develop full range of reciprocal finger flexion and extension. Since distal finger joints are resting on a supporting surface, combined flexion and extension also begins to develop with scratching. As baby continues to use scratching, especially when sitting supported in chair, fingers can be isolated so that movement of one or two fingers is differentiated from movement of all fingers together. Besides facilitating movement, scratchhing provides tactile information about different surfaces and assists with development of tactile discrimination in the fingertips. Scratching is adapted to raking movement of hand, which leads to development of crude palmar grasp.

<u>Movement Components</u>: Flexion; extension
<u>Muscle Functions</u>: Mobility; combined mobility/stability
<u>Reflex/Reactions</u>: Vertical righting reaction; support reactions
<u>Postural Control/Movement Patterns</u>: Weight bearing

Crude Palmar Grasp (Figure 5-84)

<u>Description and purpose</u>. Between 4 and 5 months, a baby reaches out with crude palmar grasp, places hand on top of an object, and rakes the object toward self. Crude palmar grasp is adapted from swiping, but can be initiated with a forward reaching pattern from either prone or supported sitting. In prone on-elbows, baby must shift weight unilaterally to reach with one extremity and use crude grasp.

Baby can partially extend fingers during reaching, due to lack of complete control over reaching. As a result, baby cannot adjust the hand to size or position of object, but only crudely places hand on the object. Palmar grasp means that the hand is in a pronated position and objects are grasped between fingers and palm of hand, more on the ulnar side at first, but later on the radial side of the hand.

<u>Movement Components</u>: Extension; flexion
<u>Muscle Functions</u>: Mobility; stability; early blending mobility/stability
<u>Reflex/Reactions</u>: Vertical righting
<u>Postural Control/Movement Patterns</u>: Beginning unilateral weight shift on elbows

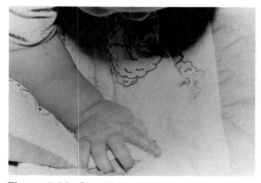

Figure 5-83: Scratching/raking

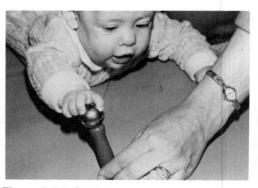

Figure 5-84: Crude grasp

Reach and Pat (Figure 5-85)

Description and purpose. Around 5 months of age, reaching becomes more accurate due to repetition of the pattern itself and increased postural control. Besides reaching to grasp objects, a baby reaches out and pats objects, such as the highchair tray, a mirror, or a face. Patting facilitates finger extension while simultaneously inhibiting effect of grasp reflex. When a baby pats on objects, there is stimulation to the palm of the hand. However, during patting a baby actively maintains fingers in full extension and does not respond to palm pressure with flexion, or flex fingers to control movement of arm. Additional facilitation to finger extensors is also occurring in prone on-hands posture and through development of upper extremity protective reactions.

Movement Components: Extension

Muscle Functions: Stability; mobility

Reflex/Reactions: Protective; support; vertical righting reactions

Postural control/Movement Patterns: None

Palmar Grasp (Figure 5-86)

Description and purpose. Crude palmar grasp is adapted to palmar grasp about 6 months of age. A baby reaches out with fingers extended and forearm pronated, contacts an object, and grasps it between flexed fingers and palm of hand. Thumb is out of palm, but does not participate much in grasp at this point in time. Forearm remains pronated, regardless of orientation of object, so that object orientation must be changed to accommodate hand position (note position of dog's tail in Figure 5-86). Grasp remains palmar regardless of size of object, so that even small objects are taken between fingers and palm, and sometimes "lost" in the palm. Palmar grasp in prone on-elbows is supported by controlled unilateral weight-shift patterns that enhance accuracy of reach and finger movement.

As baby adapts palmar grasp to a variety of situations, grasp pattern itself is modified. Between 6 and 7 months, fingers on the ulnar side of hand press object more toward radial fingers and thumb may adduct against the object. Palmar grasp is then more radial-palmar and prepares for development of prehension on radial side of hand.

Movement Components: Extension; flexion; adduction; abduction

Muscle Functions: Blended mobility/stability

Reflex/Reactions: Vertical righting reactions

Postural Control/Movement Patterns: Unilateral weight shift

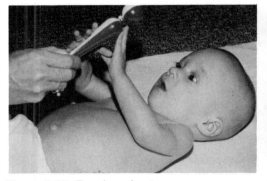

Figure 5-85: Reach and pat

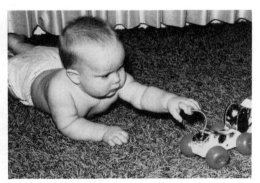

Figure 5-86: Palmar grasp

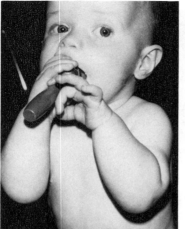

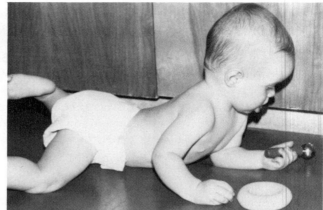

Figure 5-88: Full supination

Figure 5-87: Mouthing for object manipulation

Even though grasp functions are developing rapidly, the hand is still being used primarily in a pronated position and baby continues to take objects to mouth in order to manipulate and thoroughly investigate the objects (Figure 5-87). Once a child can bring hand and object to midline and secure object in mouth, the object can then be manipulated, transferred, or released more easily than using hands alone. Manipulation of objects in mouth requires movement through ranges of forearm supination-pronation and wrist flexion-extension. Baby uses mouth to stabilize objects while rotating forearm to change grasp on object and simultaneously combines mobility and stability functions in forearm.

Hand to mouth also assists baby with release of small objects, such as cereal, which baby has secured between fingers and palm. In order to remove small object with mouth, baby must supinate forearm and extend fingers as hand reaches mouth. Combinations of supination and finger extension modify palmar grasp at higher levels of development.

Active supination of forearm is developing, however, and can be adapted to baby's reaching and grasping patterns (Figure 5-88). Supination develops as functions within upper extremity are differentiated so that forearm can rotate in and out of supination and pronation while upper arm remains stable and provides control for forearm rotation. Active forearm rotation usually appears in an on-elbows posture first, since weight bearing on-elbows enhances stability of more proximal joint functions. In prone on-elbows, supination allows baby to visually investigate objects held in hand. Visual information about objects is integrated with tactile information obtained by mouthing objects. During this time, babies are often observed to visually inspect an object, then "mouth" the object, then look at object again, seeming to compare information from both sources. Besides enhancing visual-tactile integration, supination also significantly changes child's ability to direct grasp patterns.

By about 7 months, visual perception of hand and object, as well as ability to release objects, is enhanced by baby's ability to transfer objects from hand to hand (Figure 5-89). During transfer, a baby becomes engrossed in glancing from hand to object and object to hand in preparation for visual guidance of movement. Visually scanning during transfer, as well as during other grasping activities, allows baby to identify distinctive features of hands in relation to objects. Transfer also enhances release of grasp on objects, since baby can take object from one hand with the other hand with only minimal finger extension required for release. When supination is adapted to transfer, child is able to manipulate objects between hands. Bilateral use of hands for manipulation, as well as maturation of neuromuscular functions within the hand itself, facilitates differentiation of finger and thumb functions required for manipulative prehension.

Index Probing (Figure 5-90)

<u>Description and Purpose</u>. Around 7 or 8 months of age, a baby begins to isolate index finger extension and use index finger to poke or probe objects and move small objects around. To isolate index finger extension, baby flexes fingers on ulnar side of hand and uses ulnar flexion as stability for index finger activation. Index finger is more easily isolated in extension due to additional neuromuscular capability for extension. Index finger probing allows baby to explore small objects and small spaces, and increases sensitivity of index finger in preparation for prehension.

Baby adapts components from scratching and crude palmar grasp to develop more ability with index finger. Blending flexion with finger extension allows baby to pull small objects into the palm with a raking-type movement. At higher levels of development, objects will be moved toward thumb with index finger in preparation for pincer grasp.

<u>Movement Components</u>: Extension; flexion
<u>Muscle Functions</u>: Blended mobility/stability
<u>Reflex/Reactions</u>: Vertical righting reactions
<u>Postural Control/Movement Patterns</u>: Unilateral weight shift

Instinctive Grasp (Figures 5-91 and 5-92)

<u>Description and purpose</u>. Instinctive grasp allows child to adjust position of hand to position of object in space, and thereby increase efficiency and effectiveness of grasping patterns. As child reaches toward an object with hand in pronated position, there is a tendency to direct the radial side of the hand to contact the object. Predominance of previously acquired radial palmar grasp and increased sensitivity of radial side of hand,

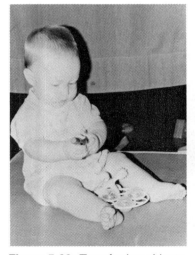

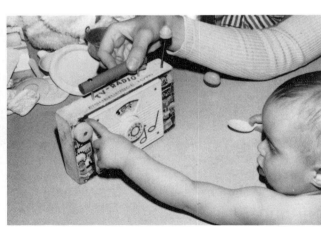

Figure 5-89: Transferring objects   **Figure 5-90:** Index probing

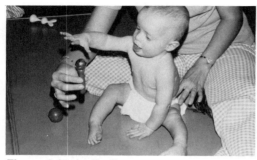

Figure 5-91: Instinctive grasp

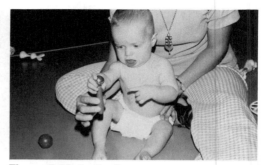

Figure 5-92: Instinctive grasp

particularly from index finger probing, influences direction of hand-to-object contact. When child contacts object with radial side of hand, tactile assimilation on side of hand facilitates a tendency for hand to adjust to position of object for grasp and integrate supination as a means for changing position of hand in relation to object. As a result, objects that are in vertical alignment in relation to pronated, palm-down hand can be grasped as efficiently as objects in horizontal alignment to pronated hand, as long as object touches radial side of hand prior to grasping. Instinctive grasp expands manipulative ability of the hand by facilitating hand adjustment to objects through touch.

<u>Movement Components</u>: Forearm supination

<u>Muscle Functions</u>: Mobility; stability

<u>Reflex/Reactions</u>: Vertical righting; equilibrium reactions

<u>Postural Control/Movement Patterns</u>: Unilateral weight shift; contralateral weight shift

By the end of the transitional phase, child has sufficient postural control from trunk and shoulders to reach accurately in any direction and from any position. Mature hand functions emerge as child uses visual information and various objects to direct and differentiate grasp patterns.

Visual Orientation (Figure 5-93)

<u>Description and purpose</u>. Visual orientation allows child to adjust position of head in relation to position of object using visual information instead of only tactile information. As a result, child can anticipate optimum hand position and adjust hand before actually touching object. Adjusting hand in anticipation smooths out patterns of reach and grasp, which enhances efficiency and effectiveness of child's manipulative abilities. Using vision to direct reach and type of grasp implies that more mature eye-hand coordination is beginning to emerge as well. With visual orientation, child adjusts hand position prior to or while in process of reaching to grasp an object. Thus, the object is grasped in the most appropriate manner and child is ready to begin manipulating object.

<u>Movement Components</u>: Extension; supination/pronation; finger flexion

<u>Muscle Functions</u>: Blended mobility/stability

<u>Reflex/Reactions</u>: Midline stability reactions; equilibrium reactions

<u>Postural Control/Movement Patterns</u>: Contralateral weight shift

Grasp patterns change from palmar to prehensive grasp when functions within the hand are differentiated, and increased sensitivity on radial side of hand encourages use of thumb and fingers on that side. Differentiation of hand functions includes isolation of

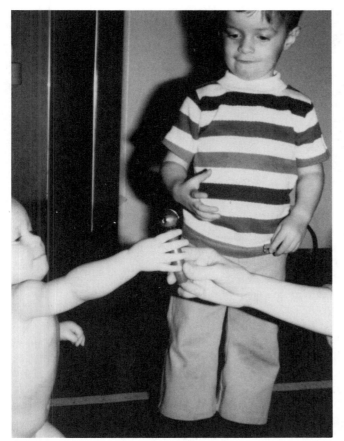

Figure 5-93: Visual orientation

finger movements and distribution of stability functions on ulnar side, and mobility functions on radial side of hand. Child is motivated to grasp small objects more precisely and adapts differentiated functions to develop prehension patterns. Description of prehension presented in this text represents basic concepts about prehension. Basic concepts include the idea that thumb and finger or fingers come together as alternate means for grasping and manipulating small objects. During first attempts to grasp between thumb and finger, thumb moves in same plane as hand (inferior pinch). As prehension matures, thumb rotates to a position perpendicular to palm of hand (superior pinch). Prehension requires stability as well as mobility in hand, including finger joints, in order to manipulate small objects held between thumb and fingers.

Inferior Pinch (Figure 5-94)

<u>Description and Purpose</u>. Inferior pinch describes pattern used to grasp objects between thumb and radial side of index finger with thumb moving in plane of hand. Inferior pinch is adapted from index finger probing between 8 and 9 months of age. As the child is using index finger to move small objects, rather than using palmar grasp to obtain object, she brings thumb over to index finger and picks up object. Child's hand must be resting on supporting surface in order to use ulnar stability as background control for thumb to index finger movement. Inferior pinch initiates thumb to finger

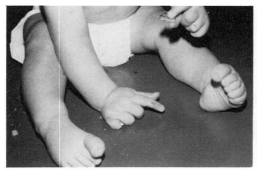

Figure 5-94: Inferior pinch.

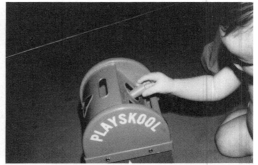

Figure 5-95: Superior pinch

patterns of movement, which are adapted to higher levels of prehension. An inferior pattern continues to be used for some activities, such as grasping a key.

Movement Components: Thumb abduction/adduction; finger extension

Muscle Functions: Blended mobility/stability

Reflex/Reactions: Midline stability reactions; equilibrium reaction

Postural Control/Movement Patterns: Contralateral weight shift

Superior Pinch (Figure 5-95)

Description and Purpose. Superior pinch describes a pattern used to grasp objects between the pad of thumb and pad of index or middle finger, or both. In order for thumb-finger pads to come together, child must be able to rotate thumb into a position perpendicular to plane of hand, which would not be possible with inferior pinch. Inferior pinch requires support from surface. But, as child gains control over thumb and finger movement, less support is required. Child rests only fingertips on surface, which creates possibility that thumb can rotate to contact finger pad and adapt inferior to superior pinch. Superior pinch is similar to radial digital grasp and usually develops by 10 to 12 months of age. Once developed, and combined with upper extremity reactions, superior pinch can be used to grasp and place objects without requiring support from surface for control. Control over finger and thumb movement depends on blending of mobility and stability functions of finger flexors and extensions, rather than external support. In order to control timing of finger movement, child tends to hold fingers extended while flexing at metacarpal phalangeal (MCP) joints. Extension of finger digits supports prehensive-type grasp, but not precise selection or manipulation of objects.

Movement Components: MCP flexion with finger extension; thumb rotation

Muscle Functions: Blended mobility/stability

Reflex/Reactions: Midline stability reactions; equilibrium reactions

Postural Control/Movement Patterns: Contralateral weight shift

Prehension (Figure 5-96)

Description and Purpose. Prehension occurs when child can bring tips of thumb and index finger together in a precise, controlled movement. Prehension is adapted from superior pinch. Superior pinch is modified to prehension when child gains control over flexion and extension of interphalangeal (IP) joints. Control of IP flexion-extension allows child to flex finger digit just enough to bring thumb-finger tips together instead of bringing only finger-thumb pads together. Tip prehension adds significantly to

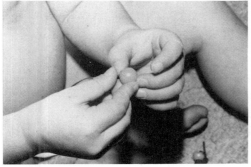

Figure 5-96: Prehension

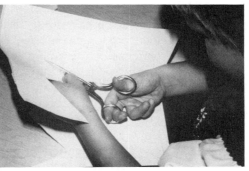

Figure 5-97: Manipulative prehension

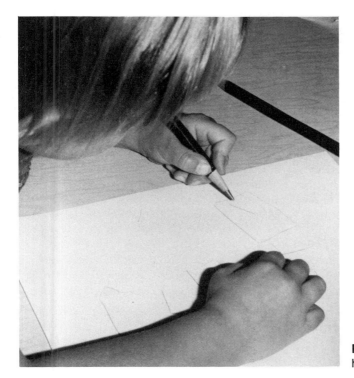

Figure 5-98: Manipulative prehension

precision for handling small objects and developing fine motor skill. The size, shape, and purpose of object determine type of prehension or pinch used by child.

<u>Movement Components</u>: IP flexion/extension; thumb rotation
<u>Muscle Functions</u>: Blended mobility/stability
<u>Reflex/Reactions</u>: Midline stability reactions; equilibrium reactions
<u>Postural Control Movement Patterns</u>: Contralateral weight shift

Manipulative Prehension (Figures 5-97 and 5-98)

<u>Description and purpose</u>. Manipulative prehension describes use of prehension to not only hold an object but also to move the object in place for a specific purpose. Examples of manipulative prehension include writing with a pencil or cutting with a

scissors. For manipulative prehension, stability through wrist and metacarpal phalangeal joints provides background, while blended mobility and stability functions in finger digits allow child to hold and simultaneously move an object in relation to another object. Exact patterns of movement related to manipulative prehension are learned according to specific purpose—for example, the precise movement required to form a certain letter or cut along a specific line.

Movement Components: All components working together
Muscle Functions: Blended mobility/stability
Reflex/Reactions: Midline stability reactions; equilibrium reactions
Postural Control/Movement Patterns: Contralateral weight shift

Prehension and manipulative prehension patterns continue to mature during the first 5 to 6 years of life. Patterns are developed according to sensorimotor-sensory and cognitive demands of activities requiring prehension. Through repetition of purposeful prehension sequences, patterns emerge which encompass essential components of prehension, but are unique to the individual using the pattern.

Summary

The spiraling process of adaptation has been illustrated by exploring progressive development of five basic developmental behaviors. The behaviors were related to child's potential and drive to achieve an upright posture, and explore and manipulate the environment. Development of locomotion and manipulative prehension represent culmination of child's development quest. Principles of adaptation, including adaptation of new-to-old and old-to-new behaviors, and effect of spatiotemporal stress on development, were evident throughout discussion of development sequences.

Figures 5-99 and 5-100 provide a pictorial summary of behaviors discussed and chronological relationships.

Key Points

1. Developmental sequences leading to upright functioning not only facilitate components required for standing and walking, but also contribute to development of reaching and, hence, grasping.
2. The hard-wired aspect of the human nervous system is comprised of certain genetic endowments that are "pre-programmed" with specific behavioral drives.
3. The soft-wired system contributes to ways in which a child can smooth out and time movements in purposeful sequences of adaptation and, eventually, in skill performance.
4. In general, strategies used for developmental sequences leading to upright are adapted to purposeful sequences used for gross motor skills; strategies used for reach and grasp are adapted to purposeful sequences used for fine motor skills.
5. Key behaviors signify an identifiable point at which a child is adapting previously acquired behaviors to achieve a new behavior, or modifying a previously acquired behavior because of environmental transactions.
6. Posture and movement strategies used during primitive development are often part of abnormal behavior that accompanies CNS dysfunction.
7. As a basic developmental behavior, the sequence for creeping provides a means for locomotion and enhances the development of extension against gravity.

8. Key behaviors associated with creeping include protective head turning, primary crawling, head lift-primitive support, head control-on elbows, on hands, prone extension, pivoting, crawling, and creeping.
9. Sitting provides a means for assuming and maintaining a vertical, antigravity posture before standing in an upright posture is possible; sitting also frees the upper extremities from their support role.
10. Key behaviors associated with sitting include primary sitting, head lag, head align, pull to sit, hands to feet and feet to mouth, supported sit, and sitting.
11. Rolling provides a means for changing position in space, or moving through space before forward progression develops in the prone posture, and leads to the development of <u>rotation</u> between body segments.
12. Key behaviors associated with rolling are primary turning, spontaneous turning, deliberate rolling to prone, deliberate rolling to supine, sidelying, and rolling.
13. As a developmental behavior, the sequence for standing and walking provides a means for locomotion in an upright posture, utilizing lower extremities for support and freeing upper extremities for carrying objects and development of skill capabilities.
14. Key behaviors associated with development of standing and walking include primary standing, primary walking, pull to stand, supported standing, supported walking, squatting, standing, and walking.
15. As a developmental sequence, manipulative prehension develops from an innate motivation to explore and manipulate the environment; reaching provides abilities for exploration, and grasping/releasing promotes object manipulation.
16. Key behaviors associated with the development of reaching, grasping, and releasing are primary grasp, primary release, swiping, scratching, crude palmar grasp, reach and pat, palmar grasp, index probing, instinctive grasp, visual orientation, inferior pinch, superior pinch, prehension, and manipulative prehension.

Self-study Guidelines

1. Differentiate "hard-wired" and "soft-wired" aspects of human nervous system maturation as described with development sequences.
2. Define "key behavior" as used with sensorimotor development.
3. Give two or three purposes for learning the sequential development of key behaviors.
4. Briefly describe the purposes of the primitive and transitional phases of developmental sequences.
5. State a major outcome for each of the developmental progressions; for example, creeping provides a means for locomotion prior to the development of standing.
6. List and describe key behaviors for the primitive, transitional, and mature phases of each of the development sequences.
7. List the movement components, muscle function, reflex/reaction, and postural control for primitive key behaviors of each of the sequences.
8. In early infancy, upper extremities are needed to support the body. Describe the developmental progressions to illustrate how a child acquires the ability to free extremities from their support role to be available for environmental exploration.
9. Compare and contrast crawling and creeping.

Figure 5-99 Developmental Sequences*†

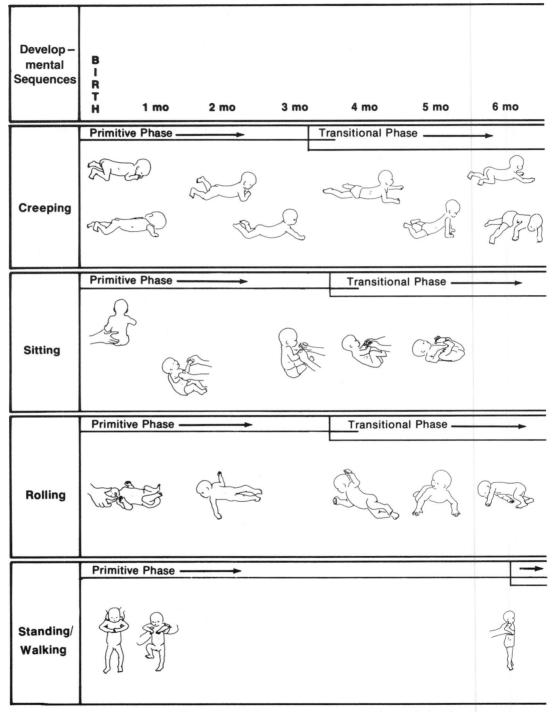

* The names of the behaviors illustrated by drawings on this chart can be found accompanying the photographs in Chapter 5.

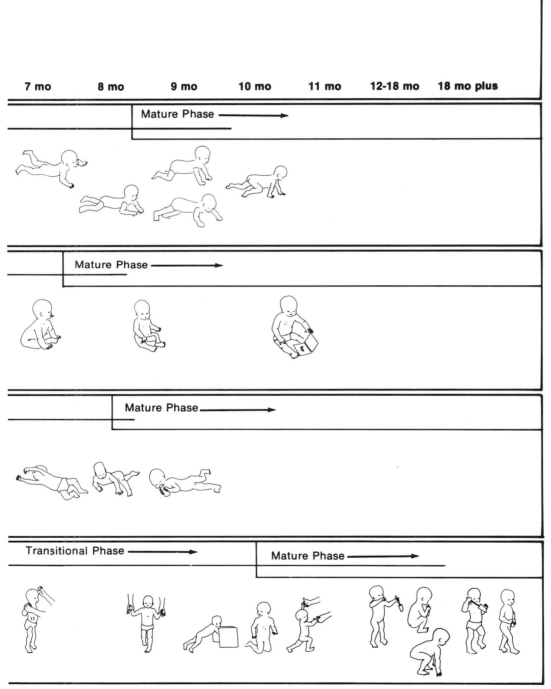

| 7 mo | 8 mo | 9 mo | 10 mo | 11 mo | 12-18 mo | 18 mo plus |

Mature Phase ————→

Mature Phase ————→

Mature Phase ————→

Transitional Phase ————→   Mature Phase ————→

† The primary purpose of this chart is to illustrate the relationships between the key
behaviors of each spiral. The specific ages cited for each behavior represent an average
age within the normal range for acquiring the behavior.

Figure 5-100: Developmental Sequences—Upper Extremity Functions

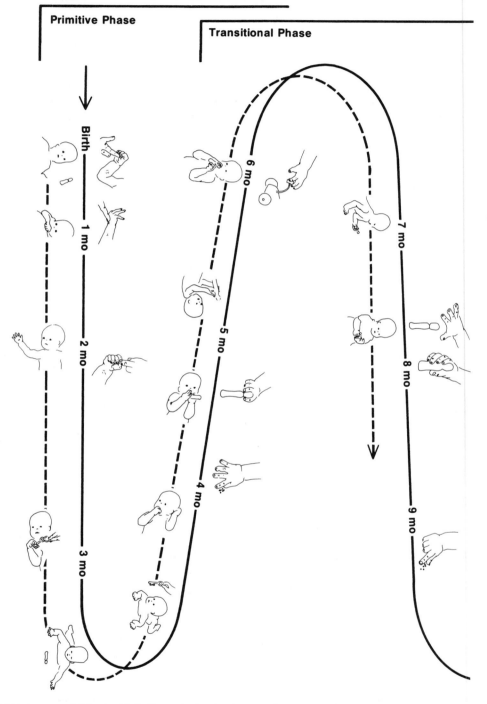

† *The purpose of this chart is to illustrate the developmental sequence of grasp and its relationship to developing behaviors. The specific ages cited represent an average age within the normal range for acquiring the function.*

Mature Phase

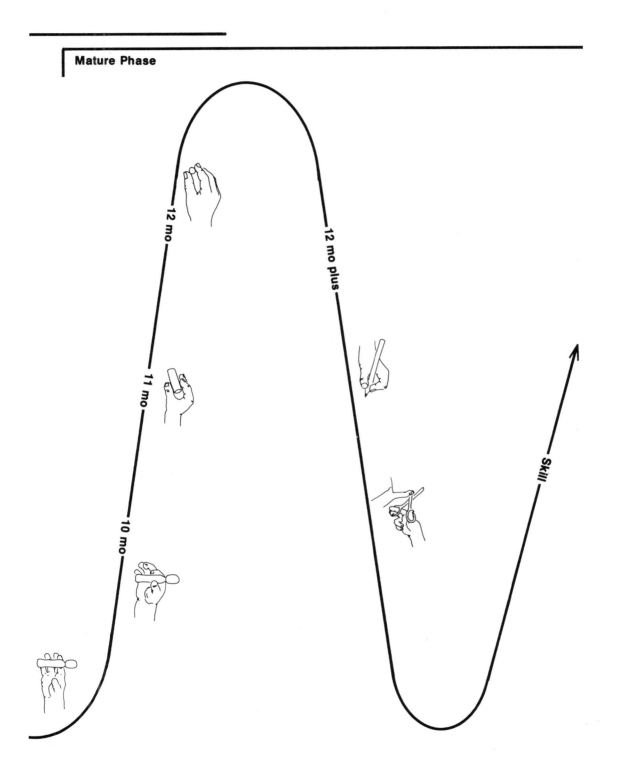

12 mo

11 mo

10 mo

12 mo plus

Skill

10. Why would intervention programs designed to remediate abnormal development be designed to facilitate aspects of transitional strategies of developmental progressions?
11. Why are symmetry and head control in space characteristic of behaviors that mark initiation of the transitional phase for prone?
12. Illustrate principles of spiraling by discussing a child's repeated use of the "high guard" position in upright in early sitting, standing, and walking.
13. Describe "pivoting" as a key behavior.
14. Compare and contrast bilateral and unilateral crawling by explaining differences in weight-shift patterns.
15. Compare and contrast spontaneous, deliberate, and automatic rolling.
16. Describe "squatting" as a transitional key behavior.
17. In early attempts for independent standing, upper extremity patterns change; arms come down from high guard to readiness-to-protect. What does this indicate?
18. Reaching begins with "swiping" at objects; swiping contributes to development of what muscle function and what movement pattern?
19. During the rolling sequence, what key behavior contributes to reaching?
20. Describe why "mouthing objects" contributes to development of release patterns.

Bibliography

Andre-Thomas: The Neurological Examlination of the Infant. Clinics in Developmental Medicine. Philadelphia, JB Lippincott Co, 1964, No. 1.

Ayers AJ: Sensory Integration and Learning Disorders. Los Angeles, Western Psychological Services, 1972.

Beintema JD: A neurological study of newborn infants. Clinics in Developmental Medicine. Philadelphia, Lippincott, 1968, No. 28.

Bly L: The components of normal movement during the first year of life and abnormal motor development. Neurodevelopmental Treatment Association Inc. Birmingham, Alabama: Pittenger & Associates, Pathway Press Association Inc., 1983.

Bobath B, Bobath K: Motor Development in Different Types of Cerebral Palsy. London, W. Heinemann Med. Books, 1975.

Bobath K: The motor deficit in patients with cerebral palsy. Clinics in Developmental Medicine. Philadelphia, Lippincott, 1966, No. 23.

Bobath B: Abnormal Postural Reflex Activity Caused by Brain Lesion. London, W. Heinemann Med. Books, 1975.

Bower TGR: Infant perception of the third dimension and object concept development, in Cohen L, Salapatek P (eds): Infant Perception: From Sensation to Cognition. New York, Academic Press Inc., 1975, vol 2, pp 33-50.

Bruner J: The growth and structure of skill, in Connolly K (ed.), Mechanisms of Motor Skill Development, New York, Academic Press Inc, 1970, pp. 63-92.

Chandler L, Andrews M, Swanson M: Movement assessment of infants, A manual. Child Development and Mental Retardation Center, University of Washington, Seattle, 1980.

Cohen LB, Salapatek P: Infant Perception: From Sensation to Cognition, Basic Visual Process. New York, Academic Press, Inc., 1975.

Connolly K (ed.): Mechanisms of Motor Skill Development. New York, Academic Press, Inc., 1970, pp. 3-18.

Ehrhardt R: Development Prehension Assessment. Baltimore, RAM Publications, 1984.

Erickson J: Activity, Recovery, Growth. New York, WW Norton & Co Inc., 1976, p. xi.

Fantz RL: Visual perception of the third dimension and object concept development, in Cohen L, Salapatek P (eds): Infant Perception: From Sensation to Cognition. New York, Academic Press Inc, 1975, vol 2, pp 33-50.

Fantz R, Faga J, Mirand S: Early visual selectivity, in Cohen L, Salapatek P (eds): Infant Perception: From Sensation to Cognition. New York, Academic Press Inc, 1975, pp 249-340.

Fiorentino MR: Reflex Testing Methods for Evaluating C.N.S. Development. Springfield, Illinois, Charles C. Thomas, 1965.

Gibson EJ: Principles of Perceptual Learning and Development. New York, Appleton, Century, Crofts, 1969.

Gilfoyle E, Grady A: Posture and movement, in Hopkins H, Smith H (eds): Willard and Spackman's Occupational Therapy. Philadelphia, JB Lippincott Co, 1977, pp 58-81.

Hirt S: The tonic neck reflex mechanism in the normal human adult. Am J Phys Med, 46, 362-368, 1967.

Holt K: Movement and child development. Clinics in Developmental Medicine. Philadelphia, Lippincott, 1975, No. 55.

Hopkins H, Smith H (eds.): Willard and Spackman's Occupational Therapy, 5th edition, pp. 58-80. Philadelphia, Lippincott, 1978.

Jones B: The importance of memory traces of motor efferent discharges for learning skilled movements. [incomplete]

Karmel B, Maidel E: A neuronal activity model for infant visual attention, in Cohen L, Salapatek P (eds): Infant Perception: From Sensation to Cognition. New York, Academic Press Inc, 1975, Vol 1, pp 78-125.

Knoblach H, Stevens F, Malone A: Manual of Developmental Diagnosis. New York, Harper & Row, 1980.

Milani-Comparetti A, Gidoni E: Routine developmental examination in normal and retarded children. Dev Med Child Neurology, 9, 631-638, 1967.

Moore JC: Proceedings of the sensorimotor symposium: Movement and learning. San Diego, California, San Diego State University, 1975.

Nash M: Neurodevelopmental treatment course syllabus. Unpublished manual, 1987.

Pearson PH, Williams CE (eds.): Physical Therapy Services in the Developmental Disabilities. Chapter 4, pp. 186-222. Springfield, Illinois, Charles C. Thomas, 1972.

Peiper A: Cerebral Function in Infancy and Childhood. New York, Consultants Bureau, 1963.

Stockmeyer S: A sensorimotor approach to treatment, in Pearson B, Williams C: Physical Therapy Services in the Developmental Disabilities. Springfield, CC Thomas Pubs, 1972, pp 186-222.

Touwen B: Neurological development in infancy. Clinics in Developmental Medicine. Philadelphia, JB Lippincott Co, 1976, No. 58.

Twitchell TE: Attitudinal reflexes. The child with central nervous system deficit. Children's Bureau Publication, US Dept Health, Education, and Welfare, Washington DC, Government Printing Office, 1965, No. 432.

Twitchell TE: Normal motor development. The child with central nervous system deficit. Children's Bureau Publication, US Dept Health, Education, and Welfare,

Washington DC, Government Printing Office, 1965, No. 432.

Twitchell TE: Reflex mechanisms and the development of prehension, in Connolly K (ed): Mechanisms of Motor Skill Development. New York, Academic Press Inc, 1970, pp 25-47.

Wells K: Kinesiology. Philadelphia, WB Saunders Co, 1963, ed 3, pp. 327-412.

White B, Castle P, Held R: Observations on the development of visually directed reaching. Child Dev 35:349-364, 1964.

CHAPTER 6

Developmental
Sequences to Stand

Objectives

The reader will be able to

1. list in chronological order the developmental sequences used to assume vertical postures;
2. describe the posture and movement patterns used with each sequence; and
3. compare and contrast key and transitional sequences.

Introduction

Most children are pulling up to a standing position by 12 months of age. Although some children begin as early as 7 months, others may not show an interest in standing until 14, or even 18, months of age. The pull-up sequences to stand and initial attempts at assuming standing independently were described in Chapter 5. Getting to stand independently without holding on for support appears after the child has some balance in squat, has already maintained standing independently, and probably walked. These patterns change significantly during the first six years of the child's life. The infant who begins pulling up to stand by using upper extremities for support can assume standing from supine by 6 years of age with little or no upper extremity support assistance. The change in pattern for getting up reflects increased efficiency in range, strength, and sequencing of movements which comes with maturation of neural mechanisms, development of muscle functions, and adaptation to the most efficient path to a goal. An infant uses righting reactions, support reactions, and combined mobility-stability muscle functions to pull up, while a 6-year-old can sequence the pattern by adapting equilibrium reactions and blended mobility-stability actions. The 6-year-old's pattern is quicker, smoother, and more directly oriented toward the goal of standing.

Observing the sequence of movements and weight shifts used to assume standing is another method for recognizing maturation and use of neuromuscular functions in action. In addition, identifying the child's pattern changes at various stages of getting up affords another opportunity to further explore the spiraling continuum concept of development. The material presented in this chapter will describe the key and transitional sequences to stand that are used by children from 1 to 6 years of age, or from the time they are able to assume standing independently until about 6 years. Posture and movement strategies and previously acquired developmental sequence skills will be identified as they are being adapted to higher level or more mature sequences, and the progression of key and transitional patterns will be related to the spiraling continuum concept.

In the first edition, six developmental sequences to standing were identified and termed: (1) pull-up sequence, (2) complete rotation sequence, (3) partial-complete rotation sequence, (4) partial rotation sequence, (5) symmetrical-partial sequence, and (6) symmetrical sequence. These six sequences were an expansion of the three levels originally reported by Florentino.[1,2] The reason for expanding to six sequences was to include three transitional sequences along with the three levels originally reported. In the interest of clarity, further differentiation and classification of sequences are appropriate.

The sequences to assume standing now include only those patterns used by a child to get to standing independently, without the use of external support for holding and pulling up. The change in classification of patterns eliminates the pull-up sequence. The pull-up sequence presented in the first edition described ways the baby used the upper extremities to hold on to objects in order to shift weight back over lower extremities or to place one lower extremity forward in weight-bearing position and pull up to the standing position, using the arms for support and initial thrust. The pull-up sequence is adapted from patterns developed with creeping behavior, occurs prior to independent standing in the progression of standing/walking skills, and is more appropriately classified with the skills that develop prior to independent standing (see Chapter 5). Although the pull-up sequence is no longer being included in this classification of independent standing sequences, it is important to note that the tendency to use the upper extremites for support during weight shifts, or to push off from floor or knee while getting up, is adapted from the original pull-up sequence to the independent sequences. This adaptation of upper extremity patterns to independent standing will be further elaborated throughout this chapter.

The five remaining sequences, complete rotation to symmetrical sequence, are subject to this classification of independent standing. Complete rotation, partial rotation, and symmetrical sequences are considered the key sequences, while partial-complete rotation and partial rotation-symmetrical sequences are considered transitional sequences. In chronological order, the sequences are as follows:

1. Complete rotation.
2. Partial-complete rotation.
3. Partial rotation.
4. Symmetrical-partial rotation.
5. Symmetrical sequence.

A sequence is considered key when the child is adapting and integrating previously acquired strategies with newly developed strategies so that a new behavior is emerging and is being consistently used. For example, partial rotation is considered a key sequence because the child using the pattern is integrating righting and equilibrium reactions and consistently rotating toward one side or the other, both to get from supine to sitting and to get from sitting to standing positions.

Transitional sequences include partial-complete rotation and partial rotation-symmetrical sequence. A sequence is considered transitional when the child begins using newly acquired strategies to initiate a sequence, but calls forth previously acquired strategies to complete the sequence. For example, partial-complete rotation is considered transitional because the child initiates the standing sequence by getting from supine to sitting by rotating toward one side, signaling the emergence of equilibrium reactions as an underlying neural mechanism for the supine-to-sit sequence. But the child completely rotates from sitting over toward a prone orientation to get from sit to stand, indicating that righting/support reactions are still being used to achieve the higher level behavior of sit to stand.

The sequences to stand will be described in chronological order. The progression from key to transitional to key sequences will be further clarified during the discussion of the relationship between the spiraling continuum and sequences to stand.

All of the sequences described begin with a child in the supine position. Key sequences have been termed according to direction and extent to which a child rotates around the body axis in order to get into a position to begin standing up. Only approximate age ranges for each sequence are available and will be included here. However, data on age ranges are insufficient for use in judging children's performance unless the discrepancy is fairly obvious, such as a 3- or 4-year-old using a complete rotation pattern to sit and stand. More important is the usefulness of information about the sequences themselves. Recognizing the way a child is using righting reactions versus equilibrium reactions to sequence posture and movement patterns at higher levels, or observing whether the patterns are well enough established to be used consistently, regardless of spatiotemporal stress, gives insight into the child's state of developmental health.

Key Sequence: Complete Rotation

The child uses a complete rotation sequence (Fig. 6-1 A-1) to come from supine to prone and get into sitting and creeping, to pull up to stand, and to get to standing independently. The complete rotation pattern starts about 7 months of age with automatic rolling and is adapted to assuming the higher level postures, including standing, until about 18 to 25 months of age.[2] Completely rotating the body from supine to prone in order to get up from supine into standing seems an indirect and inefficient approach in terms of the number of steps and range of moovements required to get from supine to prone and shift weight appropriately to get up onto feet. However, development of flexor components in supine is not sufficiently advanced to support movement against gravity from supine directly to sit or stand, even though head-righting with neck and trunk flexion is well enough developed in supine to allow the baby to pull to sit or pull to stand. In order to come to sit or stand from supine without pulling with arms, a child needs more development of the flexor muscle groups, especially abdominal muscles, before she is prepared to move directly from supine into standing. Until flexor groups are further developed, a child must roll to prone because in prone the extensor muscle groups are prepared to act against gravity at higher levels of development. In addition, in prone the extremities can be more easily positioned for support and push-up into standing.

The complete rotation sequence makes use of righting and support reactions to coordinate movement and weight shift. By the time the child is using complete rotation to get into standing, rotational and vertical righting reactions have been integrated to the extent that the child rolls using rotational righting (body on head and body on body) reactions and simultaneously begins to move head and trunk toward vertical orientation, activating lateral flexor and then extensor components of neck and trunk, using vertical righting (labyrinthine) reactions. As soon as vertical righting reactions come into play, extremity support reactions are activated to help maintain the interim positions between prone and standing. The following steps describe the sequence and maturation that occur with the sequence, from the point at which a child begins to use complete rotation until she moves into transition between complete and partial rotation.

1. Child rolls over using rotational righting integrated with vertical righting reactions. Blended muscle functions help sequence the movement from supine to prone.

2. Once in prone, upper extremity support reactions are integrated with vertical righting reactions as the child supports on hands to get up onto hands and knees. Using upper extremity support allows the child to temporarily call forth combined mobility-stability muscle functions needed to meet the demands of getting into standing.

3. Weight is shifted contralaterally between upper and lower extremities, and using an adaptation of the amphibian reaction, the child comes up on one knee and then the other. By the time the child is standing independently, the preliminary steps of rolling over and getting up onto hands and knees are executed as one smooth pattern, making use of blended muscle functions and integrated righting reactions. The child moves toward hands and knees before getting all the way over to prone, demonstrating efficiency of integrated movement sequences.

4. From the four-point position, the child shifts bilaterally onto both upper extremities in order to position lower extremities for standing. Shifting weight to the upper extremities to support lower extremity movement is similar to the way the child used the upper extremities for support in the pull-up sequence to stand, and represents an adaptation of a previously acquired behavior to a new situation. In a sense, the child "holds on" to the supporting surface to get up, which is somewhat like holding on to objects to pull up.

5. Weight is shifted to lower extremities in progressively more mature patterns.
   (a) Child may place weight on both feet simultaneously by bringing both legs forward in a bilateral movement and shifting weight back over feet bilaterally, once feet are plantigrade. This pattern is similar to the child's initial patterns for assuming creeping position and pulling to stand bilaterally. With weight shifted to lower extremities, child extends knees, lets go of upper extremity support, extends hips and trunk, and stands up.
   (b) With repetition of this pattern, controlled extension into upright improves and child may let go of support as soon as weight is on feet, squat momentarily, and then stand up.
   (c) Further development of extension along the midline leads to changes in the way a child shifts weight to lower extremities in order to get up. Making use of extension and rotation around the pelvis, the child shifts weight to both arms and one knee, and frees the opposite lower extremity, which is moved forward until the foot is in plantigrade position. Weight is then shifted to the weight-bearing foot, while the other foot is brought to plantigrade position. Child then shifts weight to feet and stands up as previously described.
   (d) Repetition of unilateral lower extremity weight shifts leads to development of

a smoother, more efficient pattern based on the child's ability to adapt contralateral weight shifts between upper and lower extremities while in the process of rolling to prone. The child rolls and places the hand on the same side in weight-bearing, while bringing the opposite leg over and immediately placing the foot plantigrade. Rolling over and preparing to get up are part of the smooth motion. Meanwhile, the opposite hand and the opposite foot are placed in weight-bearing position and the child stands as before. Contralateral weight shifting makes use of rotation and counterrotation patterns and prepares for maturation of equilibrium reactions as underlying mechanisms for getting to stand. Placing the foot plantigrade while moving into the position is an adaptation of the way a baby assumed creeping eventually and the way the "half-bear" posture was used to play and change positions between sitting and creeping, together with the child's recent experience with unilateral lower extremity weight shifting to assume standing. The pattern described here becomes even smoother when it is used during the partial-complete rotation sequence.

6. The smooth, rapid way in which the child now gets from supine into four-point and on into standing prepares for the change for complete to partial rotation sequence.

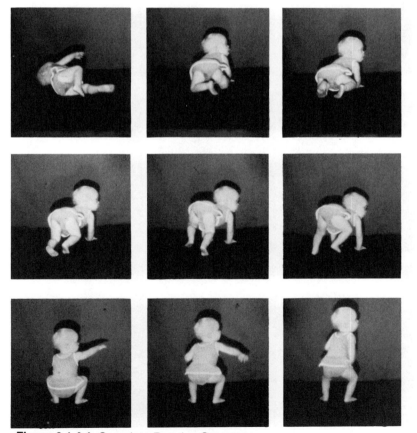

Figure 6-1 A-I: Complete Rotation Sequence

Transitional Sequence: Partial-Complete Rotation

The partial-complete rotation sequence (Fig. 6-2 A-1) introduces the concept of partial rotation. The child uses some form of partial rotation from approximately 18 to 24 months to 5 or 6 years. Partial rotation represents a significant change in a child's pattern because it allows the child to sequence movements toward the direction of standing. Partial rotation represents the beginning of an ability to select the most efficient path to the goal of standing. The change in pattern appears as a child rolls toward sidelying and starts to move toward an upright sitting position, using integrated rotational-vertical righting reactions instead of rolling completely to prone. Integration of combined righting reactions and tendency to move toward vertical more efficiently leads to adaptation of righting to previously acquired equilibrium reactions in sitting. A new developmental achievement, getting to sitting from supine, emerges. Equilibrium is

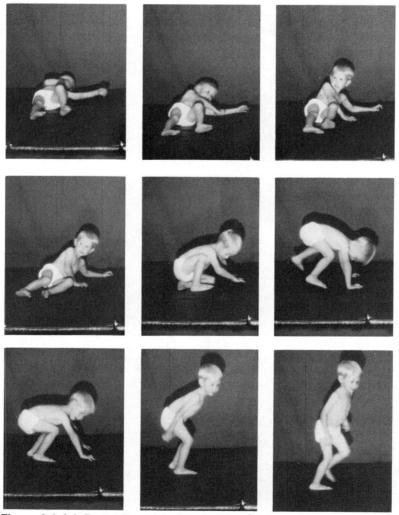

Figure 6-2 A-I: Partial-Complete Rotation Sequence

evident as a child pulls up toward the center of gravity using the head and trunk incurvation adapted from vertical righting, trunk rotation adapted from rotational righting, and use of at least one upper extremity to assist by abducting while the other upper extremity assists by pushing up into sitting. However, since equilibrium is just emerging as a mechanism for sequencing movement to achieve sitting, it is not yet available for getting from sitting to standing. A chlid cannot use partial rotation under the more stressful conditions of getting from sitting to stand. The sequence to stand is completed by calling forth the more well-established complete rotation sequence.

The following steps describe the partial-complete rotation sequence:

1. The child rolls toward prone using rotational and vertical righting reactions. As a child approaches sidelying, asymmetrical pressure facilitates more vertical righting which has been strengthened by the child's more extensive experience in getting to stand through complete rotation. The upper extremity on that side extends and supports, as vertical righting brings the child up toward sitting and interrupts the complete rotation sequence. The child has previously used vertical righting with rotational righting and upper extremity support to move from creeping into sitting position. A part of the same pattern is now differentiated and adapted to sitting from side orientation. The result is a change in the complete rotation sequence since the child only needs to partially rotate to get to a sitting position from supine.

2. From sitting, a child completely rotates toward prone in order to get to stand. By using prone, a child can make use of upper extremity support to shift weight to feet and make sure of more highly developed extensor mechanisms to stand. Patterns and variations used to get from sit to stand with complete rotation are essentially the same as those previously described in the complete rotation section.

Key Sequence: Partial Rotation

Although partial rotation (Fig. 6-3 A-G) begins with a change in the way righting reactions are used to sequence movement, it creates a pattern of movement that utilizes equilibrium reactions to control movement sequences. With equilibrium present, the partial rotation pattern matures to the extent that a child can get from supine up to standing using partial rotation, and the complete rotation pattern is integrated into a new behavior.

The following steps describe the partial rotation sequence:

1. The child partially rotates toward sidelying, but before reaching the side, begins to move toward upright. The flexion-rotation pattern that developed with equilibrium is adapted to sitting from supine. The upper extremity on the non-weight-bearing side abducts to assist with coming to sit and the weight-bearing upper extremity assists by pushing up.

2. Once in sitting, a child continues the partial rotation pattern to stand. By rotating one hip, a child can position the opposite foot in plantigrade position, move the body forward to shift weight onto that foot, and rise to the standing position, while positioning the other foot to also bear weight. Use of the upper extremities for support and push is adapted from the complete rotation sequence as a child supports and pushes off the floor with one extremity and off the knee over the plantigrade foot with the other extremity.

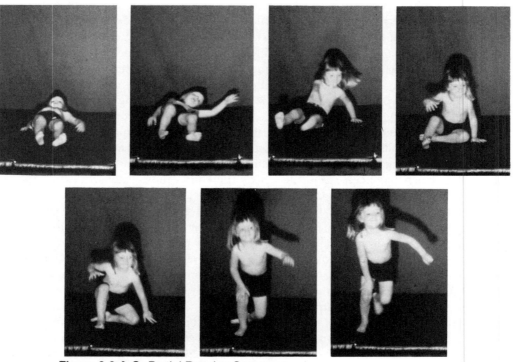

Figure 6-3 A-G: Partial Rotation Sequence

3. With repetition, the pattern becomes a smooth, coordinated sequence, making use of forward momentum to the extent that there is less rotation away from the midline before coming toward midline, less use of the arms for support and push, and more use of the arm toward the center to help lift the body from sitting to standing. The arm extends and abducts, much the way it does as the sequence is initiated from supine, again adapting an upper extremity equilibrium component to the sequence. The changes noted with repetition and maturation prepare for the advent of symmetrical sequences.

Transitional Sequence:
Symmetrical-Partial Rotation

Throughout the progressions of developing sequence skills, we noted that as midline stability and equilibrium reactions matured and mobility and stability functions were blended around midline and proximal joints, movement and weight shifting were controlled more by head and trunk adjustments and less by extremity support or pull-push patterns. The extremities were free to assist through equilibrium reactions or assistive movements, as well as being free to engage in skill activities or locomotion. Symmetrical patterns of movement from supine to upright make use of midline stability and equilibrium reactions, as well as advanced development of flexor components, particularly abdominal groups. Each time a child partially rotated and pulled back toward the center of gravity, the abdominal muscle groups were strengthened until we observed less rotation away and more tendency to come toward the center of gravity whenever the pattern was initiated. The use of partial rotation and forward momentum from sit to stand contributed to further maturation of components needed for a more symmetrical pattern to develop from supine to sit.

Using a symmetrical pattern of movement from supine up to stand requires a great deal of strength and balance. When symmetrical patterns emerge, a child can use the pattern to get from supine to sit. The spatiotemporal stress created by moving from sit to stand causes the already-established partial rotation pattern to come forth.

The following steps describe the symmetrical-partial rotation sequence (Fig. 6-4 A-H):

1. Child raises head in supine and positions both upper extremities with elbows behind shoulders in preparation to push into sitting symmetrically. Action of the arms interrupts a child's tendency to partially rotate and assists the child in activating neck and upper trunk flexors, which in turn facilitate action of lower trunk flexors. Child comes symmetrically into sitting, sequencing movement by adapting vertical righting to sitting up from supine.

2. From sitting, a child calls forth a partial rotation pattern by shifting weight to one hip, positioning the opposite foot and coming to stand. Spatiotemporal stress brought about by attempting to stand symmetrically brings out the previously acquired partial rotation pattern. However, the pattern may vary from the original partial rotation sit to stand. Experience of coming to sit symmetrically strengthens upper extremity and upper trunk reactions so that standing up, even with a partial rotation pattern, is accomplished with less support from the arms and more action of the lower trunk and hip acting on the upper trunk action. A child is preparing for the symmetrical sequence to stand by coordinating the action of upper and lower trunk along the midline and more proximal joints.

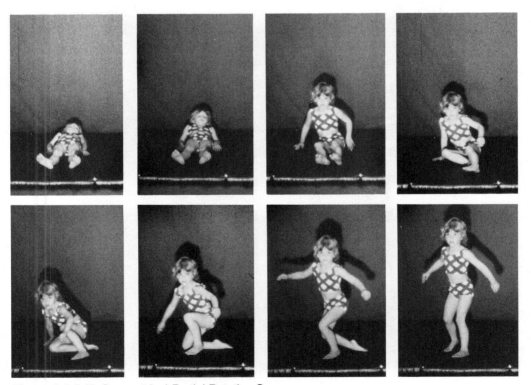

Figure 6-4 A-H: Symmetrical-Partial Rotation Sequence

Key Sequence: Symmetrical Sequence

The symmetrical sequence (Fig. 6-5 A-H) to stand represents the most mature pattern possible for children and some adults. All children may not achieve this level of development. If they attain this high level of performance, they may not consistently use the pattern, or retain it through adulthood, since it is easily affected by spatiotemporal stress. Changes in size, strength, fatigue, and motivation are all factors that influence a child's selection of sequences for standing.

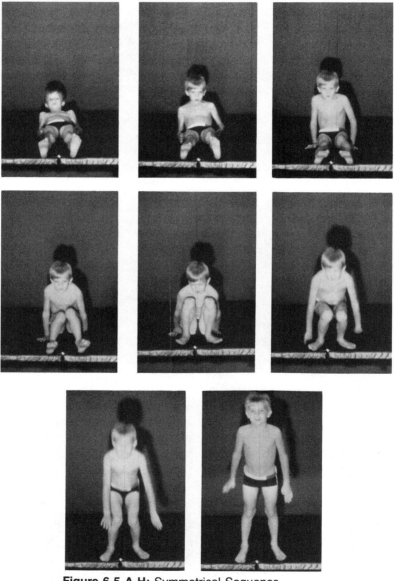

Figure 6-5 A-H: Symmetrical Sequence

The following steps describe the symmetrical sequence to standing:

1. The child raises head in supine and sits up symmetrically. Upper extremities may be used to push off lightly from the floor or to reach forward and assist with sequencing of movement along the midline. The changes in upper extremity assist patterns indicate increased blending of muscle functions at midline and established midline stability, allowing the child to move and maintain head and trunk alignment while moving. As a child is coming to sit, lower extremity preparation to stand occurs before child actually gets to sitting posture. Lower extremities are flexed at the hips and knees so that feet are plantigrade and prepared to take weight in standing. This lower extremity adaptation is similar to adjustments a child made when adapting pull to sit to pull to stand during progression of developmental sequence skills.

2. With feet prepared for weight bearing, the child uses the momentum from flexion to come up onto feet, blends flexion with extension, and stands up symmetrically. Upper extremities may be used for balance or for push-off as child extends knees and hips to stand.

Summary

The quest to stand is an innate goal for children. The change in patterns that are used to assume the standing position during the first 6 years of life reflect increased efficiency, strength, and sequencing of movements, which comes with the maturation of neural mechanisms, development of muscle functions, and the maturing spiraling adaptation process. Five distinct patterns have been presented; complete rotation, partial rotation, and symmetrical are classified as key sequences, as they reflect the adaptation and integration of previously acquired strategies with newly developed ones. The other two patterns, partial-complete and symmetrical-partial, are classified as transitional to reflect the beginning use of newly acquired strategies to initiate the sequence and the calling forth of previously acquired strategies to complete the goal. These sequences are presented here for the reader to use for observation of movement and to consider how the developmental sequences are linked together by association-differentiation into new sequences for higher level functioning.

Key Points

1. Patterns used to assume standing change significantly during the first 6 years of life.
2. The change in patterns for getting up reflects increased efficiency in range, strength, and sequencing of movements.
3. Observing the sequence of movements and weight shifts used to assume standing is one method for recognizing the child's maturational gains and use of neuro-muscular functions in action.
4. The five sequences are termed complete rotation, partial-complete rotation, partial rotation, partial rotation-symmetrical, and symmetrical.
5. Complete rotation, partial rotation, and symmetrical are considered key sequences, and partial-complete rotation and partial rotation-symmetrical are considered transitional.

6. A sequence is "key" when a child is adapting and integrating previously acquired strategies with newly developed strategies, and a new behavior emerges and is used consistently.
7. A sequence is "transitional" when a child begins using newly acquired strategies to initiate the pattern, but calls forth previously acquired strategies to complete the sequence.

Self-study Guidelines

1. List, in chronological order, the developmental sequences used to assume standing.
2. Differentiate "key" from "transitional" sequences.
3. Identify sequences as "key" or as "transitional."
4. Describe each of the five sequences.

References
1. Fiorentino MR: Reflex Testing Methods for Evaluating C.N.S. Development (sixth printing). Springfield, IL, Charles C. Thomas Pubs., 1971.
2. Fiorentino MR: A Basis for Sensorimotor Development—Normal and Abnormal. Springfield, IL, Charles C. Thomas Pubs., 1981.

CHAPTER 7

Purposeful Sequences and the Acquisition of Skilled Performance

Objectives

The reader will be able to

1. define and explain the concept of purposeful sequences, and differentiate developmental and purposeful sequences;
2. define "purposefulness" as related to movement and occupation;
3. define and discuss skill as the final stabilization of sensorimotor-sensory adaptation;
4. explain the concepts of occupation and occupational performance as used with the theory;
5. compare and contrast play, work, and self-care;
6. relate spatiotemporal adaptation theory with ecological event theory;
7. describe examples of skilled performance as outcomes for moving in space, receiving impetus, and giving impetus;
8. define and discuss the concepts of autonomy and competence as related to the theory; and
9. discuss the developmental phases of play.

Introduction

Purposeful sequences evolve through the interaction of developmental sequences with environmental events. As a youngster moves out to explore, environmental experiences are adapted with self, and developmental sequences begin to take on "new meaning." As developmental sequences are adapted with environmental events, there is an arousal of a child's intrinsically motivated behavior "to do" combined with extrinsically motivated behavior "to do something" related to events of the environment. Instead of creeping or rolling or walking for the sake of accomplishing the behavior itself, a child creeps or rolls to get a toy, or walks across the room to find "mommy." Intention or objective of actions provides the stimulus for repetition to reinforce functions needed for adaptation to higher level performance. Linking developmental sequences with environmental events results in emergence of purposeful sequences. Purposefulness of sequences adds a new dimension to the spiraling spatiotemporal adaptation process; "doing something" or actively participating with environmental events allows a child to refine bodily processes used for developmental sequences in preparation for differentiating and adapting aspects of a sequence to purposeful sequences and ultimately to skilled performances. "Doing something" becomes an occupational process for a child, and the environmental event becomes the meaningful occupation.

Purposeful sequences link differentiated components from developmental sequences into specific patterns used to interact with space, objects, and people. Both developmental and purposeful sequences make use of sensorimotor functions to produce movement, but unique to purposeful sequences is the intentionality on the part of a child that is motivated by an occupational event as a child seeks to explore and master his world, pursuing his quest for autonomy and competence. Inherent within the concepts of purposeful sequences is the interdependency or interrelationship of a child's sensorimotor-sensory actions, environmental events (occupations), and quest for autonomy and competence.

Autonomy and competence have a direct relationship with one's ability to interact with occupations; thus, the very nature of a child's spatiotemporal environment becomes a vital factor to facilitate a child to act upon innate urges. As discussed in Chapter Two, intrinsic motivation to move about, explore, and master the environment is a biologically inherent urge of one's self-system. Intrinsic motivation enhances an exploratory and experimental attitude that directs a child toward achievement of competent interactions; as a result, a child performs for the value of the occupational process and for achieving the occupation itself. As a child seeks autonomy and competence, social interactions with others add a new dimension to motivation for "doing." Purposeful sequences also become extrinsically motivated as social reinforcement enhances one's perceptions and values of "doing something." Extrinsic and intrinsic motivation to explore and master one's environment is an essential element of the purposefulness of movement and occupation. Likewise, the purposefulness of environmental interactions is central to acquisition of skilled performance.

To present the acquisition of skilled performance, the following chapter discusses purposeful sequences, occupational performance, skills, autonomy, and competence. Person-environment transactions also are explored with comparisons of spatiotemporal adaptation theory and the ecological event approach. Additionally, properties and processes of play are introduced as an example of occupation as the core media for facilitating adaptation. Chapter Seven emphasizes both occupation and the occupational process of "doing something" in relation to the event as key elements for sensorimotor adaptation of skilled performance and the achievement of competence.

Explanation of Purposeful Sequences

Through spiraling adaptation, a child moves out with previously acquired behaviors to extend self into the environment. Mere repetition of acquired actions, in itself, will not serve to facilitate higher levels of development. For maturation to occur and spatiotemporal adaptation to proceed, there needs to be an increase of demands to the self-system.

Demands are increased as a child repeats sequences and the system begins to combine specific actions of developmental sequences with spatiotemporal characteristics of occupations. Through the spiraling process, developmental sequences are adapted to events or occupations, and newly acquired goals emerge. As sequences become goal-directed toward events, the novelty and challenge of the environment arouses a child's intentionality and promotes the purposefulness of occupation. Occupation becomes purposeful when the nature of and participation with the event facilitates meaningful responses for the self-system. Responses become meaningful when feedback associated with actions provides directions and efforts that are more mature or at a higher level than those previously experienced. Thus, purposeful sequences augment sensorimotor-sensory integration and adaptation spirals to higher levels.

Purposeful sequences can be differentiated from developmental sequences by a child's goal direction. Developmental sequences are those intrinsically motivated self-starting actions that are body centered and concerned with goals innate to self (e.g., to sit, to stand), whereas purposeful sequences are directed toward goals outside the body or to events/occupations within the environment; thus, they are environment centered and motivated by the value to do something in relation to the environment. During development, children seem to utilize certain innate functions that encourage them to seek out those occupations most related to the specific developmental phase needing reinforcement and/or providing novelty and challenge for spatiotemporal adaptation to proceed to higher levels. Adaptation of purposeful sequences to skilled performance illustrates the dynamics of the theory, as the spiraling interaction of movement-environment and adaptation of self's structures, purposes, space, and time come alive. Adaptation, with its sensorimotor-sensory, developmental, and purposeful nature, is affected by the stress or distress properties of spiraling interactions.

As a child engages in purposeful sequences, association and differentiation of actions with occupations afford one aspect of sensory feedback--knowledge of the result. A child is most concerned with the objective of the event and responds to the end result of actions; for example, a toy is grasped, a shoe is tied, a ball is caught. Actions with occupations generally include social interactions with other persons; the occupational process integrates sensory feedback from self's actions with the extrinsic feedback received from others, e.g., a person smiles, words of praise are heard, a child is hugged. Therefore, knowledge of the result provides feedback for a youngster to measure success or failure of accomplishment, reinforcing both intrinsically and extrinsically motivated actions. Determination of goals, together with feedback about performance, motivates children to repeat successful experiences or experiment with alternate means to resolve problems with unsuccessful experiences. Association and differentiation of a child's intent with the end result also augment perception about space, objects, and other persons in relation to self and in relation to each other. The end result, or goal, is an essential attribute to spatiotemporal adaptation because achievement of goals challenges a child to attempt more complex occupations for the spiraling adaptation process to continue. Through adaptation of functions-to-purposes or the spiraling integration of strategies with developmental and purposeful sequences, performance skills evolve.

Performance Skills

The result of acquiring skills is the ability to (a) move the body within spatiotemporal dimensions (e.g., dancing, running, skipping), (b) receive impetus (e.g., catch a ball), and (c) give impetus to external objects (e.g., move a pencil or scissors on the paper).[1] All three desirable consequences of adapting performance skills are achieved through the ongoing function-to-purpose-to-function process of a child's active participation with environment's occupations. Therefore, occupation becomes an intervening variable for facilitating "purpose" for adaptation of performance skills.

Skilled performance is characterized by freedom of movement within spatiotemporal dimensions of the environment.[2] Skill is appropriate use of posture and movement in relation to the effort (speed, timing, exertion, space, control) used for performance of occupation. Skilled performance adds a quality of natural responsiveness or an unconscious, automatic element to actions. Natural responsiveness of actions results from regulation of flow or blending of postures and movement in relation to spatiotemporal dimensions. Regulation of posture and movement strategies requires temporal sequencing of strategies in relation to spatial confines of environmental events. [3]

Major outcomes that underlie blending of strategies and sequences include efficiency and accuracy of performance. Efficiency of performance is the relationship between the amount of work that is accomplished and force or energy expended to accomplish the action. Although spatiotemporal components affect both efficiency and accuracy, efficiency of movement is more dependent upon a child's ability to perceive and adapt to the environment's spatial dimensions. Accuracy is more dependent upon perception of self in relation to temporal dimensions of those actions being performed. Accuracy of performance includes perception or judgment of direction, distance, control, and timing of one's actions.

With skilled performance, sensorimotor-sensory actions are appropriate for a specific performance and there is no need for change or modification of the appropriate actions. Thus, skill can be characterized by its consistent patterns of performance and, as such, skill becomes the final stabilization of sensorimotor-sensory adaptation. However, during development, skilled performance of one event may need to be modified or expanded to achieve a higher level performance of that occupation. Thus, consistency of a skilled performance is interrupted and actions become purposeful once again. Purposefulness of actions further enhances neural integration for higher level meaningful responses. As the spiraling process repeats itself, certain elements of purposeful sequences are called up, and newly acquired skilled performance emerges. To illustrate, consider a child who has acquired skilled performance while skiing on certain intermediate slopes. The child becomes motivated to join his peer group on more advanced slopes; hence, the skilled performance acquired must be modified to handle the more difficult terrain. In the process of performing, actions become purposeful again, as the nature of and participation with skiing in the more advanced areas facilitate a meaningful response for the nervous system. To adapt to the new environment, the self-system calls forth past acquired strategies and sequences to direct efforts. Thus, the youngster's performance expands his/her repertoire of actions. As the youngster practices, by repeating skiing on more difficult terrain, newly acquired skills emerge.

As developmental and purposeful sequences culminate in skills, the self-system builds up familiarity with inherent efficiency/accuracy patterns of movement, and organized units of behavior are developed. Fowler and Turvey[4] termed the organized units "coordinative structures" that are used for specific acts. According to these motor-learning theorists, coordinative structures from one event (i.e., holding a crayon) can be called forth to adapt to another (e.g., holding a pencil or pen). Ability to transfer performance patterns from one event to another is dependent upon the perceptual process inherent within spatiotemporal adaptation.

As humans are motivated to act by the occupational event, the self-system designs the task for the body to "perform," to "do," or carry to completion.[5] Performance and occupation are interdependent and interchanging, and serve in a cause-and-effect relationship with human functioning. Performance that is appropriate to a person's level of functioning facilitates a sense of ability, and by increasing the environmental demand, challenges a person to higher level performance. Humans develop a self-awareness through their performance with occupations and develop realistic self-concepts of their own abilities and inabilities. Through occupational performance, the self-system receives feedback necessary for the association-differentiation components of adaptation. The nature of occupational performance enhances adaptation and serves to motivate for modification or change.

Occupational Performance

Occupational performance is action that is elicited and structured by the environment, including spatiotemporal characteristics of an occupation. Occupations derive their purpose or meaning from self-perceptions of the "doer;" thus, purposefulness of occupation is unique to the specific person "doing" the tasks and restricted to that person's goal direction. Although the "doer" may be the most important aspect of purposefulness, the richness of the occupational performance, due to the many spatiotemporal dimensions of the occupation being performed, is vital for facilitating the intentionality and motivation for "doing." Occupations take place in a life-long series of environmental transactions of play, work, and self-care, which form an interrelated triad that constitutes a common domain for environmental exploration and mastery. Competent occupational performance provides life satisfactions to self and others, as it is the process of performing those tasks and roles that is essential to mastery of self and environment. The interrelated triad of occupational performance can be illustrated as follows:

Play ⬅ ‑ ‑ ‑ ‑ ‑ ‑ ‑ ‑ ‑ ⮕ Work
Self-care

Play, defined as the process to achieve competence, includes a variety of occupations from infancy through the graying years. Childhood play involves exploration, imaginative role-playing, and game-like activities. Children are motivated by a need to be competent and to have an impact upon and adapt within their environment, much of this being accomplished through play.[6] The value of play as occupation is its spatiotemporal characteristics and interactive processes. (Properties and processes of play will be discussed later in this chapter.) Through playful experiences, the self-system creates efficient and effective means for organizing adaptations. Through play occupations, a "playful spark" can be ignited and meaningful experiences can be tried out, practiced, organized, and adapted. As children grow in years, they become less "ignited" by the physical characteristics of the play task and more intent toward their peer groups whose behaviors provide novelty and surprise for that "playful spark" critical to purposefulness. During adolescence and young adulthood, play encompasses sports, games, hobbies, and social recreation. As a person enters the later years of life, play becomes leisure and encompasses a wide variety of both social and solidarity-type activities that provide experiences to continue the quest for competence and dignity of self. Play provides experiences for children and youth to learn about their world and achieve abilities to manage their various roles. Thus, play can be described as the genesis for work.

Work, defined as the process to express competence, includes occupations classified as productive.[6] Productive occupations are those events that provide a product or service requested by others or occupations that provide a heritage to one's culture. Work is a major factor of one's self-identity through such roles as student, housekeeper, volunteer, amateur or professional athlete, laborer, and other careers. Work roles also serve to recreate spatiotemporal characteristics of one's experiences from playful exploration to productive living. Work activities encompass a major part of life roles once the person begins to engage in school activities because work becomes the central core for much of a person's personal-social interactions and perceptions of self-efficacy.

Self-care, or daily living tasks, includes a range of activities such as eating, dressing, hygiene, toileting, transporting self, and rest. Self-care is the process of maintaining self as prescribed by one's culture and for the promotion of healthfulness. Self-care experiences, the third component of the interrelated triad of occupations, assist the child with acquiring capacities needed to shape self and one's environment. Self-care occupations provide children with abilities to exert control and gain a perception of self-reliance and dignity. A harmonious balance of play, work, and self-care is essential for healthful development and for orderly adaptation to occur. The interrelated continuum of play-work-self care constitutes occupational performance of human beings.[6]

Occupation, as used in this text, is defined as those play, self-care, and work events that provide opportunities to promote exploration and mastery of the environment and enhance self-efficacy, identity, and competence. A person's quest to explore and master the world serves as the major motivation for engagement with occupation; therefore, play, work, and self-care occupations are action events that serve as the primary media to facilitate modification and change and promote spatiotemporal adaptation of skills. Joan Erikson states that "Without change, recovery (rehabilitation, restitution) is illusory. Without activity and change, which is life itself, there is no growth." [7] Activity or occupation, and the occupational performance associated with these tasks, are key elements within the spatiotemporal adaptation process of development, as occupational performance serves as the process inherent within environmental experiences and occupation becomes the product of the person-environmental transaction.

Person and Environment

The idea of changing demands of environmental experiences having an influence upon modification and acquisition of higher levels of occupational performance receives support from a study by Glencross and Reynolds.[8] Their study investigated "attention" demands during acquisition of repetitive tasks and demonstrated that the changing attention demands of an occupation are crucial to the attainment of higher levels of skilled performance. As a new task is learned and skill acquired, changes occur in the organization of action and more sophisticated· control strategies are developed. In meeting new environmental demands, a child not only calls forth past acquired actions, but attention given the new task reinforces organizational and control purposes.

Skill acquisition occurs through a coordinated relationship of a child's intentionality and attention to and experience with environmental occupations. The relationship of person and environment, both being of equal importance, has been termed an ecological approach to motor skill acquisition by the scientists Fowler and Turvey.[4] An ecological approach focuses on adaptation to one's spatiotemporal environment. In the ecological event theory,[4,9] environment in relation to person has two major components--affordances and structured media. Affordance is the relationship of event to person, and provides support for the activity. The affordance component of environmental events provides the support that allows a child to act on her/his own intention and engage in purposeful occupations. In the example of skiing, affordances are the spatial components of the terrain, gravity, and skis, which provide support for the process of skiing. Without the affordance, skiing would have no meaning to a child. Of equal importance is structured media, which is defined as aspects of the environment (light, air, sound, etc.) that are specific to the event and provide necessary temporal information to the person.[9]

Fowler and Turvey's[4] research with the ecological event theory further supports the spatiotemporal adaptation theory, as well as the philosophy of occupational therapy, which values the use of occupation as media to bring about change or modification. According to event theory, for acquisition of skill to take place, a child must discover an appropriate organization of coordinated structures in relation to the affordance and structured media of the event. Organization of environmental events in relation to a self-system is a key element of spatiotemporal adaptation and of occupational therapy.

Fowler and Turvey[4] proposed that a person limits or restricts the number of movable joints used so that the range of motion of some joints is decreased until a person has the means to control all movable joints in a manner demanded by the task. The theory of spatiotemporal adaptation proposes that the spiraling continuum of adapting past acquired strategies to present environmental demands is an innate process to provide stability and control for movement patterns used to achieve the task. By "calling up" previously acquired strategies, a child can control actions and respond to environmental demands in a manner appropriate for self. Through integration of past actions with events, higher level sequences or "coordinative structures" become a part of the child's repertoire of performance. Each action, by the nature of the occupation, has boundary restrictions that set possible posture and movement strategies that can be used to complete the action.[4] Affordances and structured media of the occupation inform the person of those boundary conditions for performance. Therefore, specific spatiotemporal characteristics of environmental occupations are essential for promotion of performance.

During development a child engages in a variety of new events. What happens if the initial action is not successful? Fowler and Turvey[4] proposed that a person is challenged to repeat experiences, modifying performances until one's goal can be achieved. Through the spiraling continuum of spatiotemporal adaptation, a child uses information from outcomes of previously adapted strategies and sequences to direct higher level performances. Spatiotemporal adaptation theory suggests that acquisition of performance skills occurs through the process of restricting and/or controlling one's own actions by calling up the more primitive lower level behaviors to adapt to the demands of the environment and to integrate past with present. An occupation or event becomes a key element, as the self-perceptions of one's occupations direct selection of acquired behaviors that have been adapted by performing similar activities. The ecological event approach to the acquisition of performance skills supports the importance of the "purposefulness" of environmental events or occupations as well as the interaction of movement and environment.

Skills

The dynamic interactions of movement, environment, adaptation, and spiraling are illustrated with the following examples of the acquisition of skilled performance. The result of the spiraling function-to-purpose-to-function process--moving body in space, receiving and giving impetus--is the format used to discuss and illustrate the dynamic interaction of the theory's categories and properties.

Moving Body in Space

Examples of skilled performance requiring ability to move the body within spatiotemporal dimensions include running, hopping, and skipping. All of these skills adapt movement strategies gained during development of walking. For higher level skills, components of walking are differentiated and purposefully adapted to events of the environment for moving faster, or on one foot, or in rhythm.

Increased speed and timing changes, and changes in familiar base of support, mean that a child encounters new experiences with shifting weight while maintaining or changing position in space. In running, hopping, and skipping, there are times when there is no contact with a supporting surface. Anticipation of leaving and returning to a supporting surface adds new dimensions to dynamic postural control. Control over exertion, direction, and timing needs to be further developed in order to successfully adapt patterns from walking to new skills of running, hopping, and skipping.

During the time that a child is purposefully using previously acquired walking patterns to create new skill patterns of movement, more primitive forms of established movements may be used to adapt to the new challenge; e.g., unilateral weight-shift/movement pattern observed with early walking may appear again with early running, hopping, and skipping.

In order to illustrate the spiraling continuum of adaptation from developmental to purposeful to skill behaviors for moving the body in space, acquisition of running, hopping, and skipping skills will be described. Each description includes references to previously acquired strategies that are being called forth to meet new challenges, and ways in which these strategies are being used purposefully to enhance both maturation of strategies and sequences, and adaptation to skill performance.

Running

Running is a type of forward progression through space in an upright position. Running is distinguished from walking by a phase in which neither foot is in contact with a supporting surface, and by speed of forward progression.[10] Running begins around 18 months to 2 years of age, depending on when a child started walking. Early running tends to be in a straight line, but during preschool years, a child develops movement components and perceptual abilities that support changing directions while running, dodging objects, and stopping quickly. Development of strategies used for running well depend upon further maturation of strategies used for walking. There will be a period of time when spatiotemporal stress experienced from "trying" to run brings forth more primitive components of a walking pattern for use with early running. But with repetition of running and further maturation of the nervous system, the running pattern, like walking, develops into a smooth, coordinated way of moving rapidly through space.

Early running. Child uses high-guard position of arms to increase trunk extension and bilateral upper body stability in order to stay upright and provide background tone for increased speed of lower extremity actions. A child also "calls up" the previously acquired wide base of lower extremity support for stability and moves with a more vertical up-and-down pattern of lower extremities, often landing on toes or flat foot. Increased extensor tone in the trunk and upper body holding, along with vertical up-and-down movement, decreases rotation between body segments in the trunk.

As trunk stability improves, arms come down into a "readiness to protect" position, decreasing upper trunk holding and allowing trunk rotation along its long axis. Trunk rotates as a whole and arm and leg on the same side come forward together. The pattern is similar to <u>unilateral weight shift/movement</u> patterns seen previously in early crawling, creeping, and walking.

<u>Mature running.</u> Child gains enough stability in the upright, more rapidly moving posture to adapt rotation and counter-rotation patterns to running. With rotation available, <u>contralateral weight-shift/movement patterns</u> and accompanying reciprocal arm and leg movements are possible. Base of lower extremity support narrows and arms and legs assist rotation by reaching forward. Vertical movement is decreased as length of stride and non-supported time increases and produces more horizontal movement forward for smooth running. Running is adapted to many formal and informal games, as well as for jogging in later years.

Hopping

Hopping is a form of jumping in which takeoff and landing are on the same foot.[10]

<u>Early hopping</u> begins around 2 to 2-1/2 years of age when a child can stand on one foot but cannot unweight the standing leg. Trying to propel forward without unweighting the standing leg results in taking a step with the opposite leg. There is a little bounce to the action, which indicates that a hop was intended. Even when unweighting is possible, hopping is usually done in place, adapting the up-and-down movement from running. Propelling forward on one leg is still difficult. The act of standing on one foot and/or trying to propel forward usually requires stabilization from upper portions of body. A child again uses high guard or readiness to protect with arms in order to gain needed <u>bilateral stability.</u>

As balance improves for one-legged standing, a child finds ways to increase forward thrust in order to move up and down and forward at the same time. Both arms and non-support leg assist. The non-support leg, which was held forward in flexion and used to take a step if balance was lost, now begins to assist by a forward swing or pumping action that precedes unweighting the support leg. Arms come out of stabilization posture and swing forward <u>bilaterally</u> to assist the upward motion of the body.

<u>Mature hopping.</u> By approximately 4 years of age the hopping pattern has smoothed out into its mature form. Mature hopping is sequenced by <u>contralateral weight-shift/ movement patterns.</u> The non-support leg swings forward before the support leg thrusts upward. The arm opposite the non-support leg comes forward when the non-support leg swings forward. Meanwhile, the arm on the non-support side moves backward to balance out forward movement of the body in space. Hopping is used for games in middle childhood and is adapted to skipping.

Skipping

Skipping is a pattern of forward progression using the skill of hopping and alternating weight shifts from one side of the body to the other side.[10]

<u>Early skipping</u> begins around 4 to 5 years of age when a child can skip on one foot and take a step with the other. This early stage of skipping is a modification of hopping. A child actually takes a hop with the support leg and intends to shift weight to the opposite foot for another hop, but is unable to sequence the hop and takes a step instead. During this period of uneven timing, arms may be used again in high guard to stabilize upper body while lower extremities acquire new sequencing skills, and/or arms may come forward bilaterally to facilitate a hop while weight is being transferred.

A child gains some rhythm and increased balance from repeating the hop-step pattern. The pattern also takes on some attributes from running as a child thrusts upward with the hopping leg and reaches forward with the walking. Balance and rhythm allow for increased speed to the extent that the hop-walk pattern develops into galloping. Galloping depends more on unilateral weight shift/movement patterns for control. Upper and lower extremities on the same side move forward together and the same side of the body leads forward movement.

Mature skipping. Around 6 years of age both sides of the body participate in skipping because of a child's ability to sequentially shift weight and move forward with a series of reciprocal hopping-like movements. Adaptation of rotation between trunk segments allows contralateral weight-shift/movement patterns to occur. Extremities can respond with reciprocal movements that, along with trunk control, help propel the body forward and smooth out weight shift and rhythm. For the mature skipping pattern, one arm and the opposite leg reach forward, while the other arm moves back to balance movement forward and the foot opposite pushes off to skip. Skipping provides a sense of rhythm and movement that implies a sense of mastery of movement, and children pursue skipping as part of their pursuit of competence.

Sequences and skills described above are only a few of the possibilities for moving the body purposefully in space. Running, hopping, and skipping are not only skills in a child's repertoire, but aspects of these skill patterns are adapted to higher level participation in games and sports. Further maturation of strategies occurs during development of these skills, and this maturation improves a child's walking pattern as well.

Receiving Impetus

Skills described above involve moving the body in space by shifting weight between points of control. Timing is related to movement of the body in relation to those points. Skills associated with receiving and giving impetus to objects in space require use of extremities, primarily use of upper extremity reach and grasp, although lower extremities are involved in activities such as kicking. Timing is related to coordination of extremity movements in accordance with somatosensory and visual information about self and objects in space. Visual information is particularly important for shaping movement to respond to objects that are moving at various speeds. An example of receiving impetus from objects is catching.

Catching

Catching is described as use of body and its parts, usually hands, to stop and grasp an object that is being propelled through space.[10]

Early catching. First stages of catching focus on building perceptions of the ball moving in space. As soon as a child can sit securely with upper extremities free from their support role and lower extremities generally extended and abducted, she is ready to receive a ball that is rolled toward her. The child attempts to trap the ball with her legs and may extend her arms in an attempt to grasp the ball with two hands. With more postural control from lower extremity base of support, she may lean forward in anticipation of receiving the ball and stop it with her hands. Through repetition and practice with catching, a child gains information about the changing position of a ball in space and timing necessary to adapt to the change, as well as changes in her body's position in space and timing of changes in relation to the ball.

A second aspect of developing perception of a moving ball is evident when a child can get up and chase a ball and stop the ball's movement in space by adjusting movements.

Moving in space to catch becomes more significant when catching skills mature; meanwhile, chasing and stopping a ball provides information about a ball moving away from, as well as toward, self.

Between 2 and 3 years of age, a child attempts to catch a ball moving through the air toward self. There is a sequence of changes in upper extremity actions, as well as position of body in space, in preparation for receiving the ball. The size and speed of the ball plays a significant role in a child's success with catching at particular ages. At first, a child extends arms in front of body with palms of the hands up. Generally, a ball of any size will bounce off the child's chest before arm adjustments can be made. However, the child soon learns to flex elbows and trap the ball against the chest. By the next stage, there is an attempt to encircle and trap the ball with arms, but arm action usually occurs before the ball arrives and the child claps hands instead. However, if a ball is large enough, arm actions may occasionally be timed well enough to trap the ball between hands and chest. Usually, a child will stand facing the thrower and, as arm actions become more coordinated, the child may squat slightly in preparation for receiving the ball, catching it with hands together.

Mature catching. Mature catching requires control over upper extremity movement to the extent that a child can maintain a preparatory position and still make rapid adjustments in position of hands relative to trajectory and speed of approaching ball. Ball is caught in hands, usually with elbows slightly flexed in preparation for receiving impetus of the ball. A child may take a step forward while catching, which brings in some rotation around the body axis for more flexible adjustments of body position. The step forward also prepares for initiation of a throwing pattern if catching and throwing are part of the game. Catching is adapted to many games and sports. Frequently, catching while moving in space characterizes the higher levels of catching skill.

Giving Impetus

Giving impetus to objects refers to ways in which the body, especially extremities, can be used to propel or push objects through space. Key components include ability to control movement and use visual information to direct movement. Skills based on giving impetus to objects include throwing, striking, kicking, coloring/writing, and cutting. Throwing, coloring, and writing will be discussed to illustrate the ongoing spiraling process.

Throwing

Throwing can be described as thrusting an object into space with unilateral or bilateral arm motion.[10] Throwing toward a target increases the purposeful nature of throwing. Patterns for throwing depend on the size of the object, as well as child's level of maturation and experience. Bilateral upper extremity patterns are used for throwing a large ball, beginning with downward movement of the arms, followed by underhanded front throw, underhanded side throw, and overhanded front throw. Unilateral upper extremity throwing patterns also begin with downward arm movement. Underhanded unilateral throwing patterns appear first, followed by overhanded patterns.

Early throwing. First attempts at throwing are characterized by a quick downward motion of the arm or arms, primarily using elbow extension. The pattern is adapted from movement strategies used to release objects by dropping them with enough force to elicit a full upper-extremity extension pattern. As a baby develops object permanence, dropping objects to release them is linked to curiosity about where the objects go. A baby begins to purposefully project objects into space and visually follow the object's course of movement. As others encourage a child to throw a ball, the volitional aspect of letting go of an object is enhanced as the child throws toward someone or something. Emphasis is then on planning trajectory and force necessary to reach a target. Generally, in early throwing, a child stands facing the direction of the throw and there is very little body movement accompanying upper extremity movement. However, as the drive to direct movement increases, preparatory arm movements appear. A child's arm moves out to the side and back, or above the shoulder with full elbow flexion, before the throw is initiated. Preparatory movements make use of full ranges of agonist-antagonist movement as part of increasing force and determining direction.

Between the ages of 3-1/2 and 5 years, more body movement is included as part of throwing patterns and unilateral throwing is preferred for most objects that can be held with one hand. Beginning body movement includes rotation of trunk backward as arm is pulled back, followed by rotation forward with the throw. At first, a child's trunk seems to rotate as a whole without much rotation between upper and lower body segments. However, extremities do not participate significantly at this point.

By 5 or 6 years of age, a child steps forward during throwing, using the leg on the same side as the throwing arm. The child's arm is drawn farther back before throwing and extends in follow-through after releasing a ball. As a child throws, weight is shifted forward onto the leg, utilizing a underlineunilateral weight-shift/movement pattern reminiscent of earlier reciprocal patterns that coordinated extremity movements in unilateral--before contralateral--strategies.

Mature throwing. Between ages 6 and 7, mature throwing patterns begin to emerge. One of the most significant events is a change in the forward step. With maturity, a child-- and adult--steps forward with the leg opposite the throwing arm. Essentially, a child uses a contralateral weight-shift/movement pattern to control throwing and position the body in space. Contralateral patterns require rotation between body segments. As upper trunk rotates forward with the throw, the lower trunk counterrotates to control the range of upper trunk rotation. Weight forward on the opposite leg facilitates the counterrotation pattern. The flow between rotation and counterrotation of trunk segments provides background stability for expanding movements of the throwing arm. There is increased shoulder action with elbow extension and shoulder horizontal adduction that improves both speed and direction.

Components of throwing are adapted to numerous games and sports requiring specific adaptations in accordance with the rules of the game. Increased strength and agility allow running and throwing, as well as running and catching. Maturation of contralateral strategies facilitates dynamic stability required for such complex, purposeful movement.

Writing/Coloring

Writing and coloring require giving impetus to objects requiring more fine motor manipulation than use of body as a whole. Pencils and crayons become extensions of fingers and can be moved in any way that mimic finger movement. Vision provides significant information about the direction and outcome of the movement. Cognition frequently dictates the purpose of the movement, such as writing certain letters to make a word, or coloring parts of a drawing.

Holding and manipulating a pencil or crayon requires control from the hand itself, as well as more proximal joints. Evidence of proximal to distal direction of control over movement of the arm is observed when a baby first shakes a rattle using shoulder motion alone, before being able to move the rattle with elbow movement or wrist action. Gross control over manipulative objects held in the hand--such as a crayon--begins with shoulder movement, progresses to elbow, then to wrist movement before the crayon can really be handled well within the hand itself.

Meanwhile, hand adaptations to objects change as control over both gross and fine movements progresses. For example, a crayon may be held with palmar grasp in pronated position or palmar grasp in mid-position. With increasing control over both proximal and distal movement, a child may begin to hold pencil or crayon with inferior pinch, superior pinch, and eventually with prehension. Various combinations of proximal and distal control are possible, and moving between more or less mature patterns follows principles of adaptation and stress. For example, a child may hold a crayon with some form of pinch or prehension while using predominant shoulder motion to move the crayon, but attempts to use elbow motion may mean child will have to revert to palmar grasp to hold and control the crayon. Or, prehension may be used to color, but if a child tries to write her name, she may revert to palmar grasp due to stress from cognitive aspects of choosing and making letters.

The examples above illustrate the spiraling interaction of movement and environment, which further emphasizes the importance of purposeful occupation and the occupational process in the acquisition of skilled performance.

Adaptation of Skill to Play

For infants and children much of learning, development, and adaptation are accomplished through meaningful play. Play is a primary occupation for acquisition of skills; likewise, adaptation of skills expands the world of play for a child. Implicitly within the reciprocal interaction of skills and play is the notion of play as both process and product of spatiotemporal adaptation. Inherent within the "purposefulness" of interaction is a child's quest for autonomy and competence.

Achieving competence and a sense of autonomy is the core or domain of concern for a developing child. Thus, competence is an outcome of the spiraling continuum of spatiotemporal adaptation. It is important to keep in mind that throughout the spiraling process, spatiotemporal adaptation is not adjustment simply to the physical environment, but includes an environment shared by a person's perceptions, ideas, and values. Engaging in occupations requires adapting within a physical environment whose significance is mediated through one's sense of autonomy and competence.[11]

Several developmental theories have described the importance of a sense of autonomy, or a sense of self-efficacy or self-competence. Bandura[12] suggested a social learning component to be the development of self-efficacy and stated a person's perceptions of self-efficacy are based on performance and mastery, with additional influence of modeling and persuasion by others. Erikson[13] proposed that a youngster's acquired neuromuscular maturation sets the stage for advanced social modalities as a child begins to acquire a sense of self or autonomy. Allport[14] also stressed the importance of autonomy and described acquisition of "functional autonomy" as a sign of maturity, stating that development of functional autonomy is a dynamic, organized process of interacting with one's environment.

A sense of autonomy is dependent upon one's perception of self-competence. Kielhofner defined competence as "the quality of being able or having the capacity to respond effectively to the demands of one or a range of situations."[5,p502] Competence can be defined as having adequate and appropriate actions to meet the demands of environmental events.[14] White[15] suggested that behavioral phenomena such as exploration, activity, and mastery were beyond the scope of instincts or drives. He believed these behavioral phenomena resulted from a motivation construct of "competence." White termed motivation for competence "effectance motivation" and stated that effectance motivation involves satisfaction or a feeling of efficacy. According to White,[15,p329] "Effectance motivation leads a person to find out how the environment can be changed and what consequences will result." Smith[16] explored competence and effectance motivation and stated that for a sense of efficacy to result, an attitude of self-respect and "hopefulness" toward the environment is needed. Smith proposed that competence thrives on challenge and success, and a feeling of mastery contributes to personal efficacy and to health. A person's perception of self's competence and autonomy can be gained through participation with occupations or events that are playful and exploratory, as well as provide direction and electivity for interaction with the environment.[15] Therefore, play occupations and acquisition of performance skills provide both the means and power by which children acquire a sense of autonomy and competence.

Properties and processes of play are presented here as an example of occupation as an important media to enhance spatiotemporal adaptation.

Properties of Play

According to Reilly,[17] play is a biosocial phenomenon. The biological component comes from the fact that play is an activity performed by living things, which implies that play grows more complex over time. As a child grows and develops a more complex self-system, a child becomes capable of engaging in more demanding play occupations. A more complex system both stimulates and results from the maturation and spatiotemporal adaptation process.

Play's social component arises from the fact that play is organized as a result of experiences a child has with environmental interactions. The social phenomenon of organizing environmental experiences implies perceptual, cognitive, and emotional development, and organization of these systems. Later authors[8,9] described play as a biopsychosocial phenomenon, to emphasize biological and sociological phenomena, as well as stress the psychological or self's cognitive and emotional component of play.

Play qualifies as "purposeful" when it is used to facilitate reciprocal interweaving by requiring progressively more mature responses to play's increasingly complex demands and when it is used to provide spatiotemporal dimensions that give opportunities for a child to adapt past acquired actions and experience. As a purposeful occupation, play also requires a self-system to evaluate and organize environmental experiences at increasingly higher levels of integration. Play, then, by its own biopsychosocial components, promotes more mature responses, enhancing sensorimotor-sensory integration for the adapting child.

A child's intention to and attention throughout play comes from the novelty and challenge of the environment; therefore, if the spatiotemporal dimensions of the play setting are not challenging, a child may become bored, and if the play setting is too demanding, the child may experience distress. Although intention or arousal to play is initiated from the physical characteristics, the ongoing adaptation within the physical environment is mediated through a world of social interactions.[18]

Processes of Play

Reilly[17] identified three phases of play: exploration, competence, and achievement.

Exploration is the time in which new experiences, objects, or people arouse intention and curiosity. Competence, as the second phase, is a period when play becomes an opportunity to repeat and practice newly acquired play skills and experiment with environmental interaction, and in the third phase, achievement, play emphasis is on skilled performance. To Reilly the first two phases are intrinsically motivated, in a similar sense that Ayres[19] described a child's "drive to play." Reilly[17] believed the third phase of play is measured by external standards; thus, achievement is extrinsically motivated. We agree with Reilly's proposal that play is developmental, with its purposes changing during the play processes. Comparative analysis research undertaken for the development of spatiotemporal adaptation theory has led us to modify Reilly's[17] classification of the phases of play. Within spatiotemporal adaptation theory, play has four phases, each with distinct emphasis but interrelated through the reciprocal interweaving of the spiraling concept.

The first phase of play is its intention phase, similar to Reilly's first phase in that intention is the period when the novelty of the event arouses a child's interest. Intention is the initial experience that calls upon a child's curiosity to interact. Intention is a time when the self-system "sets" the goal to act or not act upon the event.

Attention becomes the second phase, when a child is absorbed in the exploration of an event. When the novelty of an event, experienced through the intention phase, is sufficient but not overpowering, a child will explore the "good enough" environment and begin to learn about its spatiotemporal dimensions. Also, in the good enough or "just right" environment, a child begins to develop trust in an object and environmental relationships. Berlyne[20] believed a good enough or just right challenge of the environment to be a spiraling organizer. The hierarchical organization of play occupations consists of movement and spatiotemporal environmental transactions that make spiraling adaptation possible. During the attention phase, the context of the play task influences a child's ability to explore and acquire a sense of autonomy. A child begins to learn the sensorimotor rules about how the body operates. In the play arena, the developmental phase of attention provides important opportunities for a child to acquire "environment rules."[21] A child begins to learn the sensorimotor rules about how his body operates; rules of motion, which teach representation of how one's body moves through space; rules of objects, which is knowledge about the properties of environmental objects; and rules of people, which is knowledge about behaviors and meanings of the behaviors of others. Both intention and attention phases of play are intrinsically motivated and a child participates for the sake of "doing."

Mastery, the third phase, includes experiences of repeating and practicing the "doing," as well as experimenting with increased environmental interactions surrounding the play experiences gained during intention and attention. Play's third phase is a time when a child is motivated to master events of the environment. Mastery motivation includes both intrinsic and extrinsic factors and is similar to White's[15] effectence motivation described earlier in this text. Mastery is a time when a child becomes aware of self's abilities and capacities and begins to measure self's success and failure with tasks. During mastery a child is motivated to experiment with the environment to see how it can be changed and what will result. Mastery provides opportunities for curiosity, exploration, repetition, experimentation, creativity, role-playing, and problem-solving, and leads to perceptions of self-efficacy.

The spiraling impact of intention, attention, and mastery phases evolves into the fourth phase of play, which is termed competence. As the final phase, competence is an outcome of play experiences. Through the interweaving of intention, attention, and mastery, a child acquires a sense of adequacy and satisfaction in self's capacities to respond.

Through play processes, a child learns spatiotemporal awareness and social interactions, develops flexibility and adaptability, and increases knowledge and skills that can be drawn upon for future experiences. Thus, play increases a child's repertoire of information for problem-solving and expands one's repertoire of sequences and skills for the ongoing adaptation of self with environment. As play expands to sports and recreation, the increased challenge from the environment promotes further refinement of genetically endowed and purposely developed skills.

Summary

Acquisition of skilled performance evolves through the ongoing spiraling process occurring through the spiraling spatiotemporal adaptation of strategies with developmental and purposeful sequences. Implicit within the transactional spiraling process of person with environment are key elements of occupations and occupational performance. A child's sense of autonomy and competence becomes the outcome of spatiotemporal adaptation.

Adaptations of purposeful sequences added new dimensions to the "doing" behavior of a child as he or she began to adapt self to events within the environment, and the "doing something" or active participation with one's environment allowed opportunities to differentiate aspects of a sequence to adapt to higher level skills. "Doing something" in relation to the environment was discussed as an occupational process, and the event or activity as occupation. Purposeful sequences were defined as actions goal-directed toward events, with actions being both intrinsically and extrinsically motivated.

Concepts of occupational performance and of occupation as play, work, and self-care were presented as both the process and product from which a child explores the world to achieve a sense of autonomy and competence. Properties and processes of play were discussed as an example of occupation to enhance adaptation, with skilled performance and a child's sense of competence as outcomes of the spatiotemporal adaptation process. Skill was defined as the final stabilization of sensorimotor development, as skill is characterized by the consistency of performance. Skilled performance was illustrated through examples of moving the body in space, receiving and giving impetus to objects.

Chapters 1 through 7 have been organized to present the grounded theory of spatiotemporal adaptation, discuss neuroscience concepts supporting the theory, to illustrate the dynamic interaction of the theories, categories, and properties, and describe the adaptation of strategies and sequences for the acquisition of skills. The remaining Chapters 8, 9, and 10 will provide the reader with a relationship of theory to therapeutic services. Chapter 8 presents concepts of maladaptation and discusses abnormal development. Chapter 9 presents a theoretical framework by which theory can be related to practice situations, and Chapter 10 discusses this theory into the context of theory development in the field of occupational therapy.

Key Points

1. Purposeful sequences evolve through the interaction of developmental sequences with environmental events.
2. Mere repetition of sequence and skills will not increase a child's ability or facilitate

development; there needs to be an increase of environmental demands, which facilitates the purposeful process of environmental interactions.

3. As sequences become goal-directed toward environmental events, there is an arousal of a child's intentionality, which promotes the purposefulness of occupations.

4. As a child engages in purposeful sequences, association and differentiation of actions with occupations afford one important aspect of feedback knowledge of the result.

5. Purposeful sequences are both intrinsically and extrinsically motivated.

6. Skilled performance is a final outcome of the sensorimotor-sensory adaptation process and, as such, skill is characterized by freedom of movement, natural responsiveness, consistency of patterns, and efficiency and accuracy in relation to spatiotemporal dimensions of the environment.

7. Major outcomes of skill include the ability to move the body within the spatiotemporal dimensions, to receive impetus, and to give impetus.

8. Fowler and Turvey, motor skill theorists, have described an event approach to skill acquisition. The spiraling process of past with present has support from the work of Fowler and Turvey, whose theory provides an explanation of motor skill acquisition.

9. Occupational performance is action that is elicited and structured by the environment, including the spatiotemporal characteristics of the occupation.

10. Occupations take place in a life-long series of environmental transactions with play, work, and self-care.

11. Occupations derive their purpose or meaning from the self-perceptions of the "doer"; the purposefulness of occupation is unique to the specific person "doing" the task and restricted to that person's goal direction.

12. A sense of autonomy and competency is an outcome of occupational performance skills and the spatiotemporal adaptation of skilled performance.

13. Occupations and the acquisition of performance skills provide both the means and power by which children acquire a sense of autonomy and competence.

14. Play, as occupation, is a process to achieve competence, and as a process, play has four phases that are interwoven throughout the development of play skills: intention, attention, mastery, and competence.

Self-study Guidelines

1. Define the following terms: purposeful, purposeful sequences, occupation, occupational performance, play, work, self-care, skill, autonomy, competence, affordance, and structured media.

2. Compare and contrast concepts of Fowler and Turvey's ecological event theory with spatiotemporal adaptation.

3. Discuss the interrelated triad of play-work-self care as occupations for exploring and mastering the environment.

4. Give two examples of moving the body in space and of receiving impetus.

5. Explain occupation as a major aspect of spatiotemporal adaptations.

6. Differentiate developmental and purposeful sequences.

7. Explain occupational performance as the process, and occupation as the product, of person-environmental transactions.

8. Describe the development phases of play as presented by Reilly and compare

these phases to the interacting phases of intention, attention, mastery, and competence.

9. Discuss autonomy and competence as outcomes of spatiotemporal adaptation.

References

1. Wells K: Kinesiology. Philadelphia, Ed 3. W.B. Saunders Co., 1963, pp. 327-412.
2. Connolly K (Ed.): Mechanisms of Motor Skill Development. New York, Academic Press, Inc., 1970, pp. 3-18.
3. Bruner J: The growth and structure of skill. In Connolly K (Ed.), Mechanisms of Motor Skill Development, 1950, pp. 63-92.
4. Fowler CA, Turvey MT: Skill acquisition: An event approach with special reference to searching for the optimum of a function of several variables. In Stelmuch G (Ed.), Information Processing in Motor Control and Learning. New York, Academic Press, 1978.
5. Kielhofner G (Ed.): A Model of Human Occupation: Theory and Application. Baltimore, Williams & Wilkins, 1985.
6. Kielhofner G: Occupation. In Hopkins H, Smith H (Eds). Willard and Spackman's Occupational Therapy. Philadelphia, J.B. Lippincott, 1983, pp. 31-41.
7. Erikson J: Activity, Recovery, Growth. New York, W.W. Norton & Co., Inc., 1976, p. xi.
8. Glencross D, Reynolds N: Attentional strategies during the learning of a sequential skill. J Human Mot Studies 7:23-32, 1981.
9. Gliner J: Purposeful activity in motor learning theory: An event approach to motor skill acquisition. Am J Occup Ther 39:28-34, 1985.
10. Wickstrom RL: Fundamental Motor Patterns. 3rd Edition. Philadelphia, Lea and Febiger, 1983.
11. Englehardt HT: The importance of values in shaping professional direction and behavior. In Target 2000: Occupational Therapy Education. Rockville, MD, American Occupational Therapy Association, 1983, p. 42.
12. Bandura AC: Self-efficacy mechanism in human agency. Am Psych 37:122-147, 1982.
13. Erikson EH: Childhood and Society. New York, W. W. Norton, Inc., 1963.
14. Allport GW: Pattern and Growth in Personality. New York, Holt Rinehart Winston, Inc., 1961.
15. White R: The urge toward competence. Am J Occup Ther 25:271-274, 1971.
16. Smith MB: Competence and adaptation. Am J Occup Ther 28:11-15, 1974.
17. Reilly M (Ed): Play as Exploratory Learning. Beverly Hills, Sage Pub., 1974.
18. Kielhofner G, et al.: A comparison of play behavior in nonhospitalized and hospitalized children. Am J Occup Ther 37:305-312, 1983.
19. Ayres AJ: Sensory Integration and Learning Disorders. Los Angeles, Western Psychological Services, 1972.
20. Berlyne D: Conflict, Arousal and Curiosity. New York, McGraw-Hill Book Co., 1960.
21. Robinson AL: Play: The arena for acquisition of rules for competent behavior. Am J Occup Ther 31:248-253, 1977.

CHAPTER 8

Spatiotemporal Distress and Dysfunction

Objectives

The reader will be able to

1. define the concept of distress and discuss the distress process;
2. compare and contrast the concepts of "stress" with "distress";
3. describe the impact of spatiotemporal distress upon SMS factors;
4. describe the primitive signs of dysfunction;
5. discuss the effects of distress and dysfunction on the development of key behaviors;
6. compare the effects of distress upon sensorimotor performance in children diagnosed as having cerebral palsy with children diagnosed as having sensory integrative dysfunction.

Introduction

According to the spatiotemporal adaptation theory, changes in a person and his or her environment can result in more efficient and effective adaptation between the person and the environment.[1] For a developing child, changes in structure, function, and purposes of movement associated with sensorimotor development, (Figure 8-1)as well as a "good enough" environment, are critical for efficient and effective adaptation to occur. Relationships between change and adaptation were introduced in Chapter 2 when categories and properties of spatiotemporal adaptation were identified. The category termed "spiraling continuum," with its properties of stress and distress, relates most significantly to concepts presented in this chapter. Effects of spatiotemporal stress have been emphasized throughout descriptions of developmental and purposeful sequences. This chapter will elaborate on the effect of spatiotemporal distress and its relationship to some types of dysfunction that create performance challenges for children.

Stress, as discussed in Chapter 2, affects ways in which bodily structures, functions, or purposes can change to support more efficient and effective adjustment, or adaptation to the environment. Stress can produce a temporary interruption in sensorimotor developmental processes. The interruption usually occurs when a child is challenged by a new situation and calls up previously acquired behaviors to adapt to the new situation. Although stress may initially interrupt sequential development, under ordinary circumstances stress eventually facilitates maturation of structures, functions, and forms of response which allow a child to meet new performance challenges. Stress is a positive factor in adaptation as long as a child is developing typically.

Unfortunately, stress can produce a negative factor in sensorimotor development and adaptation if a child's nervous system is not developing typically, or if typical development is affected by an acquired insult to the nervous system. Instead of being able to use challenges from the environment as sources of stimulation for higher levels of development and adaptation, a child continues to use previously acquired, lower level responses in attempts to meet new challenges. Efforts to develop more efficient and effective means to adapt to a changing, more demanding environment are easily thwarted. The child is at risk for developing a persistent state of distress, which can result in some kind of dysfunction.

Spatiotemporal distress is stress out of control, which cannot be managed by normal development of posture and movement strategies, or by adaptation of strategies to developmental and purposeful sequences of behavior. The origins of spatiotemporal distress may lie within the child (e.g., a lesion within the nervous system preventing maturation of structures and functions) or within an environment that is not a positive source of stimulation for development, or both. In any case, the sensorimotor-sensory process of adaptation is interrupted, and the interruption may be manifested in a child's ability to assimilate information, accommodate to information, and associate or differentiate information affecting sensorimotor development. Distress can be a negative factor

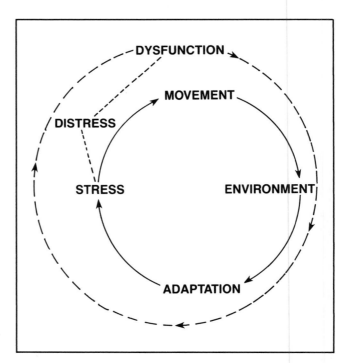

Figure 8-1: Spatiotemporal Distress to Dysfunction.

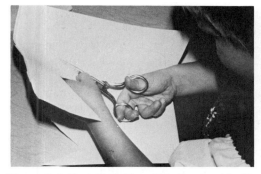

Figure 8-2: Typical Cutting: This 5-year-old with normal adaptation patterns cuts with manipulative prehension and differentiation of mobility and stability in the hand. Stability along the ulnar side of the hand provides control for radial mobility to manipulate scissors.

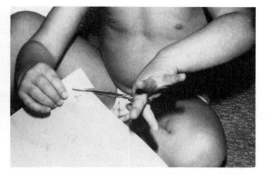

Figure 8-3: Primitive Cutting: The same child in Figure 8-2 at age 2+ used undifferentiated patterns to cut, which was a normal adaptation for her age.

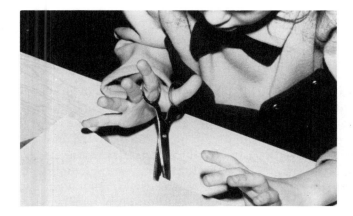

Figure 8-4: Distress in Cutting: This 5-year-old girl with learning problems cuts by adapting undifferentiated patterns (full flexion-full extension) to manipulate scissors. Her pattern reflects adaptations used by younger children with scissors.

in a child's pursuit of higher levels of functioning. With distress, as with stress, there is an alteration in the system's equilibrium. But in the case of stress, after a child adapts to the stressful situation either by calling forth previous behaviors or developing new behaviors, there is return to a state of equilibrium, or homeostasis, within the system. If distress prevents a child from using the situation to develop new, higher level responses, then a child continues to use lower level responses while trying to adapt to increasingly more complex environmental demands.[2] The system cannot return to or develop an optimum state of equilibrium. Reinforcement of purposeless rather than purposeful movement ensues. Repetition of distressful experiences that do not result in purposeful accomplishment of goals can lead to dysfunction in sensorimotor performance and perhaps in other domains of development as well. Examples of the concepts described in this paragraph are illustrated in Figures 8-2, 8-3, and 8-4.

Spatiotemporal distress results from (1) abnormal assimilations, e.g., abnormal sensory reception, sensory deprivation, or sensory overload (jamming); (2) abnormal accommodations, e.g., purposeless sensorimotor patterns, abnormal neuromuscular characteristics (tone, range, control, speed, etc.); and (3) abnormal association/differentiation, e.g., faulty sensorimotor-sensory integration.

Origins of spatiotemporal distress causing dysfunction in sensorimotor performance are numerous. There are hereditary factors; chromosomal abnormalities; unexplained birth defects; fetal distress or lack of expected development in utero; prematurity or dysmaturity; difficulties before, during, and after birth with residual brain lesions, retardation, acquired problems from trauma or disease affecting the central nervous system or peripheral systems; abuse; neglect; or environmental deprivation. Although information about origins of a child's distress/dysfunction is valuable for purposes of evaluation, prognosis, planning, monitoring progress, etc., the most valuable source of information available for analysis of spatiotemporal distress is the child.

Spatiotemporal distress affects every aspect of a child's progress toward maturity. The child's relationships within the family and world outside, his feelings of competence and autonomy, and other persons' responses to him are built upon performance expectations held by the child for himself and others for him. Since so much of early, measurable performance in children is built upon spatiotemporal adaptation, interruptions in the process, or failure to develop according to expectations has a reverberating effect upon the SMS process, neurophysiologically and emotionally.

SMS Factors

The quality and quantity of **sensory assimilations** have an obvious effect on the rest of the SMS process.

1. **Too little sensory input**, as experienced by children who are neglected or in non-stimulating situations, results in absence or poor quality/quantity of motor accommodations. Sensory feedback to self and from others from a poor response reduces the possibility of increasing quality or quantity of input. Over a period of time, the cycle may result in sufficient distress to cause dysfunction in adaptation.

2. **Too much sensory input**, which may occur in well-meaning but overstimulating situations, may overload the system, not allowing adequate accommodation and feedback for association-differentiation. The child may continue to be responsive to stimulation, but his system cannot make sufficient use of assimilations for adaptation.

3. Sensory assimilations that are **threatening** or harmful, as in child abuse, or input **perceived as threatening** due to delay in adapting protective responses, may cause the child to withdraw, physically and/or emotionally. Again, the process of accommodation-feedback is altered. Withdrawal from the initial source for modification of the system leaves the child functioning in a primitive state, or attempting to function at higher levels with primitive strategies of posture and movement.

4. Sensory assimilations may be **received but not recognized** by some children who are functioning at a lower level, or at risk for problems with sensory integration. If input is not meaningful, there may be no accommodation, or inadequate accommodation to the sensory stimulation. Neither response provides the adequate feedback for change within the system.

The quality and quantity of **motor accommodation** also affects the SMS process. It is possible that initial sensory assimilations could be considered adequate for eliciting a response, but the difficulty lies with the **motor accommodation** itself. Since accommodations play such a vital role in feedback for change, the whole SMS system is affected rapidly, even though difficulties with motor accommodation seems to be the primary problem.

1. Sensory assimilation seems adequate and appears to be recognized by the child. Due to maturational delay or trauma within the system, **motor accommodations** may be absent, purposeless, or characterized by immature strategies, including aberrations in neural and muscular functions. If accommodations are absent or purposeless, there is lack of feedback for adaptation. If responses are present, but abnormal, feedback is abnormal.

2. Sensory assimilations from abnormal feedback become the basis for adaptation with children whose problems are manifested primarily in the **motor** area. Abnormal muscle tone controlled by primitive neural mechanisms becomes characteristic of a child's attempt to adapt. Abnormal movement patterns can develop into uniquely abnormal developmental sequences which will be described later in this chapter.

Finally, for some children, the SMS process may appear to be intact for achievement of developmental and purposeful sequences. However, there may be difficulty integrating and making meaningful use of **sensory feedback**.

1. Even if assimilations are received and acted upon by the child, **feedback** must be associated and differentiated. Failure to adequately associate and differentiate feedback leads to deficits in sensory judgment, thereby interrupting the sensorimotor-sensory integrative process and development of perception.

2. Faulty **feedback** from poor association-differentiation becomes the basis for adaptation of strategies to progressively higher levels of development, activity, and skill. As a result, the child's performance may be characterized by attempts to use lower level primitive or transitional strategies to adapt to mature types of behaviors and activities. The process is further complicated because repeated immature adaptations are not meaningful for change. The child does not develop posture and movement strategies that transfer readily to skill performance.

Since sensorimotor-sensory adaptation is a spiraling process, any interruption in one aspect of the process has an effect upon the rest of the system. Outcome of distress within the system may be immediately observable or may take years to manifest full impact. Even though specific types of congenital problems may be related to a primary source of distress, effect of distress upon SMS adaptation is widespread and impacts the child and her environment totally. Knowledge of primary sources of a problem is important for assessment and intervention as long as recognition is always given to the effect of interaction between sensory, motor, and feedback components of the system.

Generally, children categorized as abused, neglected, over- or under-stimulated, developmentally delayed, or retarded have problems that originate from difficulty processing or making use of initial assimilations. Aspects of their adaptation process usually remain primitive, or may be characterized by unique posturing or repetitive movement patterns. Children diagnosed with cerebral palsy, motor delay, or a particular type of muscle tone such as hypotonia, experience initial difficulty with motor accommodation. Their behavior and activity performance may be marked by stereotyped posture and movement patterns, abnormal reflexes, abnormal muscle tone, and development of adaptations not reflective of normal development.

Finally, children with sensory integrative dysfunction, learning disabilities, or other delays may have integrative problems that begin with a failure to internally perceive initial sensory assimilations accurately,[2] thus compromising the SMS process as a basis with which to adapt. Other children with sensory integrative dysfunction may have problems that begin with failure to associate/differentiate feedback from sensorimotor experiences. Therefore, aspects of primitive and transitional strategies influence developmental and activity performance.

Children with acquired interruptions in the SMS process present other variables. If trauma or disease (for example, head injury, Reye's Syndrome, burns, amputation, juvenile arthritis) interrupts development after the basic foundation for SMS integration has been established, it is more difficult to determine which aspect of the process is most affected. Just as the SMS system functions as a whole, the system is affected as a whole. Manifestations of acquired spatiotemporal distress include regressions in adaptation; for example, calling forth primitive and transitional strategies and behaviors previously integrated. The child may also acquire some abnormal adaptations with abnormal muscle tone, especially if the central nervous system is involved in the original trauma or disease.

Whether spatiotemporal distress originates with congenital or acquired problems, the factors that tended to cause stress in normal development (i.e., gravity, combinations of movement, and complexity of behavior or activity itself) are also factors related to distress/dysfunction. In the presence of a problem within the child's system and/or environment, these stress factors lead to distress resulting in dysfunction, since the child with problems cannot make use of the stress situation to modify his responses. He tends to repeat a limited repertoire of immature or abnormal sequences without change, and dysfunction prevails. In addition, these stress factors may contribute to further progression in dysfunctional performance. The child's repeated attempts to respond to gravity with immature or abnormal muscle functions and patterns of movement, increased demands for more complex adaptations, and the child's own assessment of his competence following unsuccessful, unmodified experiences, all comprise some of the secondary factors contributing to dysfunctional performance (Figures 8-5, 8-6, 8-7, 8-8, 8-9, 8-10). Both primary and secondary stress factors impact negatively on development of strategies and adaptation of strategies to the developmental and purposeful sequences that support skill performance.

As a result of distress, posture and movement strategies are likely to be delayed or develop with deviations in quality and quantity of neural and muscular functions. Strategies may not be adapted or may be poorly adapted to developmental sequences, leaving posture and movement control to isolated stereotyped strategies rather than a

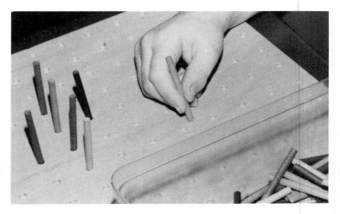

Figure 8-5: This 5-year-old boy with cerebral palsy, spastic diplegia uses a superior pincer grasp for objects requiring minimal manipulation.

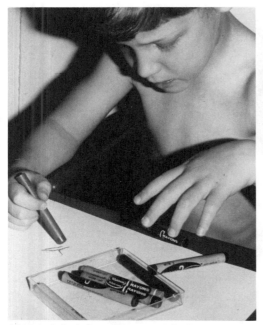

Figure 8-6: Adaptation to manipulate a crayon initially calls forth an inferior pincer grasp.

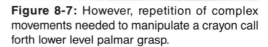

Figure 8-7: However, repetition of complex movements needed to manipulate a crayon call forth lower level palmar grasp.

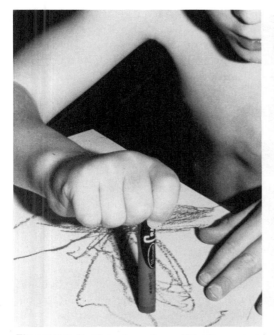

Figure 8-8: Further stress from difficulty controlling movement as well as posture results in lower level pronated grasp.

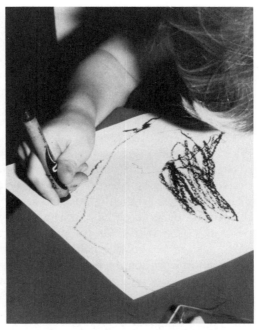

Figure 8-9: The same boy begins again, trying to maintain pincer grasp, but losing posture control due to stress.

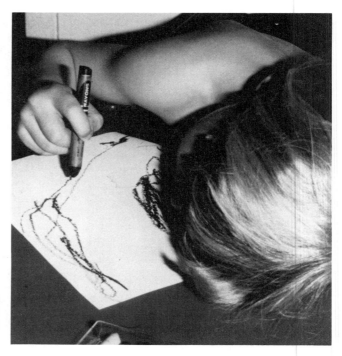

Figure 8-10: Persistent attempts to maintain pincer grasp result in disintegration of postural control over head and trunk.

variety of unfolding behaviors. The drive toward higher level developmental and purposeful behaviors may or may not be present. If the quest for development is absent or severely delayed, then purposeless, eventually abnormal, strategies can prevail. If the drive to pursue purposeful developmental behavior is intact, but if the child cannot modify strategies sufficiently for adaptation, then performance, or attempts to perform, may be goal directed, but characterized by either primitive, transitional, or abnormal patterns of movement and postural control.

Distress to Dysfunction

Primitive and transitional strategies are usually identified as dysfunctional whenever the strategies are used to adapt beyond the normal time or at higher than expected levels of behavior/activity.[2] Primitive and transitional strategies reflect early stages of normal development as described previously. The problem is usually not the strategy itself; the difficulty comes when the strategy is not modified by the association-differentiation process and is available only in the primitive or transitional form for use with mature behaviors or activities. Or, the problem may be evident when primitive or transitional strategies are too readily called forth during mature performance with the slightest provocation from spatiotemporal stress. Thus, mature functioning is so easily lost that it cannot gain from repetition. Instead, primitive and transitional strategies are repeated more often. As a result, immature neural mechanisms and muscle functions characteristic of primitive and transitional phases continue to be predominant influences on behavior, instead of being adapted to mature strategies. Evidence of primitive and transitional strategies used to adapt beyond normal periods for calling forth previous behaviors may indicate pathology in the child's adaptation process.

When central nervous system pathology is present, abnormal patterns of movements and attempts to control posture may resemble some primitive strategies, but are characterized by increased, decreased, or fluctuating muscle tone, which is never normal during the usual course of development. Or, patterns may be abnormal because they are comprised of postures or movements not observed at any time in the course of normal development. For example, some particular syndromes or developmental deviations are characterized by stereotyped postures or repetitive movement patterns unique to the particular diagnosis. Abnormal patterns of movement and control imply that the brain is not fully developed or that trauma occurred before, during, or after birth. Abnormal patterns may not be apparent in newborn infants, but can be detected in babies after approximately 4 months of age, and even before, if there is severe involvement.[3]

Abnormal patterns make use of abnormal muscle tone, either hypertonic, hypotonic, fluctuating, or combinations of these types of tone. Primitive reflexes assume control over behaviors and activities since abnormal tone interferes with normal modification of primitive reflexes. Reflexes accompanied by abnormal tone tend to control behavior in an obligatory sense. The child repeats stereotyped, reflex-like patterns, building abnormal sequences and reinforcing the effect of the reflex rather than modifying it. Patterns that appear primitive in young babies, or following trauma at any age, can develop into abnormal patterns if abnormal muscle tone, previously undetected, becomes part of a primitive strategy. Effect of gravity and demands for more complex movement at higher levels may bring forth abnormal tone when potential for abnormality is present due to brain lesions. Care should always be taken to recognize developing abnormalities by monitoring change carefully and by avoiding postures and movements known to evoke abnormal responses, even though the posture or movement maybe part of typical sequences for typical children.

Developmental sequences are interrupted whenever primitive or transitional strategies are retained and used to adapt, or whenever abnormal patterns of movement are present. The extent and degree of pathology determines lags or arrest in development of behaviors and corresponding spatiotemporal distress/dysfunction.* Each time an abnormal response is observed, or a behavioral sequence is incomplete, or an immature response is used to adapt, the occurrence should be evaluated in terms of its effect on behavior as a whole. Children with dysfunction can be analyzed by **identifying main problem** and determining **how it interferes** with function. Analysis of behavior yields information about the SMS process, distress factors, strategies retained and adapted or linked together, strategies (and hence behaviors) that have failed to develop, and abnormal as well as normal patterns that are present.

Early Signs of Dysfunction

During the normal primitive phase of development (0 to 3-4 months), only observations regarding behaviors that have failed to develop or obvious, severe abnormalities can be regarded as dysfunctional or potentially dysfunctional. The quality and quantity of behaviors developing during primitive phases may be suspect, but can be considered dysfunctional only if interfering with higher levels of development after the primitive phase. Some observations that are suspect for later problems include the following:

Note: Observations of neonates and very young infants will be particularly influenced by the baby's state at the time of observation. Factors such as prematurity will also influence posture and movement patterns. Specifically developed evaluation criteria should be used to evaluate neonates or premature babies.

1. **Poverty of movement:**[1] There is a lack of primitive movement. The baby does not make use of phasic activity for reflexive kicking, frequent head-turning, or opening and closing hands. Spontaneous movements, cuddling, movement to sight or sound may be diminished or absent. Poverty of movement deprives the child of motor accommodations that lead to development of muscle functions and key developmental behaviors. The baby may appear to be hypotonic.

2. **Stereotyped movement:**[1] If the baby develops limited movements, the movements may be linked together into stereotyped sequences. Sequences tend to be repeated, reinforcing the stereotype and interfering with development of variability needed for adaptation. If abnormal muscle tone becomes a factor, hypertonicity combined with stereotyped movements produces limited sequences repeated in serial order (i.e., the child extends neck, opens mouth, and extends upper extremities; or grasp with hands is followed by flexion of arms, neck, and trunk, etc).

3. **Static postures:** If there is inconsistency noted between ability in different postures, it may be early evidence of muscle tone problems.[4] A child may appear to be developing appropriate muscle functions in one position, but when placed in a different position requiring the same accommodation, there is a decrease in tone.[2] Early inconsistencies in primitive muscle functions may indicate that muscle tone developing in one posture is abnormal and therefore not available for transfer to another posture.

4. **Suck-swallow problems:** Feeding behavior is one of the bodily functions already established at birth which reflects synchrony of movement. Problems with suck-swallow patterns resulting in feeding difficulty may be a predictor of movement difficulties at higher levels. In addition, the baby is deprived of one of the first intact SMS cycles that can be associated with other behaviors. Feeding difficulties also interrupt early infant-parent relationships that are formed around nurturing or survival situations. Neither parent nor baby is satisfied by difficult, nonproductive feeding periods.

5. **Lack of visual responsiveness:** Visual interaction and early tracking behaviors may not be apparent during primitive development. A deficit in visual responsiveness deprives the baby of one of his more advanced methods of receiving information about his world. The deficit also eliminates one way in which the baby can attract others to respond to him. Poor visual tracking also diminishes the baby's sources of input for looking and moving, which is later adapted to visual motor coordination.[5]

6. **Lack of transitional preparation:** Failure to develop such behaviors as head lift in prone, head align in supine, and protective or spontaneous head turning in prone or supine deprives the child of necessary neural maturation and muscle development to progress from the primitive to transitional phase of development.

Signs such as poverty of movement or static postures are predictive of problems with transition due to either poor development of extension and flexion or lack of flexor development balancing extensor development. The baby needs to develop adequate flexion and extension along with the normal righting, support, and protective reactions in order to develop from primitive to mature functioning. If not, then stereotyped movement patterns controlled by persistent primitive reflexes and potentially abnormal muscle tone or problems using well-developed transitional behaviors for mature functioning form the bases of baby's adaptation to the environment.

If primitive development is suspect, the baby may not be establishing a good basis for development of strategies and behaviors necessary to adapt to higher levels. Specific areas of distress may be emerging, even though definitive dysfunction may not be identified. The origin of a baby's distress response or lack of response determines the nature of the dysfunction to follow. For example, a brain lesion occurring before, during, or shortly after birth is likely to result in some type of cerebral palsy so that dysfunction is characterized by emergence of abnormal muscle tone, interference from primitive reflex patterns of posture and movement, and compensatory behaviors used to adapt. Or, if distress occurs because of developmental delay, dysfunction may result from lack of maturation of structures and functions required for higher levels of development, resulting in delay in development and continued use of primitive strategies. The lag in development may or may not continue to influence performance, depending on the baby's potential to develop higher level structures and functions of the nervous system and to make use of facilitory environmental interaction.

Or, if distress occurs from prematurity, or from unknown origins, and observations include difficulty in developing and integrating transitional responses such as balanced flexion and extension, integrated protective support reactions, integrated vertical-rotational righting reactions, and use of rotation for equilibrium, the child's problems may be indicative of problems associated with sensory integrative dysfunction. Cerebral palsy, developmental delay, and senosry integrative dysfunction are only a few diagnoses affecting children's spatiotemporal adaptation process. Examples of cerebral palsy and some reference to effects of sensory integrative dysfunction are included for further explanation of distress-dysfunction continuum in the adaptation process.

Effects of Cerebral Palsy on Spatiotemporal Adaptation

Bax[6] defined cerebral palsy as a disorder of posture and movement due to a defect or lesion in an immature brain. In cerebral palsy, the brain lesion is non-progressive and causes varying degrees of difficulty in coordination of muscle action, with resulting inability or difficulty maintaining typical postures and performing typical movements. Since the lesion is central, there are often associated problems with speech, vision, hearing, and perceptual and cognitive development[7]. Effects of cerebral palsy may not be clinically obvious at birth, or shortly after birth, unless brain lesion is diffuse and abnormal muscle tone and postures are already apparent. Quinton[8] and Bly[7] have suggested that as many as 95% of babies later diagnosed with cerebral palsy tend to be hypotonic, or babies with low muscle tone, during the first few months of life. Low muscle tone does not provide an adequate base for development of posture and movement strategies required for developmental sequences, purposeful sequences, or skill performance.

There are a number of possible effects that can result from low tone as a basis for development of posture and movement strategies:

1. Movement components and accompanying muscle functions either fail to develop or are delayed in developing and/or combining with other movement components that are developing. One of the major problems noted is failure of adequate neck, trunk, and proximal joint flexion to develop and combine with developing extension at the appropriate time for establishing quality movement. Axial extension, unopposed by flexion, combined with the original brain lesion creates opportunity for abnormal extensor tone to influence all ensuing posture and movement patterns. Later, flexor groups that have not developed adequate muscle functions against gravity may also develop abnormal tone. Abnormal muscle tone in the

trunk and extremities may be distributed according to primitive reflex patterns, influenced by baby's position in space (TLR), or position of head in relation to trunk (ATNR, STNR).

2. Attempts to move with underlying low muscle tone and lack of combined and blended mobility-stability muscle functions means baby tends to hold postures by using only extensor patterns around proximal joints. By using extension without flexion, baby may be able to hold or "fix" in a position, but cannot move within or from the position. Primitive proximal holding patterns actually prevent combined mobility-stability, righting reactions, and equilibrium reactions from emerging and controlling posture and movement. In the presence of a brain lesion, prolonged use of extensor patterns, combined with abnormal extensor tone, leads to abnormal postural patterns and poor background tone for control of movement patterns. Movement components like neck extension, scapular stability, or pelvic mobility, intended to facilitate posture and movement strategies, instead become blocks and create distress in developmental progressions.

3. Poor quality of movement and/or abnormal postural control used to adapt to developmental or purposeful sequences creates distress and leads to compensatory patterns rather than higher level patterns of posture and movement. Repetition of compensatory or distressful strategies can lead to habitual patterns of relatively purposeless rather than purposeful movement in terms of usefulness for higher levels of adaptation. In cerebral palsy compensatory patterns, accompanied by abnormal muscle tone, can lead to muscle contractures and bone/joint deformities, further compromising the adaptation process and resulting in dysfunction in sensorimotor-sensory performance.

4. Even though the precipitating cause of cerebral palsy may be present at birth, effects are not always obvious in all segments of the body until nervous system maturation affecting development of those body segments occurs. Thus, a child whose main involvement is in lower portions of the body may seem to be developing typically, as long as development is primarily focused on upper body functions. Later, distress and dysfunction in lower body segments may bring forth compensatory patterns in upper segments as well, compromising development of higher level functions seemingly unaffected during early development. The central nature of cerebral palsy and the spiraling process of adaptation mean that interruption in development of functions affecting one segment of the body will eventually affect other segments of the body as well.

Bly[7] has focused on effects of abnormal holding or fixing patterns in proximal segments that prevent movement and higher level automatic reactions from developing. These holding patterns around the neck, shoulders, pelvis, and hips interrupt progressions of developmental and purposeful sequences and often lead to abnormal sequences of development. Effects of cerebral palsy on developmental sequences of spatiotemporal adaptation are summarized here.

Prone-Creeping Progression

1. If the baby is initially hypotonic, there may be a delay or absence of primitive behaviors such as frequent head turning, primary crawling, or head lift. The baby continues to assume a flexed posture in prone due to influence of tonic labyrinthine reflex and adaptation of fetal flexion. In the presence of a central nervous system lesion, the tonic labyrinthine reflex is accompanied by abnormal tone, increasing flexion and further preventing development of extension.

2. If baby does not begin head lift with neck extension, but neck flexion does not develop shortly afterwards in supine progression, then neck extension is basically unopposed. Neck flexion ordinarily balances extension and allows elongation of long and short neck extensors. With the stress created by lack of flexion, baby assumes neck hyperextension pattern and uses neck retraction to keep head raised in space. Shoulder elevation is sometimes added to help stabilize head on shoulders (Figures 8-11 & 8-12).

Distress: Continued use of neck hyperextension and retraction is a distress response that results in dysfunction by interfering with development of stable head control, by preventing head turning from side to side (which ordinarily develops neck rotation components), and by preventing vertical righting reactions from emerging and further developing neck and upper trunk extension. Neck hyperextension also limits downward eye gaze and mouth closure. Prolonged use of neck hyperextenion, accompanied by abnormal tone, may also prolong influence of symmetrical tonic neck reflex on prone behavior (Figures 8-13 & 8-14). An abnormal symmetrical tonic neck reflex, retained beyond its normal course and accompanied by abnormal muscle tone, becomes an obligatory posture and movement pattern characteristic of cerebral palsy. With neck hyperextension, the baby experiences increased extensor tone in upper extremities and increased flexor tone in lower extremities. The reflex-based symmetrical posture only allows child to shift weight bilaterally in prone or on hands and knees, leading to "bunny

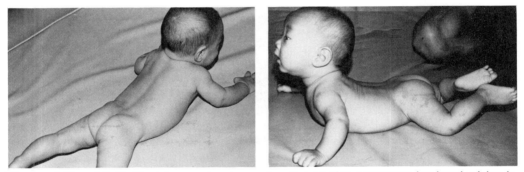

Figures 8-11 and 8-12: Neck hyperextension and neck retraction accompanying head raising in baby with low tone and delayed development of flexion.

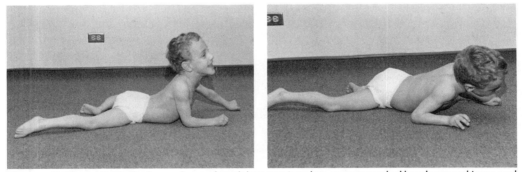

Figures 8-13 and 8-14: Prolonged use of neck hyperextension, accompanied by abnormal tone and symmetrical tonic neck reflex.

hop" prone progression pattern and tendency toward "w-sitting" (Figures 8-15 & 8-16).Unilateral and contralateral weight shift patterns cannot emerge.

3. If there is an imbalance and delay in development of neck control, shoulder development and related behaviors are also affected (Figure 8-17). When neck extension does not facilitate enough upper trunk extension to allow baby to free arms for weight bearing, and if upper trunk flexion is not developing sufficiently to assist with bringing arms forward, then baby tends to keep elbows behind shoulders. With elbows behind shoulders, baby retains a primitive upper extremity position characterized by shoulder protraction, internal rotation, and abduction along with elbow flexion, forearm pronation, and finger flexion. When spasticity occurs due to cerebral palsy, the same upper extremity flexor components are usually involved. Tightness may develop between scapula and humerus since elongation and separation between scapula and humerus cannot develop when upper extremities do not come forward to assume weight-bearing positions.

Distress: Continued interference from scapulo-humeral tightness is a distressful response that results in dysfunction by interfering with development of upper extremity support reactions, protective reactions, use of upper extremities for early locomotion, and development of all upper extremity reaching patterns. Shoulder movement components and muscle functions, as well as differentiation between upper extremity components, provide control for upper extremity support, protection, and reach and cannot develop when upper extremities retain primitive posture and movement patterns. In addition, hand functions that are dependent on early weight bearing and reaching are affected. Weight bearing on hands helps to desensitize grasp and avoidance reflexes, and elongates wrist flexors, finger flexors, thenar eminence, and intrinsic hand musculature. Upper extremity reaching places hand in contact with objects which significantly influence shaping of hand functions. Lack of controlled reaching, in addition to retention of primitive grasp patterns and possible increase in muscle tone, limits development of hand functions through decrease in environmental interaction. Finally, development of vertical and rotational righting reactions and equilibrium reactions is affected when baby cannot assume upper extremity supported positions which allow expansion of trunk extension and flexion, or use upper extremity support to change positions which facilitate development of upper trunk rotation and leads to development of components required for equilibrium.

4. If arms do not come forward into a weight-bearing position and combine extension with flexion around shoulder, then scapular adduction as a means for

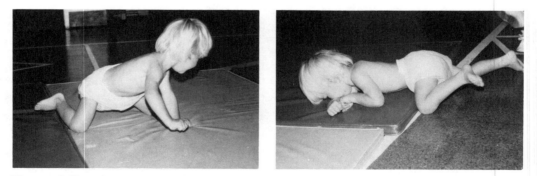

Figures 8-15 and 8-16: Effects of symmetrical tonic neck reflex on attempts to creep.

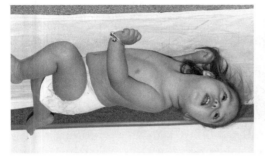

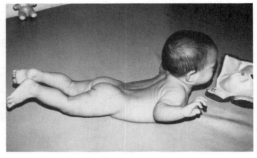

Figure 8-17: Lack of head control and shoulder development to hold head in space and bring arms forward.

Figure 8-18: Early evidence of block from neck hyperextension, neck retraction, and scapular adduction in prone.

facilitating upper trunk extension remains unopposed and upper extremities are pulled into retraction with flexion (Figure 8-18).

Distress: Scapular adduction-upper extremity retraction that is not balanced by shoulder and upper trunk flexion is a distressful response that results in dysfunction by further interfering with development of upper extremity weight bearing. Primitive scapular adduction pattern tends to keep upper extremities flexed and held in retraction. The effects of upper extremity retraction on upper extremity function are similar to consequences described under scapular-humeral tightness. In addition, the retracted pattern of upper extremities further increases tightness between scapula and humerus. Supine reaching patterns which ordinarily facilitate separation between scapula and humerus and foster scapular control for reaching are significantly affected by prolonged scapular adduction-upper extremity retraction. In prone, combinations of neck and upper extremity retraction affect mouth closure and may result in jaw retraction as well. If baby is placed in higher level positions such as sitting, or if baby attempts to lift trunk in prone, primitive scapular adduction and upper extremity flexion and retraction will be used to facilitate trunk extension. Without balance from flexion to bring arms forward and still maintain trunk control, the primitive upper body posture will continue to be used for postural control.

Distress responses affecting upper portions of the body will affect development and adaptation in lower body segments as well. The descriptions of distress presented above identify problems that occur when extension is not balanced with flexion due to a lesion in the central nervous system and primitive patterns combined with abnormal muscle tone persist. If baby's involvement is extensive, increased extensor tone will not only affect neck and upper trunk segments as noted above, but as baby attempts to adapt abnormal extensor patterns to work against gravity, increased tone affects hips and lower extremities as well. Extensor tone through the body results in increased hip extension and adduction with knee extension and plantar flexion. Full extension patterns may be more obvious in supine due to retention of the primitive tonic labyrinthine reflex.

5. If involvement does not seem to involve upper body segments at first (e.g., diplegia), the effects of cerebral palsy may not be noticed until developmental progression involves use of lower trunk, pelvis, and hips. As extension develops in prone in lower trunk and hips, but is not balanced by development of abdominal and hip flexion in supine, an anterior pelvic tilt develops, but is not balanced by development of a posterior pelvic tilt.

Distress: Anterior pelvic tilt in prone that is not balanced by flexion is a distressful response that results in dysfunction by prolonging primitive hip abduction-external rotation posture, preventing unilateral weight shift which depends upon trunk elongation and hip adduction-internal rotation, and interferes with development of pelvic mobility and stability. If baby is able to shift weight from one upper extremity to the other, but position of pelvis and hips prevents unilateral weight shift onto elongated trunk and extended hip, then weight shift is accomplished by lateral flexion of trunk on the weight-bearing side. The primitive position of pelvis and hips provides a fixation point for the abnormal weight-shift pattern which develops with lateral flexion, prolonging use of a lower level posture to adapt to a higher level activity. Pelvic-hip fixation prevents vertical righting from expanding to include hip extension, blocks expansion of rotational righting and associated segmented rolling patterns, decreases mobilization and separation of pelvic movement from upper trunk movement, and eventually prevents equilibrium reactions from developing in lower portions of the body. Without development of higher level components and reactions, upper extremity and upper trunk development is compromised. Baby cannot function with trunk off the supporting surface or transfer stability functions to lower portions of body and free upper extremity for skill.

Distress: Pelvic-femoral tightness develops when hips remain abducted and externally rotated and create a distressful response that results in dysfunction by preventing development of hip extension and adduction in prone, separation between pelvis and femur for lower extremity weight shift and reciprocation, and differentiation between functions of hip, knee, and ankle for a variety of weight-bearing postures and development of lower extremity support and protective reactions. Early foot responses are also altered if baby cannot extend lower extremities and push against supporting surface with plantar surface of toes.

If the child is not as involved in upper portions of body and is able to move forward and back using upper extremities or assume a creeping position, increased anterior tilt and pelvic femoral tightness may still be evident, and movement is likely to utilize a bilateral weight-shift pattern, due to lack of development in unilateral and contralateral weight shifting. Crawling bilaterally or creeping with a bunny hop pattern is characteristic of continuing to adapt lower level patterns to higher level functions. If child is more minimally involved, crawling and creeping may be accomplished with unilateral weight shift, but will not be smoothed out by contralateral weight shift as long as imbalance in development of movement components and increased tone in some components continue to exist. The continued use of lower level patterns to adapt to higher level demands, such as using bilateral weight shift to bunny hop in creeping, is a good example of distress, or inability to develop and use higher level functions to meet the demands of the environment. The distress of using a lower level pattern for higher level challenges becomes dysfunctional when the child continues lower level bilateral patterns for creeping, especially if abnormal muscle tone influenced by a symmetrical tonic neck reflex becomes part of the pattern. Such distress affects not only development in prone, but child's performance in sitting, rolling, standing, and walking as well.

Supine-Sitting Progression

1. If baby is hypotonic, there may be a decrease in generalized movement in supine, such as infrequent head turning or reflexive kicking, ability to hold head in midline, and there may be exaggerated head lag if pulled to sit (Figure 8-19). If

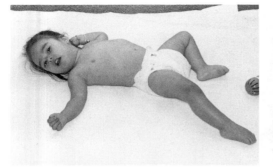

Figure 8-19: Difficulty maintaining head in midline due to lack of flexor development. ATNR is evident with head to side.

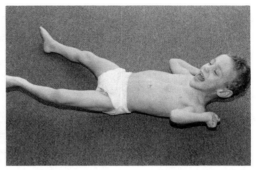

Figure 8-20: Extensor tone in supine is increased by effects of tonic labyrinthine and symmetrical tonic neck reflexes.

abnormal extensor tone develops due to lesion in brain, the tone may be distributed to a stereotyped, tonic labyrinthine reflex pattern in supine, further preventing development of flexion in supine (Figure 8-20). Without adequate flexion to align head and trunk while coming to sit or being held in sit, baby uses neck retraction and shoulder elevation to stabilize head or trunk.

2. When flexion against gravity does not develop, or does not develop at optimum time for blending with extension, most supine development and adaptation will be affected. At birth, baby's head is usually turned to one side or the other due to effect of gravity. Flexion allows baby to bring head to midline and hold it in the center. Flexion supports smooth head turning, visual pursuits, and development of symmetry. With flexion developing at midline, baby eventually aligns and then raises head when pulled to sit. Flexion is combined with extension for head control in space, and neck flexion against gravity supports maturation of vertical righting reactions, which facilitate upper trunk, then lower trunk, flexion.

Distress: Shoulder elevation is a distressful response that results in dysfunction by interfering with development of supine head raising as well as head turning. Fixing head on trunk with shoulder elevation prevents vertical righting reactions from emerging and facilitating development of neck and trunk flexion in supine and sitting (Figure 8-21). Without flexion to combine with extension, baby cannot develop head control or subsequent trunk control in any position. Lack of flexion in shoulders and upper trunk particularly limits upper extremity separation from rest of body, leads to scapular-humeral tightness, and allows scapular adduction to keep upper extremities flexed and held against supporting surface rather than serving as control for upper extremity separation and reach. Baby has difficulty bringing hands to mouth, hands to midline, hands to feet, or reaching to swipe or grasp objects in space. Development of oral-motor functions, hand functions, and both oral and manual investigation of objects is affected. Development of rolling patterns is also affected if head turning is blocked by shoulder elevation. Without frequent head turning, baby does not separate head movement from trunk movement or develop neck righting reactions which facilitate spontaneous rolling and all other rotational righting reactions.

As noted in discussion of effects of distress on prone-creeping behavior, low tone and lack of flexor development affecting upper body will eventually affect lower trunk and lower extremity development as well, since development of structures and functions

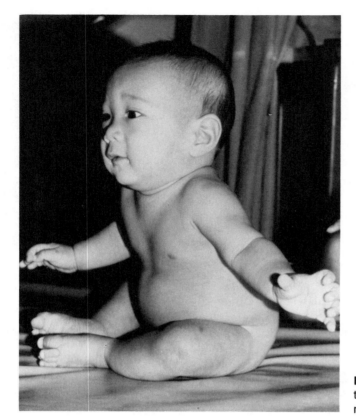

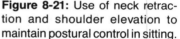

Figure 8-21: Use of neck retraction and shoulder elevation to maintain postural control in sitting.

progresses cephalocaudally. Baby will not have upper body stability as a reference point for developing lower body functions, or the mobility necessary to develop lower extremity functions. In cases of brain lesions, abnormal extensor tone may develop, increasing the difficulty of initiating flexion against gravity. For some children (e.g., children with diplegia) lack of flexion in supine may be evident only when baby reaches developmental age for using lower body flexion, although early absence of kicking, or asymmetrical kicking, may be a sign of distress.

3. If baby does not develop flexion in lower trunk and hips, ability to raise trunk and lower extremities against gravity is limited. Abdominal flexion is not available for development of posterior pelvic tilt and vertical righting reactions cannot facilitate lower trunk and hip flexion. Baby cannot explore knees or feet with hands, or bring feet together or to mouth. Oral-motor function and hand-foot function development are affected.

Distress: Anterior pelvic tilt which is unopposed in supine is a distressful response that results in dysfunction by interfering with development of lower body flexion against gravity. Vertical righting reactions cannot expand to facilitate flexion, and combination of flexion and extension, required for development of pelvic stability. Without flexion combined with extension, rotational righting reactions cannot develop. Rotation facilitates deliberate and automatic rolling, as well as separation between upper and lower body segments. Without rotation, more primitive neck righting continues to influence rolling without segmentation. With only anterior tilt available, lower extremities are

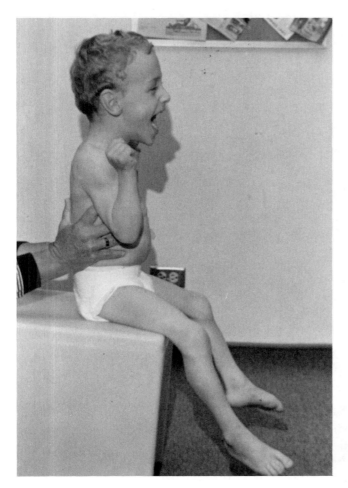

Figure 8-22: Use of scapular adduction to stabilize in supported sitting.

likely to remain in abduction-external rotation since extensions may also be blocked from combining with flexion and bringing lower extremities into more neutral rotation. Placing feet on supporting surface for foot development, or pushing with feet for bridging or turning, is also affected and decreases opportunities for foot preparation before standing.

If baby attempts to sit or is placed in sitting, lack of flexion to balance extension or counteract abnormal extensor tone leads to a number of compensatory strategies:

- Neck hyperextension and retraction for head control.
- Shoulder elevation for head control.
- Scapular adduction with upper extremity flexion to stabilize upper body in extension against gravity (Figure 8-22), or collapse of trunk over wide base of lower extremity support with upper extremities used for propping.
- Anterior pelvic tilt to fix lower trunk posture, or collapse into posterior tilt if tone in trunk is low.
- Hip flexion, abduction, and external rotation to counterbalance scapular and pelvic accommodations and provide wide base of support; or use of w-sitting to stabilize pelvis with wide base of support (Figures 8-23, 8-24).

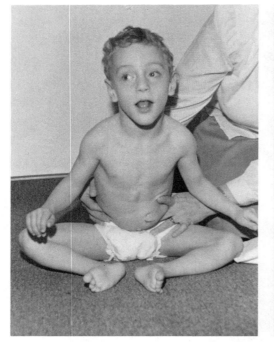

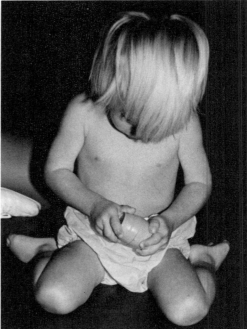

Figure 8-23: Use of neck retraction and wide base of support to compensate in supported sitting.

Figure 8-24: W-sitting to stabilize in sitting.

- In case of very strong extensor tone and influence of tonic labyrinthine reflex down through the hips, placing child in sitting may produce posterior pelvic tilt if extension prevents flexion of hips and positioning of pelvis over hips. Baby hyperextends neck, allows upper trunk to flex with gravity, and may utilize forward propping to balance effects of extension on lower trunk and extremities.

Rolling Progression

1. If baby has low tone and lack of flexor development, there may be less head turning and poor rooting associated with poor suck-swallow patterns and difficulty keeping head in midline. Asymmetry in supine continues if baby cannot bring and hold head in midline.

Distress: Asymmetry is a distressful response that results in dysfunction and interferes with development around midline of trunk and all extremity functions at midline. In addition, persistent asymmetry of head to one side or the other provides continual stimulation of an asymmetrical tonic neck reflex.[9] Child's attempts to use ATNR for spontaneous rolling may increase extensor tone and actually block rolling. If abnormal tone is present, the asymmetrical tonic neck reflex becomes an obligatory, stereotyped response that occurs whenever baby turns head, or keeps head turned. The reflex interferes with development of rotational righting and rolling, causes deformities of spine and hips, and prevents reaching from supine, hands to mouth, and hands to midline activities. The ATNR is one of the most persistent primitive reflexes to affect children with cerebral palsy (Figure 8-25).

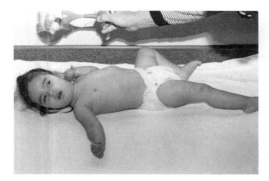

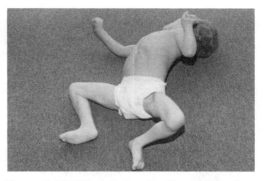

Figure 8-25: ATNR interfering with rolling from supine.

Figure 8-26: Attempts to roll with extension but no active flexion increases extensor tone and effects of ATNR.

2. If the ATNR does not interfere with rolling, but neck flexion does not develop sufficiently to combine with extension for adequate neck rotation, neck righting cannot develop to initiate rolling. Rotational righting reactions, separation of body segments, contralateral weight shift, and equilibrium reactions depend upon maturation of rotation, which begins with head turning.

Distress: Neck and trunk extension, not balanced by neck and trunk flexion is a distressful response that affects rolling. The child repeatedly attempts to roll with unopposed extension and cannot activate neck and trunk flexion to modify extension and complete the rolling pattern. Child's attempts to roll are unsuccessful, and reinforce abnormal extensor tone and tonic labyrinthine reflex. In addition, attempts to roll cannot result in combining extension and flexion around neck and trunk, which ordinarily leads to rotation and rotational righting reactions (Figure 8-26).

Standing and Walking Progression

1. Initially, primary standing or walking may be absent due to low muscle tone. If extension develops and is sufficiently affected by abnormal tone, and tonic labyrinthine reflex, later attempts to place a baby in standing result in stimulation of a positive supporting reaction to which baby cannot adapt due to abnormal extensor tone and lack of flexor development. Abnormal extensor tone may also affect lower extremity adductors, resulting in lower extremity extension and crossing one leg over the other leg.

Distress: Increased extension throughout trunk and lower extremities is a distressful response that results in dysfunction by interfering with development of lower extremity stabilization for standing and reciprocation for walking. Unbalanced extension and abnormal tone allow the positive supporting reaction to persist as an abnormal reflex so that the baby tends to stand or walk on toes. Abnormal extensor tone precipitated by positive supporting also increases use of anterior pelvic tilt and scapular adduction to gain stability in standing (Figure 8-27). Weight shift for pull to stand is also affected causing baby to use bilateral weight shift and push back over lower extremities rather than bring extremities under hip to get to stand (Figure 8-28).

If a child is able to maintain a standing position, a number of compensations may be evident as a result of compensations previously noted and effects of increased extension in standing.

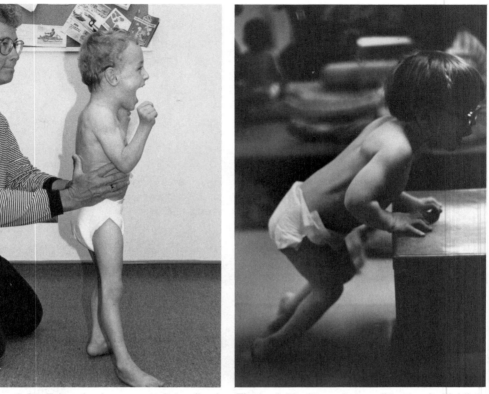

Figure 8-27: Extension in supported standing is reinforced by scapular adduction and positive support reaction.

Figure 8-28: Attempts to pull to stand with bilateral weight shift.

- Neck hyperextension and retraction.
- Shoulder elevation for head control.
- Scapular adduction and upper extremity flexion for upper trunk stability.
- Anterior pelvic tilt for lower trunk stability or posterior tilt if trunk tone is low and posterior tilt was used in sitting.
- Lower extremity flexion and adduction to lower center of gravity overcome increased extension and stabilize with knees in adduction.
- Pronation of feet due to position of hips and knees.
- Use of lateral flexion to shift weight unilaterally for locomotion.

Upper Extremity Functions

Most of the problems affecting upper extremity development have been identified and effects are summarized below:

- Lack of scapular-humeral separation and resulting tightness limits range of upper extremity movement and development of scapular control for upper extremity reach and grasp. Scapula and humerus continue to move as one segment when child attempts to reach.
- Upper extremity retraction, which accompanies scapular adduction, limits reach, opportunities for support and protective reactions to develop and decrease in experience touching parts of body and objects in space.

- Decreased opportunities exist for weight bearing and weight shifting on upper extremities required for shoulder-scapular stability and stability-mobility patterns, elbow stability, and reciprocal movement of upper extremities. Controlled reach does not develop due to decreased weight shift.
- Lack of opportunities for weight bearing on hands also eliminates source of elongation of wrist flexors, as well as elongation of structures in palm, especially thenar eminence. Weight shifting on hands facilitates differentiation between functions on radial and ulnar side of hand, and weight bearing desensitizes primitive grasp reflexes.

These descriptions of effects of cerebral palsy on development of key behaviors and possible compensations are intended to highlight only some possible effects of initial low tone status on early development. Cerebral palsy affects every aspect of a child's development, and muscle tone can range from low to normal to high tone in the form of spasticity, athetosis or ataxia (depending on the lesion), the child's state, and position.[10] Abnormally high tone is identified by presence of pathological deep tendon flexes as well.

A brief look at early signs and symptoms of cerebral palsy in the presence of low tone is presented here to illustrate problems associated with lack of development and adaptation of key postures and movement strategies, and compensations that can occur and contribute to dysfunction, especially in the presence of abnormal muscle tone.

Effects of Sensory Integrative Dysfunction on Spatiotemporal Adaptation

According to Ayres,[2] sensory integrative dysfunction comes from an irregularity or disorder in brain function that makes it difficult to organize and use sensory input for an adaptive response, learning process, or perception of self or the world. Children with sensory integrative dysfunction may be hyperactive and distractable; exhibit behavior problems related to difficulty coping with everyday stress or unfamiliar situations; have low muscle tone which provides inadequate base for developing postural tone, automatic reactions for balance, and smooth coordinated movement; or problems with speech-language development and learning. More specifically, children with a sensory integrative disorder in postural and bilateral integration exhibt poorly integrated primitive postural reflexes, immature equilibrium reactions, poor ocular control, and general lack of integration of functions of two sides of the body. Poorly integrated postural reflexes along with resulting immature righting and equilibrium reactions make a child appear incoordinated in motor activities. Child's difficulty shifting weight in contralateral patterns is evident in activities requiring equilibrium, crossing the midline of the body and even fine motor activities which require subtle shifts in background postural tone.

Less is known about early effects of sensory integrative dysfunction on the spatiotemporal adaptation process than has been observed about cerebral palsy. Perhaps early observations have not been as extensively documented because sensory integrative dysfunction tends to influence higher levels of adaptation and is not evident until demands for higher level adaptations emerge. However, developmental histories reported after diagnosis include such observations as a feeling of low tone, failure to achieve or sustain some key behaviors, poor suck-swallow feeding patterns, resistance to touch or holding, irritability, and, in some instances, feeling of stiffness and rapid movements, perhaps related to lack of sufficient postural tone to support and control movement. A type of primitive holding of body segments may be substituted for lack of postural control, as noted previously in discussion of cerebral palsy. However, with sensory integrative dysfunction, abnormal muscle tone does not become part of patterns, as noted with cerebral palsy. Instead, prolonged primitive holding or rapid execution of movements for control affect both the quality and quantity of posture and movement strategies and, hence, the child's primary means for spatiotemporal adaptation.

Some problems associated with sensory integrative dysfunction may be related to the distress experienced by a child when components of movement do not develop, or do not develop at the appropriate time to be combined with antagonist components of movement. Protective reactions may not be well enough integrated from lack of movement experience to allow the child to seek out and accept new sources of stimulation. Reflexes and reactions related to postural control, which appear with maturation of the nervous system, need movement components ready for activation in order to effectively facilitate and support protective righting and equilibrium reactions required for control of movement.

The effects of timing in development of components of movement and/or combining and blending the mobility and stability functions of movement, as well as maturation of automatic reactions that control posture and movement, are key to providing postural background tone and smooth, coordinated movement.

Movement and postural control patterns observed in children with diagnosed sensory integrative dysfunction support the idea that distress in early development of posture and movement strategies, and adaptation of strategies to developmental and purposeful sequences, may be reflected in child's later attempts to perform activities requiring skilled movement.

- **Extension** not sufficiently balanced with **flexion** in vertical postures affects some children's rapid or directed movement in upright (e.g., a child who is walking fast or running and experiences an increase in extension through upper trunk, perhaps including **scapular adduction**, in order to reinforce postural extension and maintain upright). Because extension may not have been sufficiently integrated with flexion, undifferentiated patterns of extension may be allowed to emerge under stress and child comes up on toes for fast walking or running.

- **Neck hyperextension** and shoulder **elevation** may be used to control head and neck posture, especially when child is engaged in an activity requiring postural control in sitting, like drawing or writing. In addition, child may try to control fine movement by increasing tone around shoulder. Grasping an object tightly for control over shoulder and hand movement is similar to the way a baby used fisted hands to control on-elbows or on-hands posture before proximal shoulder mobility and stability was sufficiently developed.

- **Prolonged use of righting reactions, support**, and **protective reactions** instead of **equilibrium reactions** to control posture and movement also results in distress when child is trying to perform play and academic activities. Progression from righting, support, protection to equilibrium (with protective reaction when necessary), for control of balance depends upon development and blending of extension, flexion, lateral flexion, and rotation, as well as maturation of neural mechanisms for equilibrium. If child does not develop sufficient equilibrium reactions, then development and use of rotational patterns of movement are also affected. Rotation accounts for smooth, coordinated sequences of movement, which make use of contralateral weight shift and equilibrium reactions. Rotation and equilibrium also support crossing the midline and use of a dominant extremity. If equilibrium reactions are not well developed, child may continue using righting and support reactions to change position during activity. Righting reactions tend to facilitate complete ranges of movement, so differentiating part of a sequence of movement for an activity is difficult at times. A child may intend to move only partially out of a posture, but instead changes position completely. Or, a child's equilibrium reaction may be so insufficiently developed that the slightest move away from center of gravity elicits a protective reaction rather than an attempt to regain equilibrium (Figure 8-29).

A child who does not develop adequate equilibrium with accompanying rotation and contralateral weight shifting tends to use unilateral weight shift and lateral flexion to adapt to developmental and purposeful sequences. As a result, walking is not a smooth forward progression, but rather a side-to-side weight shift, more like a two-step process of shifting and moving. Child's attempts to adapt this unilateral pattern to fast walking, running, or any upright activities requiring balance and movement results in distress, producing uncoordinated performance or lack of ability to perform. Timing of movement in relation to spatial demands is especially affected when equilibrium and rotation are not optimally developed and adapted.

- **Difficulty developing and blending muscle functions affecting development of hand functions.** The stress of fine manipulation, plus concentration on a cognitive or perceptual activity, means that stability-mobility blending within the hand may not be sufficiently adapted to higher level hand functions. Child may grasp objects too tightly in an attempt to control object and upper extremity, making smooth, coordinated movement of objects, such as following a line with a pencil, more difficult. Or, movements in hand may be undifferentiated for some activities; for example, using full extension followed by full flexion patterns to manipulate an object such as scissors, or using full flexor palmar grasp or immature pinch to manipulate a pencil.

Sensory integrative dysfunction affects many performance areas in children. Only some manifestations are in the area of development and adaptation of posture and movement strategies to developmental and purposeful sequences and, hence, the development of skill. However, those sensory integrative functions affected, such as

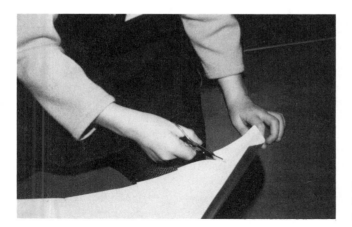

Figure 8-29: Difficulty integrating sides of body to perform fine motor task.

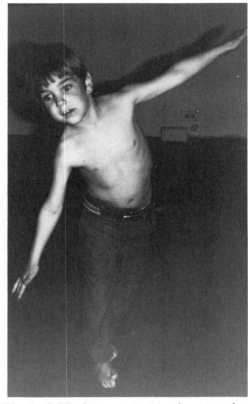

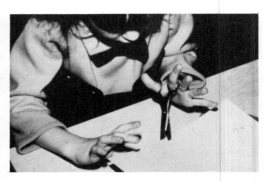

Figure 8-31: Use of undifferentiated extension to manipulate scissors.

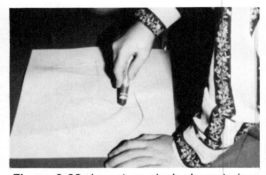

Figure 8-30: Attempts to stand on one foot results in loss of balance around mid-line of body and elicits a protective response.

Figure 8-32: Immature pinch characterizes child's manipulative prehension.

postural security and praxis, reflect spatiotemporal distress that can result in dysfunction.

Summary

The theory of spatiotemporal distress and dysfunction has been presented and applied to the examples of dysfunction in children. Spatiotemporal distress was presented as persistent use of lower level, more primitive strategies to adapt to higher level demands for developmental or purposeful performance. Distress may produce dysfunction if adaptation process is interrupted and the interruption becomes a block to further sequential development, or development of mature strategies that support effective and efficient sequential development. If distress results in continued use of primitive and transitional strategies to adapt, dysfunction in related performance areas results. If primitive strategies and attempts to use transitional strategies are accompanied by abnormal muscle tone due to brain lesion, child's adaptation process is further compromised.

Special acknowledgment and appreciation is extended to Lois Bly, MA, PT, for her meticulous observations and careful reporting of components of normal and abnormal movement in children.

Key Points

1. Stress can produce a negative factor in sensorimotor development if a child's nervous system is not developing typically, or if typical development is affected by an acquired insult to the nervous system.

2. Spatiotemporal distress is "stress out of control" that cannot be managed by normal development of posture and movement strategies, or adaptation of strategies to developmental and purposeful sequences of behavior.

3. With distress, the SMS process of adaptation is interrupted, resulting in abnormal assimilation, accommodations, and/or association/differentiation.

4. Distress may prevent a child from using the environmental situation to develop higher level responses; thus, a child continues to use lower level responses while trying to adapt to increasingly more complex environmental demands.

5. Sensorimotor-sensory integration is a spiraling process; therefore, any interruption in one aspect of the process has an effect upon the rest of the system.

6. Regardless of the origin of spatiotemporal distress (congenital or acquired), factors that tended to cause stress in normal development (gravity, combinations of movement, complexity of behavior/activity) are also factors related to distress/dysfunction.

7. Spatiotemporal distress affects every aspect of a child's progress toward maturity.

8. As a result of distress, posture and movement strategies may be delayed or develop with deviations in quality and quantity of neural and muscular functions. Strategies may not be adapted to purposeful behaviors and the "drive" toward purposeful behaviors/activities may not be present.

9. Primitive and transitional strategies are usually identified as dysfunctional whenever strategies are used to adapt beyond the normal time or at higher than expected levels of behavior/activity.

10. When CNS pathology is present, abnormal patterns of movements and attempts to control posture may resemble some primitive strategies, but are characterized also by increased, decreased, or alternative muscle tone, which is never normal during the usual course of development.

11. Movement patterns that appear primitive in infancy, or following trauma at any age, can develop into abnormal patterns if abnormal muscle tone becomes part of a primitive strategy.

12. Developing sequences are usually interrupted whenever primitive or transitional strategies are retained and used to adapt, or whenever abnormal patterns of movement are present.

13. During the primitive phase of development (0 to 3-4 months), only observations regarding behaviors that have failed to develop, or severe abnormality, can be regarded as dysfunctional or potentially dysfunctional.

14. Observations that are suspect for pathology include poverty of movement, static postures, and inconsistent patterns, such as swallowing problems, lack of visual responsiveness, and/or lack of transitional preparation.

15. Distress and dysfunction affect the development of key behaviors, resulting in spatiotemporal maladaptation.

16. Low muscle tone does not provide an adequate base for development of posture and movement strategies required for developmental sequences, purposeful sequences, or skill performance.

17. Low tone may be present in babies later diagnosed with cerebral palsy.
18. Cerebral palsy causes difficulty in coordination of muscle action with resulting difficulty maintaining typical postures or performing typical movements.
19. Sensory integrative dysfunction comes from an irregularity or disorder in brain function that impacts the system's capacities for organization and use of sensory input for an adaptive response.
20. Sensory integrative dysfunction impacts the child's learning process and perception of self or the environment, thus interfering with spatiotemporal adaptation.
21. Some problems associated with sensory integrative dysfunction may be related to the distress experienced by a child when components of movement do not develop, or do not develop at the appropriate time to be combined with antagonistic components.
22. Movement and postural control patterns observed in children with diagnosed sensory integrative dysfunction support the idea that distress in early development of posture and movement strategies and adaptation of strategies to sequences may be reflected in child's later attempts to perform activities requiring skilled movement.

Self-study Guidelines

1. Define spatiotemporal distress and compare it with spatiotemporal stress.
2. List seven observations of behaviors manifested in the primitive phase that may be suspect for pathology.
3. List three or four examples of abnormal assimilation and abnormal accommodations.
4. Chromosomal abnormality is one basic origin of spatiotemporal distress; list five other factors that may be the primary sources of distress and dysfunction.
5. When can primitive and transitional strategies be identified as dysfunctional? Is the strategy the problem that leads to dysfunction? If so, explain; if not, explain.
6. Define and describe abnormal muscle tone.
7. Describe "stereotyped movement" and "static postures."
8. Discuss the effects of cerebral palsy on the prone-creeping progression of spatiotemporal adaptation.

VIGNETTES

Twins K and G

Two sets of twins have been chosen to illustrate the effects of distress on performance. The photographs compare the children's performance during one session. Photographs and information do not comprise a complete case study but illustrate selected behaviors and activities.

One set of twins (K and G) are illustrated with the first vignette, Figures 8-a through 8-t. Twin K demonstrates performance affected primarily by delayed developmental sensory integrative dysfunction. The second vignette illustrates twins M and T with photographs 8-aa through 8-pp. Twin M has been diagnosed as spastic cerebral palsy and demonstrates the effect of abnormal patterns upon performance.

Background Information

K was the second of identical twins born approximately 32 weeks gestation. His birth weight was 890 grams. K was transferred to an intensive care newborn nursery shortly after his birth. He was hospitalized in the nursery for approximately 2 months. Diagnosis included prematurity, small for gestational age, respiratory distress syndrome, hyperbilirubinemia, and growth retardtion. At 2 years, 2 months of age K was referred for evaluation because of developmental delay. According to the evaluation he was functioning at approximately 15-16 months in fine motor, gross motor, and social-language development. Following the evaluation K was treated in a coordinated occupational therapy, physical therapy, and speech language program.

The photographs were taken when K was 3 years, 2 months. At that time a re-evaluation indicated that he was functioning at approximately a 3-year-old level in gross motor skills, 2½-year-old level in fine motor skills, and a 3-year-old level in social-language development. However, skill performance was affected by poor joint stability and trunk rotation, difficulty with balance, and incoordinated movements. Participation with behaviors and activities that exceed his ability to perform at his highest level produces distress.

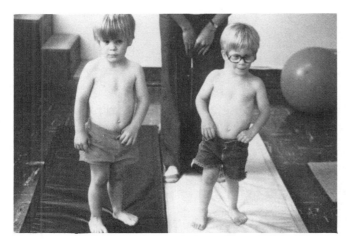

Figure 8-a: Twin "G" (on left): Twin "K" (on right). Age 3 years, 2 months.

Adaptive Behaviors: Supine to Standing

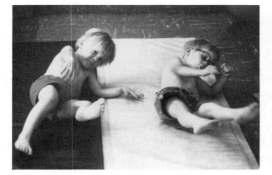

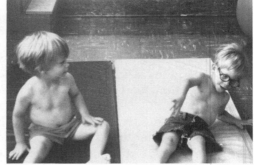

Figure 8-b: Twin G on the left and Twin K on right are in the process of assuming standing from supine with an age appropriate partial rotation pattern. Twin G shifts weight to one side, makes use of equilibrium to pull toward midline, and differentiates between upper and lower body segments. Although Twin K can initiate the partial rotation pattern, he is unable to differentiate between body segments for rotation and makes use of generalized tonal increases throughout the trunk, upper, and lower extremities.

Figure 8-c: Twin G has already achieved sitting while Twin K is adapting primitive undifferentiated patterns to weight shift, thus affecting temporal sequencing of adaptation.

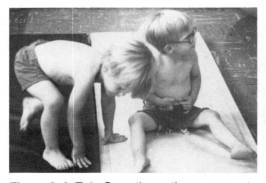

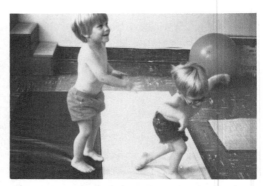

Figure 8-d: Twin G continues the sequence to assume standing by adapting support reactions to stabilize the upper portions of the body and shifts weight to move toward standing. Twin K gains postural reinforcement in sitting before proceeding to stand.

Figure 8-e: Twin G transfers weight back to lower extremities, freeing hands from support and stands erect. Twin K is unable to call forth appropriate upper extremity support reactions and thus experiences difficulty shifting weight to one leg. He attempts to adapt to the distress by stabilizing with neck retraction and scapular adduction.

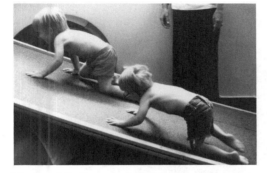

Figure 8-f: Creeping. Twin G demonstrates good postural stability evidenced by contralateral creeping pattern. Twin K adapts primitive neck retraction, poor upper extremity support reactions, and utilizes unilateral weight shift set to creep.

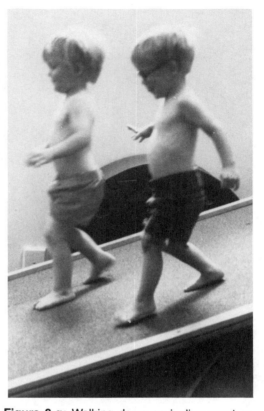

Figure 8-g: Walking down an incline requires high level adaptations. Twin G maintains his heel-toe reciprocal gait while reinforcing his balance with a readiness to protect. Twin K watches his feet, adapts with shoulder protraction, scapular adduction, and a flat-footed gait.

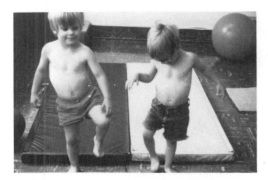

Figure 8-h: Standing on one foot requires weight-shift and realignment of the midline with gravity. Although Twin G is not well aligned with gravity, he can shift weight and balance appropriately for his age. Twin K has difficulty shifting weight and maintaining balance. He attempts to adapt arm postures to assist as well as monitor his process visually.

Equilibrium Reactions

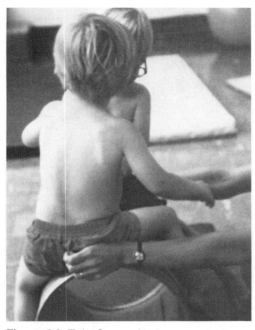

Figure 8-i: Twin G experiences a normal equilibrium reaction in response to movement of the barrel.

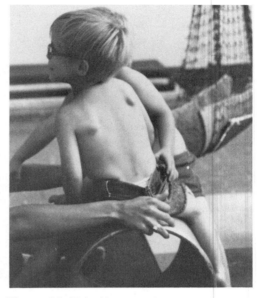

Figure 8-j: Twin K responds with a variety of abnormal responses. He adapts with neck retraction to reinforce stability.

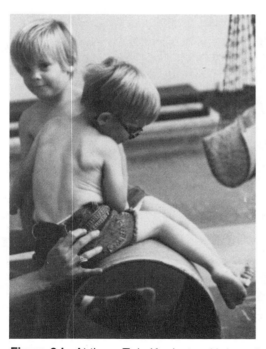

Figure 8-k: At times Twin K adapts with lateral trunk flexion instead of rotation.

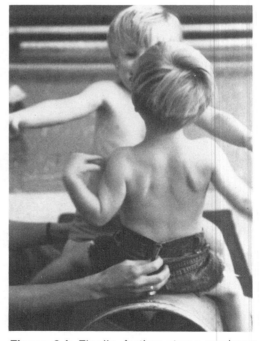

Figure 8-l: Finally, further stress produces asymmetrical upper extremity retraction for stabilization. Twin G can call forth an appropriate upper extremity equilibrium reaction.

Adapting Activities

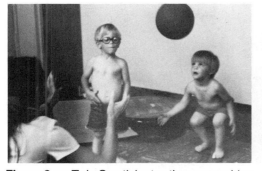

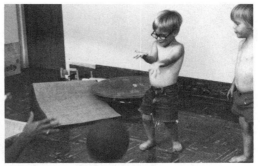

Figure 8-m: Twin G anticipates the approaching ball by adjusting body position in space, preparing arms for catching and visually monitoring the speed (temporal) of the on-coming ball.

Figure 8-n: Twin K's primitive response is to concentrate on the spatial adaptation of his hands. He places them in a primitive catching posture. K visually monitors his hands but is unable to simultaneously monitor the temporal component of the on-coming ball.

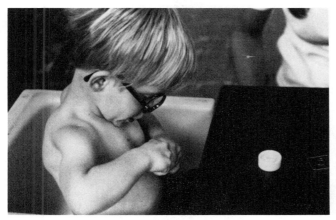

Figure 8-o: Manipulative Activity: Activities of the upper extremities call forth increased coactivation from proximal joints in response to distal fixation used to control movement.

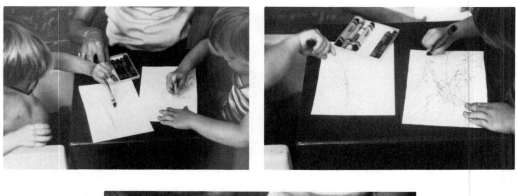

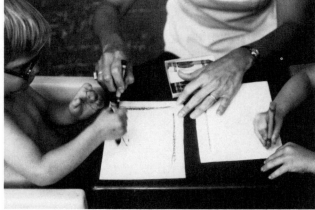

Figures 8-p to 8-r: Adaptation to Crayon: In 8-p, K's adaptation to a crayon calls forth a variety of primitive hand functions and a need to switch hands frequently. Development of skill is impeded by his inability to use consistent hand functions and one hand predominantly. Note that Twin G consistently uses his right hand and adapts with a superior grasp even though activity seems stressful to him also.

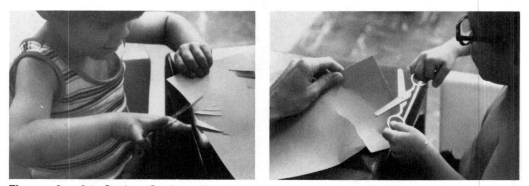

Figures 8-s, 8-t: Cutting: Cutting with scissors is stressful to both children. Twin G succeeds in snipping the paper with the scissors by calling forth undifferentiated finger flexion and extension to manipulate the scissors. G's response is an appropriate spatiotemporal stress response for his age and experience with scissors. Twin K calls forth a lower level bilateral attempt to manipulate the scissors. K's response indicates spatiotemporal distress.

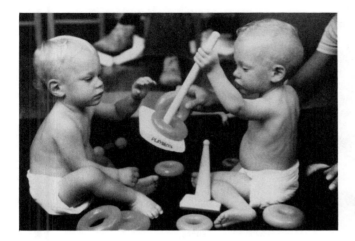

Figure 8-aa: Twin "M" (on left); Twin "T" (on right). Age 18 months.

Twins M and T

Background Information

M was the second twin born at 28 weeks gestation. His birth weight was 1100 grams. He was transferred to an intensive care newborn nursery shortly after birth and hospitalized approximately 2½ months. Diagnosis included prematurity, hyperbilirubinemia, and respiratory distress syndrome secondary to Hyaline Membrane Disease. M was evaluated by occupational therapy and physical therapy when he was 5 months corrected age. The evaluation was initiated at the request of his parents who noted that M was not using his right upper extremity well. At that time increased flexor tone of the right upper extremity and increased extensor tone of right lower extremity were noted. In addition an asymmetrical tonic neck reflex was present. There were stretch reflexes noted in both right upper and lower extremities. The developmental landmarks achieved by M were at the 2 to 3 month level. Following the evaluation the parents were given a home program, followed periodically by occupational therapy and physical therapy.

Supine Behaviors

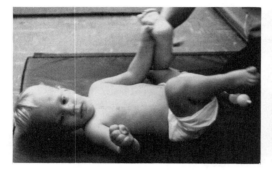

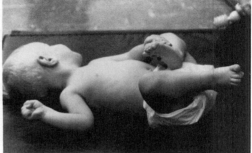

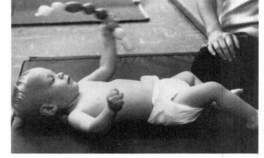

Figures 8-bb to 8-dd: Abnormal patterns influence M's supine behavior. The more affected right side is influenced by increased tone, asymmetrical tonic neck reflex, and insufficient sensory awareness from contact with self or toys.

Rolling

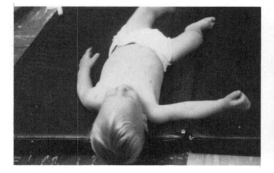

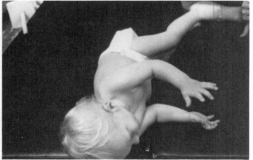

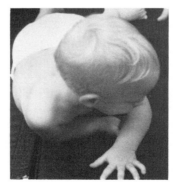

Figure 8-ee to 8-gg: M rolls toward his right, more affected side, using his left upper extremity to compensate for poor rotation within the body axis. Lack of rotation between body segments and difficulty with spontaneous adaptive upper extremity movements produce abnormal rolling as well as difficulty adjusting posture in prone.

Moving in Prone

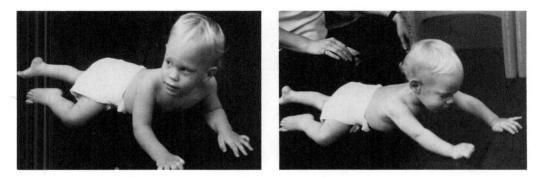

Figures 8-hh to 8-ii: Use of amphibian crawling and "pushing back" in prone represent significant delay in M's development of locomotion. The patterns are influenced by increased tone in the right side and lack of development around the midline for trunk stability. Compare the effect of upper extremity weight bearing on the development of finger extension and upper extremity support reactions. The right upper extremity remains under the influence of primitive and abnormal patterns.

Sitting

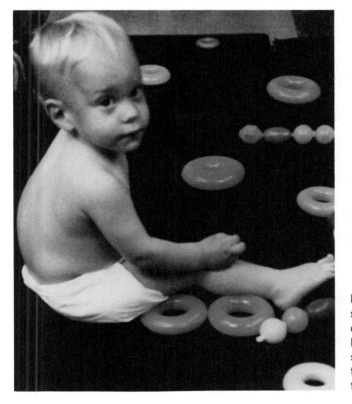

Figure 8-jj: Neck retraction, shoulder protraction, posterior tilt of pelvis, collapse of trunk, and lower extremity internal rotation in sitting represent abnormal patterns and inadequate adaptation to perform activities.

Pulling to Stand

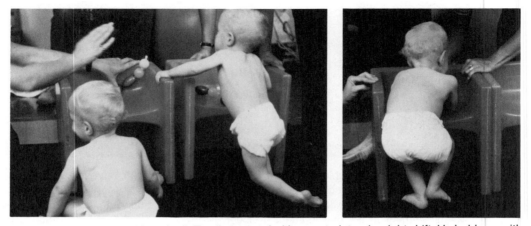

Figures 8-kk, 8-ll: In 8-kk and 8-ll, T pulls to stand with a contralateral weight shift. He holds on with his upper extremities while he shifts weight to one lower extremity, bringing the other extremity into weight bearing. M (illustrated in Figure 8-ll) is under the influence of abnormal patterns. He utilizes neck retraction, pulls down with his upper extremities because of the influence of flexor tone, and adapts an abnormal bilateral weight shift pattern to stand.

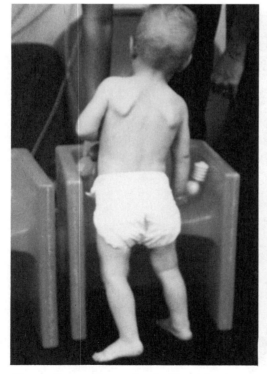

Figure 8-mm: T can stand with minimal or no support from his upper extremities while he engages in activity.

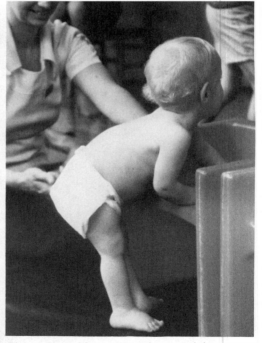

Figure 8-nn: M cannot attain an upright posture due to influence from flexor tone and dependency on upper extremity support. He attempts to compensate for lack of extension with abnormalneck hyperextension.

Adaptation to Activity

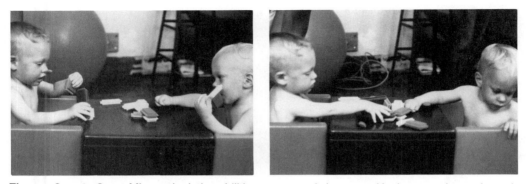

Figures 8-oo to 8-pp: M's manipulative abilities are severely hampered by increased tone through associated reactions in his upper extremities which prevent bilateral coordination. His highest levels of manipulative activities include mouthing to manipulate and throwing to watch object movement.

References

1. Bobath B, Bobath K: Motor development in the different types of cerebral palsy. London, Wm. Heinemann Books, 1975.

2. Ayres J: Sensory integration and the child. Los Angeles, Western Psychological Services, 1979.

3. Bobath K: A neurophysiological basis for the treatment of cerebral palsy. Philadelphia, J.B. Lippincott Co., 1980.

4. Drillien C M: Abnormal neurologic signs in the first year of life in low-birthweight infants: Possible prognostic significance. Develop Med Child Neurol 14:575-584, 1972.

5. Fanti R, Fagan J, Miranda S: Early visual selectivity. In Cohen L, Salapatek P (Eds): Infant perception: From sensation to cognition, Vol. 1. New York, Academic Press, 1975, pp. 249-343.

6. Bax M: Terminology and classification of cerebral palsy. Developmental Medicine and Child-Neurology 6:295-297.

7. Bly L: Components of normal movement during the first year of life. Chicago, Neurodevelopmental Treatment Association, Inc., 1983.

8. Quinton M: Notes from neurodevelopmental treatment course. Seattle, 1978.

9. Fiorentino M: Normal and abnormal development. Springfield, C. Thomas, 1972.

10. Wilson J: Cerebral palsy. In Campbell S (Eds) Pediatric neurologic physical therapy. New York. Churchill Livingstone, 1984.

CHAPTER 9

Relationship of Theory and Practice

Objectives

The reader will be able to

1. describe the relationship between theory and practice;
2. identify and describe the six components of a theoretical frame of reference for practice; and
3. relate the theory of spatiotemporal adaptation with its theoretical frame of reference.

Introduction

As a set of ideas, theories are organized to explain phenomena and provide strategies for further research. Research and theory are bases for scientific inquiry that ultimately lead to rational knowledge. Theories also provide strategies for practice application; however, theories do not provide an automatic transition to practice because application of theory to practice requires more than a set of ideas, concepts, organized assumptions, and hypotheses.[1] Practice also must reflect a profession's heritage and philosophical base, and is influenced by unique interpersonal relationships within a specific practice situation. Thus, relationship of theory and practice may have variations unique to a specific discipline and practice situation.

In health- and education-related professions, practice is concerned with the nature of change. Analysis of theory cannot provide information that can be directly applied to change processes; rather, theory's ideas must be translated into assumptions about assessment and intervention strategies for practice.[1] Theory becomes a key element in delineation of practice processes, as theory provides logic and language to identify (name) the problem and plan means for altering the situation (frame). Relating theory to practice gives practitioners the abilities to "name it and frame it," as theory allows us to explain what we see and determine how to facilitate desired change or modification.[2]

To relate spatiotemporal adaptation theory to health- and education-related services, a theoretical frame of reference is presented. A system for activating the conceptual frame of reference is discussed.

Frame of Reference

A theoretical frame of reference becomes the mental plan of how to do something. As a plan, the frame is based upon a set of ideas, beliefs, and assumptions inherent within theory, and within the philosophy of a profession. The purpose of a frame of reference for practice is to guide thinking and suggest processes for identifying (naming) problem(s) and implementing solutions to solve problem(s). A frame of reference cannot be developed independently, as it must have a direct link to an organized set of ideas and philosophical beliefs to provide an overview and broad perspective for explaining phenomena. Theory becomes the springboard for practice, as theory provides the gestalt or overview of phenomena and the frame of reference serves to link theory to practice[2,3,4] by guiding processes to change phenomena.

According to Williamson,[3] a frame of reference provides guidelines for therapeutic approaches to be taken to produce a desired change and achieve an expected outcome. A frame uses concepts of theory to develop rationale for assessment and intervention strategies. Generally, a frame of reference addresses a specific domain of concern emanating from a profession's philosophical base or model and having a direct link to theories.[3,4] Simply stated, a frame of reference relates theory with the philosophy of a profession and suggests principles and guidelines for assessment and intervention. Spatiotemporal adaptation theory with its spiraling framework provides a frame of reference on which practitioners can base their therapeutic actions. A framework provides basis for therapeutic reasoning and implies a mode of action. Spatiotemporal adaptation theory has its foundation in the spiraling continuum of development; therefore, the mode of action within a practice session is based upon the spiraling process of adapting strategies and sequences to facilitate adaptation.

Therapeutic reasoning respects the law of "Individual Differences" that prevails with human behavior; thus, a frame of reference for intervention must be adaptable for each individual and his or her assessed needs. A theoretical frame of reference based upon spatiotemporal adaptation theory does not provide a structured formula or "step-by-step" intervention program. Because each self-system is unique, a frame provides only an organized system by which clinical reasoning can be guided and a variety of intervention processes applied to meet individual needs.

The System

To link spatiotemporal adaptation theory to practice, a system has been designed. There are six components within the system (Fig. 9-1): (1) theoretical orientation, (2) domain of concern to be addressed, (3) expected outcomes or desired results, (4) processes for assessment, (5) postulates for change, and (6) intervention strategies to bring about change. The first three components comprise a frame of reference's theoretical or conceptual base and the last three the technical or practice base.

Theoretical orientation, the first component, contains those elements of theory pertinent for specific practice situations. Elements may include concepts, properties, assumptions, and/or hypotheses to conceptualize the process and guide action. A theoretical orientation can be likened to a "cause-and-effect" relationship, as it provides ideas and language to communicate what is observed, as well as an understanding of phenomena being observed. Further, a frame's theoretical orientation establishes boundaries by defining the domain of concern to be addressed. The second component, domain of concern, dictates such boundaries as the behavior or performance to be addressed, age ranges for which the theory is applicable, delineation of specific problems or conditions along the function-to-dysfunction continuum, and the focus for implementing change as addressed by the profession. Also, theory directs practitioners' thinking to communicate expected outcomes or predicted results that may occur through an intervention process. Just as domain of concern provides boundaries for addressing specific problems on the function-to-dysfunction continuum, expected results guide one's thinking to predict realistic changes that may occur along the dysfunction-to-function continuum. These three components (theoretical orientation, domain of concern, and expected results) form a theoretical base to "name" and "frame" the problem to be addressed.

From a theoretical base, practitioners can translate concepts and assumptions into

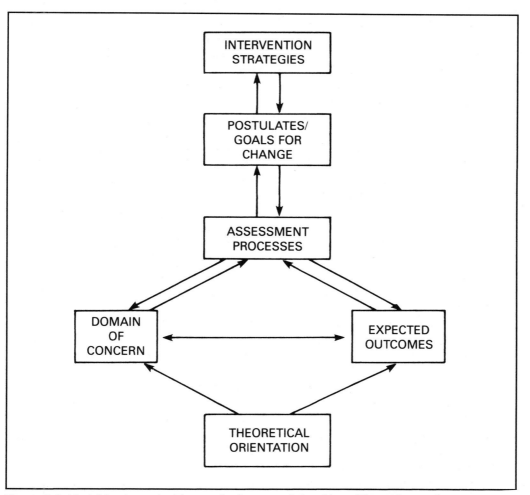

Figure 9-1: Model for theoretical frame of reference relationships of theory to practice.

assessment processes to identify appropriate problem(s) to be solved. Identifying problem(s), suggests Schon,[5] requires an artistry and ability to sort out, from the multiple and complex human behaviors, those problems important for attention. Parham[2] proposes that identifying the appropriate problem is a conceptual process termed "problem-setting." She states that in problem-setting, a clinician names the problem(s) to be addressed in practice, and then "frames the context for intervention—'name it and frame it' in the words of Schon."[2,p20] Having identified or set the problem(s), problem-solving can take place.

Data from assessment and delineation of expected results are used to guide problem-solving processes, which begin with beliefs regarding predicted change. Postulates for change articulate these beliefs and values subscribed in theory, including environmental interactions that will affect change toward the direction of higher level function.[3] Postulates guide one's selection of goals and objectives, and ultimately govern selection of media and methods used to produce change. Selecting intervention strategies is the final component in the frame's problem-solving process. Strategies are specific plans to bring about change and include the delineation of goals, objectives, media, and methods. Development of goals is a collaborative process with child, family, and clinician. Although a child's needs, wants, and desires are paramount, they must be addressed realistically. Theory provides the necessary knowledge base to guide development of realistic goals. A clinician has the ethical responsibility to collaborate with the child and family to develop realistic goals that are based upon beliefs and values regarding change and appropriate intervention to affect desired change.

Goals provide a direction for intervention, as goals link the theoretical base with practice. Delineation of performance objectives is the next step of intervention strategies. Performance objectives are specific behavioral statements representing measurable guidelines toward achievement of established goals and, as such, guide selection of media and methods to achieve objectives. Media and methods available for a clinician include tools and approaches that reflect philosophy of the profession and may be dictated by stated regulations such as licensure.

Components of assessment processes, postulates for change, and identifying intervention strategies form the frame's practice base. An overview of the six components and their relationship, which comprise theoretical and practice basis, is illustrated in Table 9-1.

Selection of assessment instruments, media, and methods are profession specific and make up the technical aspects of a theoretical frame of reference that must have a direct link with the conceptual aspects. A practitioner must engage in an ongoing dialogue of comparing results of intervention processes with the original description of the problem, expected outcomes, and domain of concern. Schon[5] terms this dialogue a "reflective conversation with the situation," as it is the going back and forth between conceptual and technical processes of the frame.

A theory and its theoretical frame of reference provide both rational and intuitive knowledge to plan, appraise, and make decisions in response to complex problems and ever-changing circumstances. Frequently in practice situations, a clinician must act without having time to reflect or consciously plan actions. Schon[5] terms the process "reflecting-in-action" to describe the flexibility in clinical decision-making brought about by the clinician's intuitive knowledge. Implicit in one's abilities for "reflecting-in-action" is the valuing and use of theory, as theory and one's theoretical orientation provide the rational knowledge to direct intuitive clinical practice actions for facilitating change.

Table 9-1
Analysis of Theoretical Frame of Reference

Theoretical Orientation	Domain of Concern	Expected Outcomes	Assessment Processes	Postulates for Change	Intervention Strategies
Elements of Theory: • Concepts • Properties • Assumptions • Hypothesis • Philosophy • Perspective of profession	Boundaries to be addressed: • Components of behavior • Ages • Specific problems of function-dysfunction continuum • Focus of profession	Predicted results: • What can be expected— • Dysfunction to function continuum	Instruments and methods to identify problems	Statements that describe beliefs and values based upon theory and profession	Goals/objectives and media-method to be used to achieve these goals

Theoretical Base ⟷ **REFLECTION-IN-ACTION** Practice Base

The relationship between theory and practice is examined further in the following discussion of spatiotemporal adaptation theory's frame of reference.

Theoretical Orientation

To relate spatiotemporal adaptation theory to practice, those elements making up the theoretical orientation include the four categories of the theory, their properties, and corresponding assumptions. The following narrative provides a detailed listing of the four categories, their properties, and corresponding assumptions that relate spatiotemporal adaptation theory to practice. To discuss the relationship, certain assumptions from spatiotemporal theory have been used, although possibilities have not been exhausted with this illustration. The following presents specifics of spatiotemporal adaptation theory; however, it is important to keep in mind that a frame of reference may have more than one theory from which it draws its orientation, and/or parts of a theory might be selected for specific practice situations.

Theoretical Orientation for Spatiotemporal Adaptation Frame of Reference
 Conceptual Category: Movement
 Properties: Structures, Functions, Purpose
 Assumptions:
   1. Acquired or congenital pathology, resulting in handicapping conditions, impacts the spiraling process of adapting functions-to-purposes-to-functions, resulting in meaningless movements.
   2. When lower level functions are not modified through the spiraling adaptation process, blocks to normal sequential development of movement emerge and higher levels of development are compromised.

3. In the presence of pathology, blocks to normal sensorimotor development are characterized by combinations of abnormal postural tone, abnormal patterns of movement, and abnormal reflex behavior, resulting in persistent use of primitive strategies or developmental sequences beyond the normal or expected period of adapting those actions.

4. There is a similarity between movement patterns used by older children with dysfunction and movement patterns used by normal children during their primitive phases of development.

5. Children with dysfunction continue to perform at primitive/transitional levels, or they continue to attempt higher level activities by using lower level functions.

6. A therapeutic program must consider the relationship of a child's ability to move, motivation to move, and acquisition of performance abilities. Participation with the environment is both extrinsically and intrinsically motivated.

7. A therapeutic program can be designed to facilitate the spiraling process of functions-to-purpose to functions using neurobehavioral approaches most appropriate to the child's problems.

Conceptual Category: Environment
Properties: Space, Time
Assumptions:

1. When development of higher level functions are compromised and abnormal movement patterns used, a child's interactions with the environment may be purposeless.

2. Environmental situations that promote purposeless actions are distressful transactions for a child, resulting in spatiotemporal maladaptation.

3. Methods of intervention consider the process of structuring the spatiotemporal characteristics of the environment so that a child's transactions with those events will provide experiences that are purposeful and directed toward a goal.

4. Purposeful, goal-directed actions are meaningful for the self-system when active participation with the environment enhances maturation by directing adaptive responses to higher level functions.

5. The spatiotemporal environment may be "too harsh," thus placing demands that require responses that are "out-of-sequential-reach," causing a child to experience distress and maladaptation of movement in environmental transactions.

6. When the holding, facilitating, challenging, and interacting functions of the environment are not in balance with each other or out of balance with a child's functional abilities, the child will not be able to direct purposeful movements.

7. When the transactional process between movement and environment is compromised, a child's spatiotemporal orientation is disrupted.

8. Difficulties with one's spatiotemporal orientation is characterized by an inability to produce a response coincident with an external event that may be manifested by (a) one's accuracy problems visualizing the event, (b) efficiency problems with initiation and control of movement, (c) memory problems concerning past performance or failure to adapt past experiences, and/or (d) lack of experiences.

Conceptual Category: Adaptation
Properties: Developmental nature, Purposeful nature
Assumptions:

1. Maladaptation is characterized by altered SMS interpretation resulting from abnormal assimilations, abnormal accommodations, and abnormal association-differentiation processes.

2. Spatiotemporal maladaptation of environmental transactions is a process of repeated dysfunctional performances that is meaningless for adaptation, and results in further dysfunctional performance.

3. A program to facilitate the adaptation process in children with central nervous system deficits must consider the developmental and purposeful nature of adaptation.

4. Therapeutic programs that enhance spatiotemporal adaptation of strategies, and developmental and purposeful sequences, will enhance a child's acquisition of performance skills.

Conceptual Category: Spiraling Continuum

Properties: Stress, Distress

Assumptions:

1. A tendency for children to "call up" previously acquired patterns to adapt under stress is also evident with children who have disabilities, but a child with dysfunction is frequently unable to make use of stress to move to higher levels of development.

2. An intervention program designed to facilitate adaptation has, as its core, the spiraling process of modifying a child's purposeless actions by facilitating higher level functions for adaptation to purposes. The principles of "spiraling" provide a framework for the development of intervention programs so that modifications of dysfunction can occur.

3. Spiraling makes its therapeutic impact through a process of "reciprocal interweaving" or reincorporation of several sequential levels of development that consider specific aspects of actions that are one level below the child's present functional level and facilitation of specific aspects of performance that are one level above the child's present functioning level.

4. Interweaving of lower, present, and higher levels of activity performance enhances association-differentiation processes of adaptation for the modification of lower and higher levels of functions.

Domain of Concern

Spatiotemporal adaptation's domain of concern includes (a) sensorimotor skills as major behavioral component being addressed, (b) newborns to age 5 as the appropriate age range, (c) children with central nervous system insult and resulting handicapping conditions as the problems to address, (d) spiraling adaptation as the process to facilitate change, and (e) spatiotemporal environmental events as the focus for intervention strategies. At times practitioners may select to use concepts of theory for situations outside the stated domain of concern. Extrapolating theory ideas and concepts to another domain must be done with caution and attention given to deviations from the original intent.

Expected Outcomes

Having determined the boundaries or domain of concern for spatiotemporal adaptation, expected results can be articulated. Due to individual differences and uniqueness of each person, expected results and intervention strategies cannot be standardized or categorized to fit a given population. Practice must be individualistic in nature, just as each person is. Therefore, spatiotemporal adaptation theory, as presented in this text, provides underlying concepts and principles by which expected results can be articulated and individual intervention programs can emerge. The spiraling continuum process of spatiotemporal adaptation theory provides a clinician with a clear understanding of what should be expected from intervention strategies. Using strategies, developmental sequences, and purposeful sequences as guidelines, higher level behaviors that should emerge from the spiraling process of integrating previously acquired actions with new situations can be predicted. Properties of the environment category, as well as properties of adaptation, stress, and distress, also guide thinking processes for communicating expected results of neurobehavioral performances being observed. For example, expected results, using a spatiotemporal adaptation frame of reference, could include such statements as

(a) When environmental demands exceed a child's functional capacities, you would expect the child to use a lower level function; however, if the environment is "good enough," the lower level functions would be integrated with the present situation and a higher level movement pattern should emerge.

(b) During the course of development, the sequential nature of adaptation will persist; therefore, "next steps in the developmental process" can be predicted and facilitated.

(c) Using play activities or events of the environment as media will facilitate the child's intrinsic motivation to move and adapt movement patterns with a purpose, e.g., to feed oneself, to grasp a toy, to use scissors, etc.

(d) By engaging a child in a "doing" process—one that elicits active participation with the "good enough" environment— you can expect adaptation of purposeful sequences, and through repetition of purposeful sequences, skilled performances will evolve.

Expected results also may be specific to a particular child and situation, and thus affected by the child's specific problems and history. Even though each child is unique, the spatiotemporal framework can provide a broad perspective and overview of what might be expected as a result of intervention, as well as guide decisions regarding the selection of assessment processes, media, and methods. Expected results also may include practical outcomes of an intervention program, such as the self-care or play activities that a child may be able to achieve as a result of spatiotemporal adaptation.

Delineating those actions or results that might be expected provides a point of departure for the conceptual theoretical base to relate practice situations with daily life experiences. Expected results guide decisions for problem-solving processes of assessment, postulates for change, and intervention strategies. Communicating expected results with the child and family also promotes an understanding of what will take place through intervention programs. Understanding of an intervention program enhances a child's and family's active participation with the program and promotes parent-professional collaboration.

Assessment

Assessment processes selected may include test instruments, clinical observations, and other data-gathering methods, such as interview to gather information about a child's neuromuscular functions, how functions are adapted to purposes for environmental interactions, as well as information about the family unit and daily activities important to the child's functioning.

There are many standardized and criterion-referenced instruments to assess a child's neuromuscular functions and developmental status. However, data from assessment instruments provide only the "skeletal" view of a child; to see the "whole" child, assessment must be supplemented with other problem-solving processes, such as clinical judgments made from personal interactions with the child, observations of performance and environmental interactions, interviews with the child and family, and records of the child's history. For example, decisions regarding postural and/or muscle tone come from clinical experiences and judgments. Effects of environmental demands upon stress-distress can be made through observations. Because the focus of spatiotemporal adaptation theory centers around spiraling adaptation of movement and environment, assessment processes also must include interviews with family members to determine important characteristics of a child's everyday activities and life. To "name" and "frame" the problem, assessment processes need to gather information about a child's motivation, interests, available toys, play and interpersonal relationships, family's use of time, and their desires, needs, goals, and concerns for the child and family unit. A child with central nervous system deficit has multiple problems and the complexity of these problems is exacerbated further by the complex web of social problems in today's culture. To problem set and problem solve, the clinician must be aware of not only the clinical problems of the child, but also the child within the family and community units. Intervention must address the varied scope of problems faced by the child and family. Outcomes of intervention may be jeopardized when technical solutions focus on one small piece of the whole, particularly when that piece may be insignificant in comparison to the web of complexities that have a profound impact upon the life situation of the child.[2] Focusing on one small piece of the problem ignores the broader context, and shortsightedness can occur when one's practice includes techniques and technical procedures alone, and fails to employ conceptual processes based upon a well-articulated theoretical base.

Appendix 9-A provides a listing of suggested assessment processes that are appropriate for use within the spatiotemporal frame of reference. The listing is not conclusive, but presented as examples of both norm and criterion-referenced evaluations that might be used within the spatiotemporal frame of reference. Additionally, no endorsement, preference, or value judgment of the listed assessments are intended by the authors.

Postulates for Change

The fifth component, postulates for change, is influenced by a profession's philosophy, a theory itself, and the theoretical frame of reference, which are integrated into the basic belief system from which a practitioner guides decisions to establish an intervention plan. The spatiotemporal frame is based on beliefs that each child is unique, the value of movement-environmental transactions, or "doing" process, adaptation of functions-to-purposes within the context of a child's daily life, facilitation of developmental and purposeful sequences, and the inherent "reciprocal interweaving" process of spiraling adaptation. These beliefs and values influence the development of an intervention plan that includes overall goals, objectives, media, and methods that reflect a profession's philosophy.

To facilitate a child's potential to achieve his highest level of performance is the ultimate purpose of spatiotemporal adaptation. Achievement of performance abilities is an individual matter; some children may progress to higher levels or at a faster pace than other children. Paramount within postulates for change are two primary factors: (1) a child is a unique individual who responds to treatment in his or her own unique manner and who has his or her own unique potential, and (2) acknowledgment and acceptance of realistic expectations for a child's potential. Consideration of a child's uniqueness and realistic expectations, guided by the theoretical base, provides a climate for healthy intervention; thus, an ideal practice situation ensues.

Intervention Strategies

Within the intervention process toward achieving the ultimate purpose of facilitating a child's potential, there are several overall goals. To implement an adaptation program, overall goals include prevention, modifications, remediation, compensation, and maintenance. **Prevention** occurs when the child engages in activity that is designed to keep distress from occurring or to hinder secondary complications from the initial identified problem. **Modification** occurs when a child facilitates change within the self-system which is brought about by his or her own participation with actions/activities. **Remediation** is the process of engaging a child with activity that is designed to correct, remedy, or improve skills. **Compensation** occurs when intervention programs are designed to promote other aspects of performance or substitute a different form of action. **Maintenance** in a practice situation is that activity that helps a child keep in condition and retain the acquired, appropriate functions. Repetition of appropriate functions augments adaptation of performance skills.

Within the adaptation framework, any one or all of the above-stated overall goals may be considered. Working toward a goal will be dependent upon a child's assessed needs and specific program plan. Spatiotemporal adaptation frame of reference permits flexibility for incorporating overall goals into a specific program at any given time. For example, during early childhood, it may be realistic to implement a program designed to prevent and modify, whereas during later periods, such as elementary school years or adolescence, it may be more realistic to emphasize activities and techniques for employing compensation and maintenance. In addition, any one practice session may include several of the overall goals, depending on assessed needs and session objectives. Decisions for emphasis must consider a variety of variables, including age, degree of disability, priorities of the child's educational program or overall health care, impact upon the family, and availability of equipment or characteristics of the milieu where the session will occur.

Intervention strategies are specific to each child, although the base of strategies is influenced by beliefs, value judgments, and ethical concerns of practitioners emanating from the unique perspective of their profession. Strategies within the spatiotemporal theoretical frame of reference would include statements of performance objectives that reflect the categories and properties of the theory. Media and methods selected to achieve objectives may reflect a variety of neurobehavioral approaches. Neurobehavioral approaches suggest that the intervention focus is on human behavior and not just on developmental or physiological processes. Within the spatiotemporal adaptation frame, neurobehavioral approaches are concerned primarily with sensorimotor behaviors. Other performance components, such as psychosocial, cultural, cognitive, and sensory integrative, are important and relate to neurobehavioral, but these are not the focus of the theory. Media and methods selected that reflect neurobehavioral intervention approaches emphasize positioning and handling; selected activities/events; active participation with the environment; adaptation to enhance self-care, play, and education/work skills; use of technology and adapted equipment to enhance a child's access to the environment; and child-family interactions.

Application of spiraling principles, as presented in Chapter 2, serves as guidelines for implementing an intervention program. Spiraling makes its therapeutic impact through a process of "reciprocal interweaving" or reincorporation of several sequential levels of development.[6] Spiraling of actions that are goal-directed toward the events of the environment facilitate association and differentiation for completion of the adaptation process. Interplay of spiraling actions within therapy is based upon a child's homeostasis and activities being performed. By applying spiraling principles for directing/controlling a child's accommodations, accuracy of feedback is more likely to occur. The nature of activity itself, and clinician-child interpersonal relationship to direct activity performance, promote active participation for appropriate adaptations.

Spiraling occurs when the practice situation enables a child to participate with activity that may be designed to call forth certain elements of posture and movement strategies for incorporating the immediate behavior being elicited, as well as aspects of higher level performances being facilitated. Preparing the practice environment to facilitate spiraling is a most demanding task for the practitioner. Care and judgment must be taken in the selection of activity tasks to enhance spiraling and ensure some success pleasing to a child.[7]

For preparation of the practice environment, clinicians may ask themselves several questions to assist with decisions regarding the spiraling process. Using initial and ongoing assessment findings as the foundation for clinical reasoning, practitioners should ask themselves, "What do I wish to change and why; and what does the child/family want to change and why?" In order to promote meaningful therapy, both internal and external systems may need to be modified. The content of this book has emphasized modification of the self-system; however, intervention must also consider the possible need to modify the external systems with which the child interacts. A child, family, clinician, and other persons involved may need to modify their expectations of the child's performance abilities. Demands and expectations of the environment must complement a child's potential so that the child can achieve success and be stimulated to engage in a variety of realistic activities. A child, family, and significant others become principal sources for direct involvement with intervention.

Another question to be considered is the method of documentation, as ongoing planning and reordering of performance objectives and program priorities depend upon results of intervention. A process for documentation is imperative for success; therefore, practitioners must decide how they will rate or determine a child's progress. Rating progress is an ongoing process and serves as the ultimate guideline for altering programs when necessary, as well as collecting data to document the effectiveness of intervention.

Having specified performance objectives, which have been determined by answering the questions of what it is that the intervention program will attempt to change and why, a clinician then monitors the session by asking several questions regarding outcomes. For example, Is the child becoming involved with the activity? Are the expected results being elicited? Does the environment facilitate stress or, in fact, is distress resulting?

The adaptive social involvement of the child with activity is an essential element for modifying actions and facilitating change within the self-system. Adaptive social responses add meaning to movement. Movement is in close connection with perceptions, feeling, and attitudes.[7] Should the activity require either too high- or too low-level accommodations or efforts, a child is not likely to become involved. A therapy process cannot force activity upon the child; rather, the child must guide or direct his own actions.[8] Each child is the best judge of the appropriateness of an activity, as children seem to have an innate sense of their needs for adaptation.

A prerequisite to social involvement may well be the element of success experienced by activity involvement. Therefore, it is imperative to constantly ask, "Does the activity provide a success experience for the child?" As stated by Ayres, "There is no reward that has quite the enduring qualities that success holds."[8,p276] Success is the most powerful reinforcer available, and success occurs through appropriate adaptations of movement-environment transactions.

During an intervention program, a clinician observes responses and reactions, and attempts to assess the child's ability to interpret feedback from posture and movement stimuli. Appropriate sensorimotor stimulation is therapeutic only when feedback is appropriate and when the child is aware of that feedback. A clinician should constantly be alert to a child's involvement with, interest in, and improvement of actions. The degree of involvement and self-direction from a child provides valuable clues to assess the child's awareness of feedback.

Repetition of actions is another area for monitoring and providing guidelines for intervention. Achievement of appropriate performance provides success experience, which further motivates a child to repeat performances. Repetition can be likened to the overall goal of maintenance and becomes a vital aspect of intervention, particularly with planning and implementing programs that can take place outside the clinical situation. Once an appropriate behavior has been acquired, it is necessary to practice the performance to augment adaptation and enhance the transfer to performances with similar activities. Providing a variety of activities gives a child an opportunity to not only repeat actions but apply performances for transference and expand his or her repertoire of performance skills.

Principles and concepts of the spiraling continuum of adaptation provide guidelines for clinical reasoning. Using spiraling as a framework for eliciting adaptation does not imply that an intervention program perfects the achievement of one behavior or skill before going to the next. Instead, spiraling stresses the overlap of performances and serves as a major aspect of intervention. A child with dysfunction can benefit from a program based upon the spiraling adaptation of strategies, developmental and purposeful sequences; however, intervention programs do not recapitulate the normal process. Caution must be taken not to mirror each strategy or sequence, as some aspects of the normal process may only augment the already present dysfunction.[9] For example, facilitating some posture and movement patterns of infancy may only enhance continued participation in undifferentiated or fixation patterns. Within normal development, a baby frequently calls forth elements of prone extension to reinforce needed trunk stability; to recapitulate that process may only enhance the abnormal pattern by increasing extension tone and repeating the undifferentiated pattern. Facilitation of neck extension or primitive fixation patterns may augment an abnormal retraction pattern. Recapitulating primitive kicking patterns may produce scissoring, increase extension tone, and prevent the development of hip flexion.[9] Caution also must be taken regarding the speed and repetition of movement; e.g., too fast may increase tone, facilitate an excitatory state, or produce sensory overload. Another factor for consideration includes the temporal aspects of activity performance; e.g., activities requiring a quick reaction time or fast movement may elicit a less mature response and present distress. The clinician should not force activity nor present activities at too high or too low a level for a child to adapt. A good guide is to call forth aspects of performance one level below the child's present functioning level with a specific performance and pull out those appropriate aspects one level above, to facilitate association and differentiation for modification. Awareness of sensory input and feedback that a child's system is assimilating is vital, as sensation is a powerful therapeutic means. It is important to observe the signs from the autonomic nervous system as a guide for the effect of sensory input. Throughout an adaptation intervention program, a child is the best indicator of the effect of activity, as a child's performance is a functional expression of the self-system. Observations and clinical judgments must be guided by rational knowledge emanating from theory base, as well as knowledge concerning the biopsychosocial systems.

Mode of Therapeutic Action

Preparation, facilitation, and adaptation are viewed as primary processes for those intervention strategies designed for the purpose of augmenting development through adaptation. Preparation, facilitation, and adaptation constitute the mode of action for intervention, as the process is inherent within the theoretical frame of reference and relates spiraling principals to practice. The mode has its own threefold spiraling process, with each being called forth when needed during an intervention session.

Preparation is both a preliminary and ongoing process of enhancing the neural and muscular functions for their readiness and use as posture and movement strategies. Preparing strategies for use is necessary for a child's self-system to achieve a state of homeostasis. Preparation within a therapy session attempts to do for a child what strategy development accomplishes within the normal adaptation process. Preparation includes normalizing postural tone, e.g., increasing, decreasing, or stabilizing tone, increasing range of motion, strength, promoting subcortical attention, securing a balance of the inhibitory-facilitory state, as well as controlling sensory input. In addition to preparation of a child's internal environment, the process also considers the structures of the external environment to assist in bringing the strategies forth for purposeful use.

Facilitation is the continued successive application of necessary stimuli and/or assistance given to elicit an adaptive response. A facilitory process includes the use of external means applied during the intervention situations for enhancement of an appropriate reaction. Stimuli and assistance may include movement, holding, activity, child, and/or what the clinician may provide directly to a child in order to enhance both stability and mobility components, automatic reactions, and sequences of movement. The major purpose of facilitation is to provide needed and appropriate input to enhance association and differentiation. When dysfunction and/or distress is present, a child's system may not associate/differentiate pertinent elements of one action for adaption to another; thus, stimuli applied in a practice session must attempt to facilitate appropriate sequences and opportunities for the association/differentiation components to occur. Vital components of adaptation are best facilitated through the therapeutic control over a child's accommodations so the self-system can associate/differentiate elements of the action being facilitated with previously acquired behaviors.

Adaptation as a therapeutic mode within a practice session gives purpose to performance. Adaptation is the process of promoting a child's abilities to differentiate those aspects of a developmental sequence pertinent for purposeful sequences. Adaptation considers connecting or linking movement with environmental events; thus, adaptation is the process of "making use" of movement to apply to events outside the body. Linking movement and environment promotes association and differentiation by structuring and guiding the child's active participation. A clinician must have knowledge of those components or patterns from developmental sequences that a child needs to "call forth" for adapting to the demands of an environment. Therapeutic adaptation promotes positive use of spatiotemporal stress and prevents distress.

Summary

Relationship of spatiotemporal theory and practice, as presented above, provides the reader with an abbreviated illustration of the use of theory behind clinical decisions and the basis for practice, as well as how theory provides the broad perspective for problem-setting and problem-solving, and how theory becomes the key element for the practitioner's "reflection-in-action process." Professionals who direct their services to human behavior and the nature of change are confronted with a multitude of problems and clinical decisions. Theory brings a perspective for seeing, analyzing, and discovering ways for dealing with problems. Programs based on well-articulated conceptual frameworks provide the practitioner with both rational and intuitive knowledge to frame the context for intervention and direct the nature of desired change.

Key Points

1. Analysis of theory cannot provide information that can be directly applied to practice; rather, theory ideas must be translated into assumptions about assessment and intervention strategies for practice.
2. Relating theory to practice provides a broad perspective to explain what we are seeing and to determine how to facilitate desired changes or modifications.
3. A theoretical frame of reference is a mental plan of hoow to do something, as it provides guidelines for the therapeutic approaches to produce desired change and achieve expected outcomes.
4. Theory concepts provide rationale for therapeutic actions.
5. The model for spatiotemporal adaptation theory's frame of reference has six components: theoretical orientation, domain of concern, expected outcomes, processes for assessment, postulate for change, and intervention strategies.
6. The first three components comprise the theoretical base; the last three have a direct relationship to the practice base.
7. A theory and its theoretical frame of reference provide practitioners with rational knowledge to guide clinical reasoning and actions in response to complex problems and ever-changing circumstances presented in practice situations.

Self-study Guidelines

1. Explain theory as the base for practice.
2. List the six components of the theoretical frame of reference.
3. Discuss the theoreticaal orientation of the spatiotemporal frame of reference. Relate two or three assumptions to each of the four categories.
4. Describe the component "postulates for change" as used with the frame of reference's components and differentiate from the "expected results."
5. Discuss the relationship of the profession's perspective or model, theory, and theoretical frame of reference.
6. Describe the domain of concern for the spatiotemporal frame of reference.
7. Discuss assessment as a problem-setting process.
8. Discuss the mode of action that serves as a process to implement the spiraling continuum framework.

References

1. Reed K: Understanding theory: The first step in learning about research. Am J Occup Ther 38:677-682, 1984.
2. Parham D: Applying theory to practice. In Target 2000: Promoting Excellence in Education. Rockville, MD, American Occupational Therapy Association, 1987, pp. 119-122.
3. Williamson GG: A heritage of activity: Development of theory. Am J Occup Ther, 36:716-722, 1982.
4. Mosey A: Occupational Therapy, Configuration of a Profession. New York, Raven Press, 1981.
5. Schon D: The Reflective Practitioner. New York, Basic Books, 1983.
6. Ames L, Ilg F: The developmental point of view with special reference to its principle of reciprocal neuromotor interweaving. J Genetic Psych 105:195-209, 1964.
7. Stockmeyer S: A sensorimotor approach to treatment. In Pearson P, Williams C (Eds.), Physical Therapy Services in the Developmental Disabilities. Springfield, Charles C. Thomas, 1972.
8. Ayres AJ: Sensory Integration and Learning Disorders. Los Angeles, Western Psychological Services, 1972.
9. Bobath K, Bobath B: Cerebral palsy. In Pearson P and Williams C (Eds.): Physical Therapy Services in the Developmental Disabilities. Springfield, IL, Charles C. Thomas Pubs., 1972. Chapter 3, pp. 31-185.

Appendix 9-A
Assessment Instruments

Alpern, G. & Boll, T.: Developmental Profile. Psychological Development Publications, Indianapolis.

Ayres, A.J.: Southern California Sensory Integration Test. Western Psychological Services, Los Angeles, CA. Ages 4-11 years.

Bayley, N.: Bayley Scales of Infant Development. Psychological Corporation, New York. Ages 2-30 months.

Beery, K. & Buktenica, N.: Developmental Test for Visual-Motor Integration (VMI). Follett Educational Corporation, Chicago, IL. Ages 2-15 years.

Brazelton, B.: Brazelton Behavioral Assessment Scale. J. B. Lippincott Co., Philadelphia. Age neonate.

Brigance, H.: Diagnostic Inventory of Early Development. Curriculum Associates, Inc., Woburn, MA. Ages 0-7 years.

Bruininks, R.: Bruininks-Oseretsky Test of Motor Proficiency. American Guidance Service, Circle Pines, MN. Ages 4-14 years

Chandler, L., Andrews, M., Swanson, M.: Movement Assessment of Infants. Rolling Bay, WA. Ages 0-12 months.

DeGangi, G.: Assessment of Sensorimotor Integration in Preschool Children. ERIC Clearinghouse, Arlington, VA. Ages 3-5 years.

Doel, E.: Vineland Social Maturity Scale. American Guidance Service, Inc., Circle Pines, MN. Ages 0-25 years.

Fiorentino, M.: Reflex Testing Methods for Evaluating CNS Development. Charles C. Thomas, Springfield, IL. Ages 0-4 years.

Frankenberg, W.: Denver Developmental Screening Test. Ladoca Project and Publishing Foundation, Denver. Ages 0-6 years.

Frostig, M.: Developmental Test of Visual Perception. Consulting Psychological Press, Palo Alto, CA. Ages 3-8 years.

Gesell, A., et al.: The Gesell Developmental Schedules. The Psychological Corporation, New York. Ages 4 weeks to 6 years.

Goodenough, F., & Harris, D.: Goodenough-Harris Drawing Test. Harcourt Brace Jovanovich, Inc., New York. Ages 3-15 years.

Hurff, J.: A Play Skills Inventory in Play as Exploratory Learning. Sage Publications, Beverly Hills, CA.

Knox, S.: A Play Scale in Play as Exploratory Learning. Sage Publications, Beverly Hills, CA.

Koppitz, E.: Drawing Scale of Developmental Maturity. Grune and Stratton, New York. Ages 5-12 years.

McCarthy, D.: McCarthy Scales of Children's Abilities/MSCA. Grune and Stratton Publications, New York. Ages 2.5 -8.5 years.

Milani-Comparetti, A. & Gidone, E.: Milani-Comparetti Testing Procedure. University of Nebraska Medical Center, Omaha. Ages 0-2 years.

Miller, L.: Miller Assessment for Pre-school Children (MAP). Foundation for Knowledge in Development. Littleton, CO. Ages 3-6 years.

Montgomery, P. & Richter, E.: Fine Motor Development Test. Western Psychological Services. Los Angeles, CA. Ages 0-4 years.

Nihira, K., Foster, R., Shellhass, M. & Leland, H.: AAMD Adaptive Behavior Scale. American Association of Mental Deficiency, Washington, DC. Ages 3 to adulthood.

Rogers, S. et al.: Early Intervention Developmental Profile. The University of Michigan Press, Ann Arbor. Ages 0-36 months.

Slosson, R.: Slosson Drawing Coordination Test. Slosson Educational Publications, E. Aurora, NY. Ages 1 through adult.

CHAPTER 10

A Theory for Occupational Therapy

Objectives

The reader will be able to

1. relate spatiotemporal theory with occupational theory;
2. discuss the philosophy and values of occupational therapy;
3. link spatiotemporal adaptation theory's frame of reference with occupational therapy; and
4. discuss "occupation" as therapeutic media.

Introduction

Concepts of occupation and the occupational process, as introduced in Chapter 7, interwoven with the theoretical frame of reference (Chapter 9), become the basis for relating spatiotemporal adaptation theory to occupational therapy. Purposeful occupation and the occupational process, used therapeutically to enhance a person's performance and life satisfaction, are the domain of occupational therapy. As a profession, occupational therapy's philosophical beliefs are based upon the notion that goal-directed occupations that are meaningful to a person can promote a state of healthfulness, influence development, remediate dysfunction, and elicit maximum adaptation.[1] Spatiotemporal adaptation theory contributes knowledge that parallels occupational therapy's philosophical beliefs and serves to guide the use of its body of knowledge and professional behaviors. Providing occupational therapy for children for the purposes of promoting adaptations is a clinical reasoning process of acting within the boundaries of the profession's values and philosophy and relating theory with values and philosophy.

Spatiotemporal adaptation theory is but one theory within a system of theories appropriate for use in guiding clinical reasoning and providing strategies for practice application. The clinician's use of theory as a springboard is essential for competent practice; however, practice also must reflect one's philosophy, as a profession's value system is the unifying core and a significant element for defining and differentiating a profession.[2] To relate theory with occupational therapy and explore the use of spatiotemporal adaptation with pediatric occupational therapy practice, it is essential to have an understanding of the values of the profession, as those values are the foundation from which a clinician develops professional identity and practice competency.

Philosophy and Values of Occupational Therapy

Occupational therapy is defined as "therapeutic use of self-care, work, and play activities to increase independent function, enhance development, and prevent disability."[3] Implicit within the dictionary definition are values of occupational therapy that emerge from the profession's heritage and philosophic beliefs. Within the philosophy, the most fundamental values for occupational therapy are the meaning of occupation as a vital component for all change and growth, active participation—or the "doing" process—within the boundaries of the occupation, and a person's right to acquire his or her own unique capacity to achieve productive living and experience life satisfaction. Pediatric occupational therapy is grounded in the theoretical concepts that the use of play, schoolwork, and self-care tasks, together with enhancement of family-professional collaboration, can promote purposeful experiences for a child.

Environmental experiences become purposeful for a child when the process to achieve a task is adapted by the self-system. The nature of and/or process to achieve the occupation and a child's active participation or "doing something" with the event are necessary components for facilitating purposefulness of actions for adaptation within the self-system. Adaptation assists organization of neural mechanisms by providing controlled sensory feedback. Sensory feedback includes the interaction of (a) the product or event itself, including the child's intention and attention given to the stimulus and self-perception of the end result, and (b) the sensorimotor-sensory and psychosocial processes to achieve the event, which requires subcortical attention and organization. The process or manner in which the child participates provides the desired sensory feedback to enhance maturation. Through active participation with purposeful occupations, the self-system organizes actions of the event at a subcortical level. Organized actions are integrated into the self-system for use in directing automatic skilled performances.

In addition to purposeful occupations as the technology of occupational therapy, interpersonal relationships that emphasize family-clinician collaboration are vital to occupational therapy. Through ongoing family-professional collaboration, a child's capacities for experiencing life satisfaction and for being integrated into the "mainstream" of society can best be achieved. The use of technology and enhancement of family-professional communication can promote normalization, biopsychosocial development, and primary prevention—principles implicit within the concept of "mainstreaming." The principle of normalization, although initially derived from application from the field of mental retardation, has been broadly redefined to fit child management in general. Wolfensberger[4] proposes that normalization involves implementation of therapy and/or services in a manner complementary to a child's life experiences so that therapy can be as culturally normative as possible. Involving the natural networking of community personnel and families is inherent in the important principle of normalization. Because occupational therapy uses activities of daily life as therapeutic media, the profession can become a central discipline in the promotion of "normalization" for children with special needs. Activities of daily life can serve as a natural organizing process with occupational therapy environments organized to facilitate behavior for "meaningful cultural contexts."[5,p26]

Biopsychosocial developmental theories are grounded in the belief that both prevention and intervention of problems are most successful when a program is carried out with individuals, groups, families, or communities directly involved with the problem situation.[5,6] The key component of biopsychosocial development is the implementation of services *with* children that incorporates *their* community. An effective system of intervention must be based upon goals and strategies that are negotiated between those persons responsible for implementation of services and those persons in the community who have control of resources, as well as the legal mandates, including the family and significant persons associated with community resources.

Community-integrated services designed to promote normalization and development may take place in a variety of environments, including medical care facilities, as the actual setting is not the primary factor. Rather, community-integrated programs are those services designed to promote normalization and development to assist children's achievement of their endowed capacities to participate with play, work, and self-care tasks and experience life satisfaction. This goal can best be accomplished when an occupational therapy program considers a child's community and integrates individuals, families, and community resources involved with the child and the problem situation.

The theoretical concept of primary prevention is basic to spatiotemporal processes. According to Bloom,[7] primary prevention involves those environmental events that are directed toward reducing potentially harmful configurations of one's biopsychosocial environment and, at the same time, promoting beneficial configurations. The process is a therapeutic process of structuring the environment to be "good enough" to present novelty and challenge for the promotion of adaptation through a child's active participation with play, work, and self-care tasks, and to avoid an environment that may facilitate distress.[5] Occupational therapy programs for children with special needs must be designed to promote adaptation and prevent secondary complications that would occur during development. The beliefs inherent in spatiotemporal adaptation theory are complementary to the concepts of normalization, biopsychosocial development, and primary prevention.

Although parts of the above philosophy can be applied to other health-care disciplines, particularly physical therapy, the distinguishing features or uniqueness of occupational therapy is inherent within its set of values and in the manner in which technology is used in a practice situation to facilitate "purposefulness" of experiences for adaptation to higher level actions. Pediatric occupational and physical therapy have similar philosophies and practice techniques. Both professions have the common goal of facilitating a child's highest level of functioning to enhance development and maturation. Both professions use activity as a part of their media. Both professions are necessary for the totality of health care for many children with handicaps. Similarities are multiple, and the overlap of philosophy and practice a known factor among practitioners. However, the distinction between the two professions is paramount and essential for implementing the best possible health-care program for many children.

Within the theoretical framework of spatiotemporal adaptation, we view the role of physical therapy as facilitating adaptation of postural and movement strategies to developmental sequences and facilitation of "purposefulness" of these actions through use of body-centered goals (e.g., to sit, to stand, to reach), whereas the role of occupational therapy is facilitating adaptation of strategies and developmental sequences to purposeful sequences through active participation toward environment-centered goals that are experienced in one's natural daily life (e.g., to feed oneself, to color a picture, to catch a ball).

The therapeutic process for both professions proceeds in the development of sensorimotor-sensory order from automatic functions or reflective-like performances through purposeful adaptive interactions with one's physical and social environment. Therapeutic programs are individualized by the uniqueness of both the patient and the therapist's own beliefs and style. The therapeutic relationship is respectful and caring, with a desire for collaboration with child and family toward achieving adaptation and competence.

Because evolution of sensorimotor-sensory order toward the adaptation of performance skills is on a spiraling continuum, collaborative occupational and physical therapy programs can be most effective for a child. Therapists can work together in planning their separate but interrelated goals, and by working together, appropriate strategies and sequences can be facilitated and appropriate environmental events designed to provide needed motivation to encourage a child's quest for autonomy and competence.

Occupational Therapy's Value System

An occupational therapy value system is a blended synthesis of a clinician's own values and values of the profession that are expressed in one's therapeutic style of behavior. Occupational therapy's value system has been identified in the literature [1,2,8-11] and synthesized by us into the following set of value statements:

- Each individual is a unique and highly flexible creation who is trying to adapt to life by progressing and, at times, retrogressing along his or her own spiraling continuum.
- Occupation is a central aspect of a person's transactions with the environment and through which individuals fulfill a basic need and accumulate a repertoire of subjective experiences.
- Humans are complex, open systems who can influence their own state of health through active participation with purposeful occupations.
- An occupational therapy process is a collaborative and interactive relationship between patient, family, and therapist within their biopsychosocial environments.
- One's state of healthfulness can be influenced by a harmonious balance of self-maintenance activities with playful and productive participation in society.

The philosophy of occupational therapy is holistic, with its science based upon the therapeutic use of occupation to bring about positive change or modification of human behaviors. The art of therapy includes the purposefulness of the occupation and the caring, respectful relationship of serving each human as a unique entity who is attempting to adapt and progress along his or her own spiraling continuum. A fundamental value or belief for occupational therapy is the notion and purposefulness of occupation and the occupational process. Purposefulness or the meaning of occupation is a quality of inner experience; thus, a therapeutic situation must be individualized for each child.

Spatiotemporal Frame of Reference and Occupational Therapy

Spatiotemporal adaptation's theoretical frame of reference has as its core the spiraling process of modifying a child's actions by facilitating higher level functioning. The primary objective of the intervention services is linking strategies and sequences to be adapted for skilled performance with play, work, and self-care tasks. Inherent within the evolution of skill is subcortical organization of neuromuscular functions, which becomes part of the self-system to be called forth for purposeful performance. Appendix 10-A provides a listing of the theory's premises that provide assumptions for occupational therapy, and Appendix 10-B lists the general principles for occupational therapy intervention strategies. These two appendices are presented to provide a basic framework for linking spatiotemporal adaptation theory and occupational therapy.

A spatiotemporal frame of reference considers the impact of nervous system attention and transactions of the child with his environment. Maturation is dependent upon the child's attention to and active participation with events of the environment. Thus, learning and memory (including "subcortical learning") are enhanced and performance modified through the child's attention and active participation with goal-directed purposeful behaviors.

A prime responsibility of an occupational therapist is an ongoing process of structuring the environment, including a child, in such a manner to promote opportunities for a child to attend to and participate with events that facilitate a meaningful response for the self-system. Cortical attention, directed toward the end result of an event, and subcortical attention, directed to the process to achieve the event, are key factors for an occupational therapy spatiotemporal adaptation program. Active participation with play, work, and self-care occupations can facilitate meaningful or purposeful responses when the environment, including a child, is structured in such a manner to direct higher level functioning adapted from appropriate, acquired lower level performances. An occupational therapist's clinical reasoning guides decisions on "how" to structure the therapeutic environment to be "good enough" or "just right" to facilitate a purposeful adaptive response.

To provide occupational therapy to children with special needs, therapists need to know "why" they are doing what they are doing, as well as "what" it is they are attempting to achieve. To understand "why," therapists need to think in terms of what is going on— biologically, psychologically, and sociologically. The more clearly the biopsychosocial processes underlying human behavior are understood, the more effectively a holistic concept can be applied to therapeutic programs. The totality concept, in relation to how a child functions, and the enhancement of normalization are paramount for occupational therapy programs.

To provide knowledge of "what" is being attempted through therapy, therapists need to think in terms of adaptation processes, particularly the effect of sensory feedback from a child's therapeutic performance and the impact of association and differentiation of occupational performances. Sensory feedback with association and differentiation are vital for "subcortical learning." The knowledge of "why" and understanding of "what" provides needed information for the therapeutic decision of "how" to implement an individualistic intervention program. Implementation process may include a variety of media, methods, techniques, and/or approaches; however, the technology selected must be applied to a child's needs and uniqueness, with the ultimate goal of facilitating a child's adaptation to the spatial and temporal components of his world.

Purposeful occupation is the point of departure for occupational therapy intervention programs. The effect of therapy depends upon the change or modification that a child can elicit within self by adapting the occupation being experienced into the self-system. Adapting purposeful experiences depends upon the competence of the child's internal environment (the mastery level of performance directed by the self-system), together with the expectations of the external environment (the system with which the child interacts) including space, objects, and persons within the child's milieu. Therefore, occupational therapy becomes a multidimensional service program; the child, family, therapist, other persons involved with the child, and those physical settings in which a child participates must be a part of the intervention plan.

During intervention processes, the primary role of an occupational therapist is to structure the environment in a manner to promote the "purposefulness" of experiences for the child that the self-system has not been able to do for itself. Therapists guide those appropriate actions/occupations so that the child can explore the environment with "meaningful experiences." Occupational therapy provides an appropriate environment that motivates a child to engage in purposeful experiences for adaptation. Adaptation occurs when a child's level of competence is in harmony with the environment's expectations of the child. When there is a discrepancy between competence and expectations, spatiotemporal distress occurs.

According to Ayres, therapy brings out the child's "inner urge" for action, thus eliciting a child's potential for self-directing responses that will augment maturation.[12,p256] Self-direction of actions/occupations that are purposeful provides success experiences that are pleasing to a child. Self-direction leads to a feeling of "mastery" over one's environment, augmenting the acquisition of autonomy and competence.

Occupation as Therapeutic Media

Occupation that brings meaning to a person can be used for therapeutic media as a means to restore or enhance the development of life skills; therefore, the uniqueness of occupational therapy "is its role as custodian of meaning."[13,p727] Occupation, as defined in Chapter 7, includes those play, work, and self-care action events that provide opportunities for exploration and mastery of the environment. Occupation is the basic media for spatiotemporal adaptation processes, as it is essential to both sensorimotor development and acquisition of competence, as well as being essential to the therapeutic process to facilitate or restore productive living for individuals with special needs. Because much of learning and adaptation is accomplished through purposeful play, play becomes a powerful media for therapeutic programs.[14]

Occupational therapists have always valued children's play as both a means of intervention and a measurement of abilities. A child's motivation or natural drive to play is an excellent way to facilitate active participation with environmental events and thus enhance spatiotemporal adaptation. The range of play activities and events are vast; many are grounded in years of tradition and have cultural significance.[14] Today's scientific advancements in electronic technology have opened up opportunities for children with handicaps to access their world of play and learning. Personal computers, the vast range of software programs, electronic switches for toys, and robotics have expanded the repertoire of playful occupations available to elicit maximum adaptation for each child. Today's technology has added exciting new dimensions for occupational therapy but, more importantly, electronic technology used as media to elicit spatiotemporal adaptation has enlarged the scope of play for a child with a handicapping condition. High technology, used for therapeutic media to enhance a child's occupational process, provides occupational therapy with unique opportunities to actualize its values to promote life satisfaction and social integration for persons with special needs. Occupational therapy's historic roots are founded in the profession's commitment to persons with chronic and profound disabilities.[15,16] Today's technology used to elicit play, work, and self-care occupations opens up new avenues for occupational therapy intervention programs for children with significant disabilities. Technology in play is an integral part of pediatric occupational therapy.

Evoking play is actually a major therapeutic task, and a therapist must have a playful attitude, as well as knowledge and skills in determining how to create a playful environment to facilitate a child's adaptation through purposeful play. Purposefulness of play is elicited when the environment provides interest and excitement within a child to promote intentionality of actions.[17] Consequently, a major challenge for the therapist is designing the play space and play time that can facilitate a child's ability to use his or her body effectively to interact with others competently and to use problem-solving approaches to environmental problems. A therapeutic environment becomes effective when it is conveyed to a child for the purpose of play and generates a meaningful contact from which behaviors can be tried out, practiced, and organized. A child's initiative and active involvement are critical to the therapeutic play process and are dependent upon the "good enough" challenge of the environment. The self-direction of a child is primary in guiding therapy to achieve the ultimate goal of competence in daily life activities.[14] Therefore, an occupational therapist must prepare a play environment by balancing the structure and freedom of the situation in such a way that active participation with a "good enough" environment will enhance reciprocal interweaving.

Spatiotemporal adaptation occurs within the context of childhood play, and thus the adequacy of spatiotemporal adaptation facilitated in therapy will be a major factor for influencing a child's ability to explore and master the environment. A play program would consider a child's life roles and related skills, as well as the spiraling levels of play competencies. A therapeutic program would include opportunities for curiosity, exploration, and repetition of playful behaviors; decision-making; and a balance between play, schoolwork, and self-care. The value of play is in its characteristics and properties, which provide experiences to learn the rules of motion, rules of objects, and rules of people, which are acquired through sensorimotor play, constructive play, and social play.[15,16] Sensorimotor play is pleasurable activity involving sensation and movemnt, constructive play is the sequencing of objects in spatiotemporal relationships, and social play is both physical and verbal interaction with others.[16] Spiraling organization of sensorimotor, constructive, and social play considers a person's movement-environment transactions that make adaptation possible.

Play is considered central to the intervention process employing spatiotemporal adaptation theory, as play is a mode of action, a means to both develop and support occupational performance skills required for life's various roles. Within spatiotemporal adaptation theory, the mode of play involves internal receiving by the child, not external giving by the therapist. Therefore, it is through internal receiving that playful occupations become purposeful. Inherent in the internal receiving process of the self-system are intrinsic and extrinsic motivational phenomena. Through play activities, the occupational therapist influences the extrinsic phenomena of the environment to contribute to realizations of intrinsic motivation of the child. Play, as used by occupational therapists, includes both an intrinsic value for a child and a therapeutic purpose for facilitating adaptation. The intrinsically motivating phenomenon for play is to say that play is engaged in for its own sake, or for the sake of one's inner consciousness. The therapeutic purpose of play is to say that play is engaged in for the sake of facilitating higher level adaptations and promoting competence.

Summary

Spatiotemporal adaptation theory has its therapeutic impact in the use of purposeful occupations and the occupational process. Play is a powerful therapeutic media for occupational therapy, as play can be used to enhance adaptation, restore function, and facilitate purpose. The spiraling continuum of spatiotemporal adaptation provides a theoretical framework for occupational therapy practice, as the theory is a "road map" for the understanding of the acquisition of performance skills. Although the theory emphasizes the consistency of the spiraling process, variabilities and differences of each individual are stressed. Each child is unique and expresses his uniqueness through his transactions with the environment. Each child develops a unique "self."

Occupational therapy is a profession whose scientific base is emerging; however, its set of values shall remain one of its most vital characteristics for defining and differentiating the profession. Accepting occupational therapy's uniqueness as the "custodian of meaning," occupational therapists will provide an important humane perspective to an expanding health-care world being influenced by high technology.[2]

Key Points

1. Concepts of occupation and the occupational process, interwoven with the theoretical frame of reference, become the basis for relating spatiotemporal adaptation theory to occupational therapy practice.
2. Spatiotemporal adaptation theory is but one theory within a system of theories appropriate for use in guiding clinical reasoning and providing strategies for practice application.
3. Within the philosophy, the most fundamental values for occupational therapy are the concepts of "occupation," "active participation," and "individual's right" to achieve productive living and experience life satisfaction.
4. Pediatric occupational therapy is grounded in the concepts of "play, school work, and self-care" tasks, and family-professional collaboration.
5. The use of occupational therapy's technology and enhancement of family-professional communication can promote normalization and primary prevention.
6. Occupational therapy programs for children with special needs must be designed to promote adaptation and prevent secondary complications that could occur during development.
7. Distinguishing features of occupational therapy are inherent within its set of values and in the manner in which technology is used in a practice situation to facilitate "purposefulness" of experiences for adaptation to higher level actions.
8. Occupational therapy's value system includes beliefs that an individual is unique and flexible; occupation is the central aspect of an individual's transactions with the environment; humans are complex, open systems who can influence their own state of health; and one's state of healthfulness is influenced by a harmonious

balance of self-maintenance activities with playful and productive participation.

9. The science of occupational therapy is based upon the therapeutic use of occupation to bring about positive change or modification of human behaviors, whereas the art of therapy includes the purposefulness of occupation and caring, interpersonal relationships.

10. To relate spatiotemporal adaptation theory's frame of reference and occupational therapy, the theory's premises and general principles for occupational therapy intervention strategies provide the foundation for that relationship.

11. Occupation is the basic media to faciltiate spatiotemporal adaptation processes and, with occupational therapy, play becomes the powerful media for therapeutic programs.

Self-study Guidelines

1. Occupational therapy's philosophical beliefs are based upon what?
2. How can theory be used to enhance competent practice in occupational therapy practice?
3. Define occupational therapy.
4. Identify the fundamental values for occupational therapy.
5. Define the terms "normalization" and "primary prevention" as concepts basic to occupational therapy intervention.
6. Discuss the value system of occupational therapy.
7. What is the primary role of an occupational therapist during intervention processes?
8. Discuss why "play" is considered a powerful medium for therapeutic programs with children.
9. Discuss the premises of the spatiotemporal adaptation theory.
10. State the principles for intervention strategies as identified with spatiotemporal adaptation theory.

References

1. American Occupational Therapy Association: Philosophical base of occupational therapy. Am J Occup Ther 33:785, 1979.
2. Englehardt HT: The importance of values in shaping professional direction and behavior. In Target 2000: Occupational Therapy Education. Rockville, MD, American Occupational Therapy Association, 1986, pp. 39-43.
3. Bing RK: Report of the president to the members. Occup Ther News, 40(6), June 1986.
4. Wolfensberger W: Normalization: The principle of normalization in human sciences. Toronto, Canada, National Institute on Mental Retardation, Leonard Crainford, 1972.
5. Vandenburg B, Kielhofner G: Play in evolution, culture, and individual adaptation: Implications for therapy. Am J Occup Ther 36:20-28, 1982.
6. Farris B: Introducing social development content into social work curriculum. Soc Dev Issues 6(1):41-52, 1982.
7. Bloom M: Primary Prevention. Englewood Cliffs, NJ, Prentice-Hall, 1981.
8. Kielhofner G: A paradigm for practice: The hierarchical organization of occupa-

tional therapy knowledge. In Kielhofner G (Ed): Health through Occupation. Philadelphia, F.A. Davis Co., 1983, pp. 55-87.

9. Mosey AC: Occupational Therapy: Configuration of a Profession. New York, Raven Press, 1981.

10. Yerxa E: The philosophic base of occupational therapy. Occup Ther 2001 A.D., pp. 26-30, 1979.

11. Yerxa E: Audacious values: The energy source for occupational therapy practice. In Kielhofner G (Ed): Health through Occupation. Philadelphia, F.A. Davis Co., 1983, pp. 149-152.

12. Ayres AJ: Sensory Integration and Learning Disorders. Los Angeles, Webster Psychological Services, 1972.

13. Kielhofner G: A heritage of activity: Development of theory. Am J Occup Ther 36:723-729, 1982.

14. Vandenberg B, Kielhofner G: Play in evolution, culture, and individual adaptation: Implications for therapy. Am J Occup Ther 36:20-28, 1982.

15. Kielhofner G, Miyake S: The therapeutic use of games with mentally retarded adults. Am J Occup Ther 35:375-382, 1981.

16. Mach W, Lindquist JE, Parham LD: A synthesis of occupational behavior and sensory integration concepts in theory and practice. Part 1, Theoretical foundations. Am J Occup Ther 36:365-374, 1982.

17. Berlyne D: Conflict, Arousal and Curiosity. New York, McGraw-Hill Book Co, 1960.

Appendix 10-A
Premises of Spatiotemporal Adaptation Theory

Premises implied in the spatiotemporal adaptation theory:

1. Development is a function of nervous system maturation, which occurs through a process of person-environment adaptation.
2. Adaptation is dependent upon attention to and active participation with purposeful events within the spatiotemporal dimensions of the environment. Without active participation the self-system is deprived of certain forms of sensation (sensory feedback) about self and the environment which, in turn, affects maturation.
3. Purposeful events (occupations) provide meaningful experiences for enhancement of maturation by directing a higher level adaptive response on the part of the "doer."
4. Higher level responses result from integration with and modification of acquired lower level functions; thus, adaptation of higher level functions and purposes is dependent upon a certain degree of association/differentiation of specific components of acquired lower level actions.
5. Adaptation spirals through primitive, transitional, and mature phases of development occurring at the same time within different body segments. The concurrent development of phases considers the adaptation of posture and movement strategies to developmental and purposeful sequences and of linking strategies and sequences for adaptation to skilled performance.
6. Environmental experiences may present situations of spatiotemporal stress. With stress, the system calls forth past acquired strategies and sequences to act upon the demands of the environment and maintain the system's homeostasis. Thus, acquired strategies and sequences are adapted with the present situation to direct higher level adaptive responses.
7. Spatiotemporal distress provokes dysfunctioning behaviors, resulting in maladaptation. With distress a child repeats purposeless lower level strategies and sequences and these actions are not linked to higher level behaviors. Repetition of purposeless strategies and sequences results in regression.
8. The developing nervous system has capacity to compensate for impairments by forming new connections during the early periods of maturation. Plasticity or flexibility of the formative nervous system enhances its capacity for sensorimotor-sensory adaptation processes to facilitate nervous system modification, e.g., changes in degree of myelination, dendritic growth, formation of new synapses.
9. An intervention program based on a spatiotemporal adaptation process of active participation with purposeful events provides appropriate sensory stimuli necessary to help mature synaptic connections.
10. An intervention program providing appropriate sensory input, motor output, and sensory feedback, and employing the spiraling process of linking strategies and sequences, enhances previously unresponsive brain cells, influences neural organization, establishes new engrams, and thus facilitates maturation.

Appendix 10-B
Principles for Intervention Strategies

---

1. Each child is a unique being who has the potential for healthful development and self-perception of competency.

2. Occupation is the vital component to elicit the adaptation for skilled performances and enhance one's competencies.

3. Within an adaptation framework, any one or all of the following overall goals may be considered: prevention, remediation, compensation, maintenance.

4. Overall goals provide the framework for delineation of intervention strategies that are specific to each child.

5. Spatiotemporal adaptation theory provides a practice framework that focuses on the enhancement of human behavior and not just on developmental or physiological processes.

6. Within the spatiotemporal adaptation frame, therapeutic media and methods are concerned primarily with enhancement of sensorimotor-sensory behaviors with a recognition of the importance and powerful relationship of psychosocial aspects of neurobehavior.

7. Media and methods selected within neurobehavioral intervention strategies emphasize position and handling; selected events/occupations; active participation with the environment; adaptation to enhance self-care, play, and schoolwork skills; use of technology and adaptive equipment to enhance the child's access to the environment; and child-family interactions.

8. The spiraling process of spatiotemporal adaptation makes its therapeutic impact through a process of "reciprocal interweaving" or reincorporation of several sequential (spiraling) levels of development.

9. Preparation, facilitation, and adaptation are viewed as primary processes for those intervention strategies designed to augment development of skilled performance through spatiotemporal adaptation.

10. Intervention strategies are influenced by the beliefs, value judgments, and ethical concerns of practitioners emanating from the unique perspective of their profession.

Glossary

Accommodation—motor response of adjusting the body to react to incoming stimuli

Accuracy—when referred to the accuracy of performance, includes perception or judgment of direction, distance, control, and timing of a person's actions; dependent upon perception of self in relation to temporal dimensions of actions being performed

Activation (mobility)—development of mobility muscle functions in undifferentiated patterns by complete shortening of agonists and lengthening of antagonists

Adaptation—continuous, ongoing state or act of adjusting bodily processes required to function/perform within the demands of environment; adaptation as a therapeutic mode within a practice session gives purpose to performance; making use of movement to apply to environmental events

Affordance—component of the ecological event theory used to describe the environment and relationship to a person, and provide support of activity or component of environmental event that provides support for a person to act and engage in activities of the environment

Assimilation—sensory process of receiving information

Association—organized process of relating sensory information with the motor act being experienced; relating present and past actions

Autonomic nervous system (ANS)—a part of the nervous system that innervates smooth and cardiac muscle and glandular tissues and governs involuntary actions; consists of the *sympathetic* nervous system and the *parasympathetic* nervous system

Autonomy—perception of self-competence or sense of self-efficacy/self-efficiency

Bilateral weight shift—movement forward and backward or up and down, using upper or lower extremities bilaterally and shifting weight from upper to lower parts of the body and vice versa

Blended mobility/stability—mature stage of muscle development to allow extremities to move freely in space and the body as a whole to move freely through space

Brain stem—levels 2, 3, and 4 of the central nervous system (medulla, pons, and midbrain)

Category—a major concept or construct of grounded theory

Caudocephalic—equals distance to proximal sequence of development

Central nervous system (CNS)—a part of the nervous system that, in vertebrates, consists of the brain and spinal cord, and to which sensory impulses are transmitted and from which motor impulses come; that supervises and coordinates the activity of the entire nervous system; CNS has seven structural levels that parallel the ontogenetic development as well as the phylogenetic appearance of the structures in evolution (see also, Triune brain)

Cephalocaudo—head to tail sequence of development

Cerebellum—the fifth structural level of the central nervous system; endows the nervous system with synergy, i.e., smooth, orderly sequencing of direction, force, timing, and tone involved in patterns of movement

Cerebral hemispheres or Telencephalon—the seventh structural division of the central nervous system (tel = distance + encephalon = brain); consists of the cerebral cortices, subcortical white fiber tracks, and deep-grain nuclei

Coactivation (stability)—simultaneous contraction of agonists and antagonists around joints in order to hold that joint in a particular position to allow the body to maintain postures

Cocontraction—simultaneous contraction of agonist and antagonist muscles

Compensation—an intervention process designed to promote other aspects of performance or substitute a different form of action

Contralateral weight shift—rotation within the body axis allows one body segment to rotate in one direction while the adjacent segment rotates in the opposite direction; makes it possible for a child to shift weight and move forward simultaneously

Cortical—involving or resulting from the action of the cerebral cortex, which is involved in higher level processes

Cranial nerves—peripheral nerves associated with cranial vault structures (brain stem and brain); 12 pairs of cranial nerves, numbered in sequence from fore to aft; first cranial nerve (cr N.I = olfactory nerve, cr N.II = optic nerve, cr N.III = oculomotor nerve, cr N.IV = trochler nerve, cr N.V = trigeminal nerve, cr N.VI = abducens nerve, cr N.VII = facial nerve, cr N.VIII = vestibulocochler nerve, cr N.IX = glossopharyngeal nerve, cr N.X = vagus nerve, cr N.XI = spinal accessory nerve, cr N.XII = hypoglossal nerve)

Combined mobility/stability—mobility functions of muscles superimposed on stability functions to allow a person to maintain a position and move within the limited range of the position

Competence—adequate and appropriate actions to meet the demands of environmental events; quality of being able to respond effectively to demands of one or a range of situations within the environment

Complete rotation—sequence within the developmental sequences of coming to the upright position, which describes the process used to attain upright; process by which a person goes from supine to prone, then to sitting, to creeping, to pull up, and then to stand independently

Coordinative structures—concept of the ecological event theory meaning organized units of behavior used for specific acts

Developmental sequences—developmental behaviors leading to upright functioning, such as creeping, walking, and running, as well as behaviors required to reach out with the upper extremity and grasp; includes developmental behaviors of creeping, sitting, rolling, standing/walking, and reaching/grasping: sensorimotor functions to produce movement

Developmental sequences to stand—sequences used by the infant and child to assume the upright position; the order of these sequences are complete rotation, partial complete rotation, partial rotation, and symmetrical standing

Diencephalon—the sixth structural level of the nervous system; also termed "thalamus" (dia = through + encephalon = brain); located deep within the brain where millions of synapses occur; concerned with viscera and/or autonomic hypothalamic regulation, growth hormone responses, and diurnal rhythms; hypothalamus and associated pathways are the master control center of the autonomic nervous control system and endocrine system.

Differentiation—process for discriminating essential elements of actions pertinent to a given situation from those actions that are not pertinent

Distress—stress that is out of control; a negative factor for development

Ecological event theory or Ecological approach—a theory or approach to motor skills acquisition developed by scientists Fowler and Turvey; describes the relationship of the person and environment as being both of equal importance

Effectance motivation—a biologically inherent urge to "do" or perform; internal to self

Efficiency—as related to performance, is the relationship between the amount of work that is accomplished and the force or energy expended to accomplish the action

Environment—complete setting or surrounding—milieu, self, other persons, objects, earth, space, and relationship with space; everything with which a person interrelates

Equilibrium reaction—compensatory movements used to regain midline stability when alignment of one's midline with gravity is significantly disturbed

Event—activity or occupation in which a person engages

Extrinsic motivation—urge to act or "do" for a reward external to self

Facilitation—refers to external stimuli aimed at specific areas of the nervous system which results in excitation; continued successive application of necessary stimuli and/ or assistance given to elicit an adaptive response

Frame of reference—set of interrelated definitions that provide a description with a particular aspect of a profession that links the model with practice; guidelines for practice; a mental plan of how to do something

Functions—bodily processes that exist within structures and are used to adapt to the environment

Generalized movement—first movements of newborn; appears to be lack of control or obvious purpose; movements generally confined to the extremities; serves the purpose of developing muscle functions and establishing neuropathways; contains incipient patterns of movement, mostly reflexive in nature but sufficient to give the baby a sense of moving in patterns of rhythms; generalized movements can be viewed as non-directive and form the basis for development of automatic righting, protection, and equilibrium reactions.

Hard-wired—concept that the central nervous system was "in place," i.e., once all the nuclei, pathways, and synapses were mature, changes that occurred during growth and maturation were the result of repeated use over time of various circuits, which resulted in the development of different skills; when lesion occurred, it was thought that many neurons and pathways involved in a functional circuit would die and permanent deficits would remain (see Soft-wired); hard-wired aspect of the human nervous system is thought to be comprised of certain genetic endowments that are "free programmed" with specific behavioral drive (e.g., getting up, walking on two feet); hard-wired system includes the developmental sequences for acquiring upright posture and reach and grasp

Hyperactivity—hyperresponsive; excessive, uncontrolled movement

Hypertonic—muscle tone higher than normal; resistance to passive movement: in extreme form, spasticity

Hyporeactive—hyporesponsive

Hypotonic—less than normal muscle tone; flabby, soft muscles

Inhibition—a decrease in neural activity resulting from a particular process, state, or external stimulation

Intrinsic motivation—effectance; a biologically inherent urge to "do" or perform; reward contained within self

Key behaviors—"snapshots" at certain points along the progression that signify an identifiable point at which a child is adapting previously acquired behaviors to achieve a new behavior, or modifying a previously acquired behavior because of a new experience

Kinesthesia—the sense by which one is aware of the position and movement of various body parts

Kinetic system—group of subcortical nuclear centers that contribute the background movement patterns that are necessary for postural adaptation and, later in development, the foundations upon which learned skills will be superimposed; mnemonic for kinetic system is PASS, which means postural adaptations that are either stereotyped (genetically endowed) or semiautomatic (learned)

Limbic system—major area of the CNS responsible for moving a person or providing a motivating force behind basic behaviors and personality traits; mnemonics for limbic system are M^2OVE (M^2 stands for motivation or basic drive and memory function, $0 = $ olfaction or sense of smell, V = vicero or automatic responses, E reflects emotional tone or emotional stability)

Maintenance—an intervention process in a practice situation that provides activity that helps a person maintain or keep the present state or condition and retain acquired appropriate functions

Maladaptation—dysfunctional adaptation process or the inability to adapt to and with the demands of the environment (see **Distress** and **Adaptation**)

Mature strategies—ultimate developmental phase which implies muscle functions are blended in such a way that posture is controlled by stability and mobility within the body axis and is not dependent upon the extremities for support of positions in space; extremities move freely in space, controlled by countermovements with the trunk or more proximal joints; midline stability reactions and equilibrium control balance between postural control and movement

Midline stability reactions—mature neural functions to maintain vertical postures and control postural adjustments within a confined area

Mobility—activation of muscles and muscle groups (see **Activation**)

Model—philosophical belief system, content, and internal structure of a profession; a profession's paradigm

Modification—intervention process that facilitates change within the self-system, which is brought about by a person's own active participation with action/activity/occupation/events

Motor—referring to muscular movement; causing motion relating to or being a nerve or nerve fiber that passes from the central nervous system or a ganglion to a muscle and conducts an impulse that causes movement

Motor planning (praxis)—ability to automatically organize and plan movement

Movement strategies—components to give rise to action; components to promote and sequence changes in position of body or body parts

Muscle tone—status of muscle to give it the "rigidity" necessary to maintain joints in defined positions; normal tension or responsiveness to stretch; quality of the muscle, health, elasticity, or resiliency

Neocortical system—consists of parietal and occipital lobes and posterior parts of the frontal and temporal lobes; mnemonic is $A^2P^2ES^3$ (A = appreciation and anticipatory behaviors, P = planning and programming, E = executing the behavioral response, S = skill, survival, and strategems)

Neo-neocortical system—prefrontal lobes and interior temporal lobes; mnemonic for these areas is JEM^2 (J = judgment, especially as judgment relates to E, emotional tone, and M, motivation and memories)

Neural—pertaining to nerves

Neurological—pertaining to the scientific study of the nervous system, its functions and disorders; especially concerned with diagnosis and treatment of disorders of the nervous system

Neuroplasticity—concepts of "hard-wired" and "soft-wired" nervous system; refers to the flexibility or malleability of the nervous system, particularly developing stages in utero or early infancy and childhood

Occupation—environmental events that provide opportunities to promote exploration and mastery of the environment: goal-directed use of time, energy, interest, and attention; is an agent for learning, development, and life satisfaction

Occupational performance—an interrelated triad that constitutes a common domain of environment exploration and mastery; triad includes play, work, and self-care occupations

Parasympathetic nervous system (PNS)—the part of the autonomic nervous system whose stimulation creates a physiological calming effect on the body; contains cholinergic fibers that tend to induce secretion, to cause dilation of the blood vessels in muscles, and that consist of a cranial and sacral part

Partial rotation—the third step in the developmental sequences to stand; child goes from supine to sidelying, pushes self to sitting, and then to stand

Partial-complete rotation—the second step in the developmental sequences to stand; child goes to supine to side rolling, pushes self to sitting, then to complete rotation, to creep, then to pull to stand or assume upright independently from the all-fours position

Perception—sensory judgment or feeling about information; internal interpretation of sensations that affects resulting behavior

Performance skills—sensorimotor-sensory behaviors that give the person the ability to move the body within spatiotemporal dimensions, to receive impetus, and to give impetus to external objects; skilled performance has a quality of natural responsiveness, an automatic element to actions with regulation of flow or blending of postures and movement in relation to the spatiotemporal dimensions of the environment

Peripheral nervous system—nerves that enable the CNS to communicate with the organism's external environment (somatosensory and motoneurons) and its internal environment (viscerosensory and visceromotor neurons) of the ANS (automatic nervous system)

Phasic reflexes—observable movement in response to stimuli

Plasticity—flexibility of the developing nervous system, particularly in utero, infancy, and childhood

Play—the process to achieve competence; includes a variety of activities from infant and childhood play to leisure activities in the adult years; involves exploration, imaginative role-playing, and game-like activities (sports, games, hobbies, and recreation) and social recreational activities

Postural strategies—components to control movement; the means for distributing postural tone needed to maintain posture

Postural tone—state added to muscle tone (mainly extension) to allow functioning against gravity

Praxis—the conscious awareness of type and sequence of movement

Preparation—therapeutic mode of action that is preliminary, as well as an ongoing process of enhancing the neural and muscular functions for their readiness and use as posture and movement strategies

Prevention—intervention strategy that engages a person in activities designed to keep distress from occurring or to hinder secondary complications from the initial identified problem

Primitive reflexes—phasic/tonic reflexes present at birth

Primitive strategies—a phase in development when movement components of flexion and extension are developing, along with accompanying functions of mobility and stability, covering birth through the first few weeks of postnatal development; support for posture is trunk-centered and comes from external sources rather than from self; primitive mobility and phasic reflexes produce undifferentiated patterns of movement; primitive stability and tonic reflexes produce holding or fixing

Prone—lying on the stomach

Property—an aspect of a category as used to explain grounded theory

Proprioception—relating to the reception of information received from nerve endings in the muscles, tendons, and joints, which gives us an internal awareness of our body parts

Purpose—that which can be done with something; identifies a specific outcome that will result; intentional action

Purposeful—having meaning to a person; enhances change or modification

Purposeful sequences—component of the developmental process which links components from developmental sequences to specific patterns used to interact with space, objects, and people; makes use of sensorimotor functions to produce movement, but unique to purposeful sequences is the intentionality on the part of the child; motivated by intentions as a child seeks to explore and master the world; purposefulness of movement adds the dimension of "doing something"

Reactions—series of responses to sensory input or combination of sensory stimuli

Reflexes—responses that are simple, predictable, and result from one or two sources of stimulation

Remediation—intervention process of engaging a person in activity that is designed to correct, remedy, or improve skills

Reticular—formation of the brain stem and hypothalamic nuclei; integrates the major functions with the sensorimotor-sensory system; located in the central core; consists of numerous recognized nerve cell groups; plays a key role in regulating a great number of functions that are critical

Rotational righting—reactions that cause the head and trunk to rotate around the central axis

Self-care—daily living tasks; a range of activities such as eating, dressing, hygiene, toileting, transporting self, and rest; process of maintaining self as prescribed by one's culture and for the promotion of healthfulness

Sensorimotor-sensory (SMS)—sensory input, motor output, and sensory feedback

Sensory integration—the interaction and coordination of two or more functions or processes in a manner which enhances the adaptiveness of the brain's response

Skill—appropriate use of posture and movement in relation to the effort (speed, timing, exertion, space, control) used for promotion of occupation; characterized by consistent patterns of performance

Soft-wired system—aspects of the nervous system that are not pre-programmed to specific behavioral drives but are influenced by transactions within the environment; includes gross and fine motor skills of the developing purposeful sequences

Spatial—space surrounding an individual; spatial dimensions encompass environment

Spatiotemporal—refers to space and timing dimensions of environment

Spinal nerves—nerves associated with the spinal cord; 31 pairs which reflect the 31 functional embryonic segments of the spinal cord and associated somites of the body wall structures; of the 31 pairs of spinal nerves, 8 are cervical, 12 are thoracic (or dorsal), 5 are lumbar, 5 are sacral, and 1 (or 2) make up the coccygeal nerves; spinal nerves form the four functional plexuses of the spinal cord (i.e., C 1-4 is the cervical plexus, C 5-TI the brachial plexus, T12-L4 the lumbar plexus, and L4-S4 the sacral plexus)

Spiraling continuum—framework to illustrate ongoing and reciprocal interlinking aspects of development

Stability—a dynamic muscle function to produce "stay-ability" or regulation of change; characterized by coactivation or contraction of agonists and antagonists simultaneously (see **Coactivation**)

Strategies—neuromuscular component parts of adaptive sequences

Stress—phenomenon characterized by alteration of the system's equilibrium; a positive factor for development

Structured media—component of the ecological event theory; equals aspects of the environment (light, air, sound, etc.) that are specific to the event; provides necessary temporal information to the person

Structures (of body)—bones, joints, muscles, and neural mechanism

Subcortical—relation to, involving, or being nerve centers below the cerebral cortex; learning that occurs on a reflex or subconscious level

Supine—lying on the back

Symmetrical—last phase of the developmental sequences to stand; a person can assume the upright from the supine position by coming to the sitting posture in a symmetrical, upright fashion and then pushing self on to stand

Sympathetic nervous system (SNS)—the part of the autonomic nervous system that contains chiefly adrenergic fibers and tends to depress secretion, decrease tone and contractibility of smooth muscle, and cause the contraction of blood vessels. Stimulation of this system creates the fight/flight reaction responsive to fear or stress; alerts the individual to action

Synergic system—cerebellum; mnemonic = SOS-DEFT^2 (i.e., synergy is the SOS reflecting smooth, orderly sequencing of the DEFT = direction, extent, force, timing, and tone of all activities in which a person engages)

Tactile—perceptible by touch

Temporal—time, duration, regulation, memory, and sequence of a person's actions; temporal dimensions encompass planned actions in relation to objects

Theoretical frame of reference—mental plan of how to do something within practice setting (see **Frame of reference**)

Theory—an interrelated set of ideas, assumptions, or constructs that presents a systematic view of phenomena to provide order for explanation

Tone (muscle)—degrees of tension normally present in the resting state of the muscle

Tonic reflexes—postures assumed to respond to position of head/trunk in place, or in relation to each other

Touch—the sensation whereby stimulus to the skin is perceived: different receptors perceive pain, temperature, light touch, pressure, and vibration, and will elicit a protective or discriminative response

Transitional strategies—phase in development which begins several months after birth and continues until mature postural control and movement patterns have developed; during transitional phases, primitive reflexes are adapted to righting reactions and support protective reactions; muscle functions are stabilized around neck, trunk, and proximal joints to support new positions in space; proximal stability is combined with mobility functions to allow movement within postures and between postures; weight bearing on extremities signifies that support for posture is extremitive center (control for posture is developing in the neck, trunk, and more proximal joints); weight-bearing support reactions, combined with vertical righting reactions, lead to bilateral weight-shift patterns of control for movement in space.

Triune brain—constant for understanding the central nervous system based upon phylogenetic subdivisions; three major areas—archi or oldest, paleo or intermediate, and neo or newest components of the nervous system

Unilateral weight shift—weight shift to one side of the midline, supported by either the trunk or extremities on that side, and then move extremities on the opposite side of the body

Vertical righting—reactions that move the midline of the body into alignment with the center of gravity

Volitional movements—movements that have some controlled purpose; developed from directed movement patterns, such as visually guided reaching or adapted walking to running

Weight bearing—maintenance of a position in space, supporting by bearing weight on specific aspects of the trunk or extremities

Weight shifting—ability to maintain positions by bearing weight on specific segments of the body and, at the same time, ability to change positions by shifting weight from one segment or combination of segments to another; provides some postural stability required to control movement

Work—process to express competence; includes occupations classified as productive or events that provide a product or service requested by others; activities that provide a heritage to one's culture; includes roles such as student, housekeeper, volunteer, amateur or professional athlete, laborer, professional, and/or other career events

INDEX